Power Eating

THIRD EDITION

Susan M. Kleiner, PhD, RD

High Performance Nutrition
Mercer Island, Washington

with

Maggie Greenwood-Robinson, PhD

HUMAN
KINETICS

Library of Congress Cataloging-in-Publication Data

Kleiner, Susan M.
  Power eating / Susan M. Kleiner, with Maggie Greenwood-Robinson. --
3rd ed.
     p. cm.
  Includes bibliographical references and index.
  ISBN-13: 978-0-7360-6698-3 (soft)
  ISBN-10: 0-7360-6698-5 (soft)
  1. Athletes--Nutrition. 2. Bodybuilders--Nutrition. I.
Greenwood-Robinson, Maggie. II. Title.
  TX361.A8K595 2006
  613.2'024796--dc22   2006024655

ISBN-10: 0-7360-6698-5
ISBN-13: 978-0-7360-6698-3

This publication is written and published to provide accurate and authoritative information relevant to the subject matter presented. It is published and sold with the understanding that the author and publisher are not engaged in rendering legal, medical, or other professional services by reason of their authorship or publication of this work. If medical or other expert assistance is required, the services of a competent professional person should be sought.

Acquisitions Editor: Jana Hunter; **Developmental Editor:** Heather Healy; **Assistant Editor:** Laura Koritz; **Copyeditor:** Alisha Jeddeloh; **Proofreader:** Erin Cler; **Indexer:** Betty Frizzell; **Permission Manager:** Carly Breeding; **Graphic Designer:** Nancy Rasmus; **Graphic Artist:** Kim McFarland; **Photo Manager:** Laura Fitch; **Cover Designer:** Keith Blomberg; **Photographer (cover):** Alloy Photography/Veer; **Photographer (interior):** Human Kinetics unless otherwise noted; **Printer:** Sheridan Books

Human Kinetics books are available at special discounts for bulk purchase. Special editions or book excerpts can also be created to specification. For details, contact the Special Sales Manager at Human Kinetics.

Printed in the United States of America   10 9 8 7 6 5 4 3

Human Kinetics
Web site: www.HumanKinetics.com

United States: Human Kinetics
P.O. Box 5076
Champaign, IL 61825-5076
800-747-4457
e-mail: humank@hkusa.com

Canada: Human Kinetics
475 Devonshire Road, Unit 100
Windsor, ON N8Y 2L5
800-465-7301 (in Canada only)
e-mail: info@hkcanada.com

Europe: Human Kinetics
107 Bradford Road
Stanningley
Leeds LS28 6AT, United Kingdom
+44 (0)113 255 5665
e-mail: hk@hkeurope.com

Australia: Human Kinetics
57A Price Avenue
Lower Mitcham, South Australia 5062
08 8372 0999
e-mail: info@hkaustralia.com

New Zealand: Human Kinetics
Division of Sports Distributors NZ Ltd.
P.O. Box 300 226 Albany
North Shore City, Auckland
0064 9 448 1207
e-mail: info@humankinetics.co.nz

Power Eating

THIRD EDITION

Contents

PART III   Plans and Menus

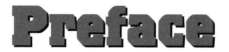

Preface

The science of sport nutrition is moving at an astronomical pace. The third edition of *Power Eating* is virtually a whole new book, and it's bigger and better than ever. The input from readers of the last edition has been invaluable, and I have added new sections and menus for novice strength trainers, as well as staying on the cutting edge of the science of nutrition for competitive athletes.

Power Eating has held its place at the top of the bookshelf because it gives not only the latest published research but a play-by-play report of what research is currently being conducted in laboratories around the world. Finally, it tells you how to put it all together to reach your goals. It's a true insider's view of the latest news on muscle-building supplements like beta-alanine as well as state-of-the-art diet and supplement strategies for gaining energy, getting cut, enhancing mood, and tightening mental focus.

Power Eating is the leader in guiding you through all your training periods throughout the year. The *Power Eating* menus are unsurpassed in their level of detail, yet they're practical to customize and follow in your busy life. Whether you are trying to maintain muscle, build muscle, lose fat, or cut, the *Power Eating* diet plans will get your body where you want it to be when you want it to be there while keeping you healthy, safe, and legal. You can have it all. Just train hard and Power Eat!

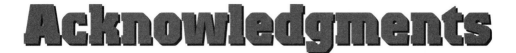

Acknowledgments

To Maggie Greenwood-Robinson, once again, thank you for an extraordinary job. I always look forward to working with you. Many thanks to Martin Barnard, our acquisitions editor, who has always shared our *Power Eating* vision; to Jana Hunter, for coming on board and helping us bring the third edition to life; to Heather Healy, our developmental editor; and to Alisha Jeddeloh, our copyeditor, for your keen eyes and high standards. To Al Zuckerman, my agent, thank you for your encouragement, intelligent advice, and great laugh. To the many teams, athletes, and clients whom I've worked with over the years, your passion to excel has challenged me to keep growing in my knowledge and practice. To my readers, your e-mails are thoughtful and uplifting. Thank you for all your suggestions and kind words. To my whole family, thanks for always being in my corner.

PART I

Foundation

Nothing is more important than a good foundation. A house must be built on a strong foundation to remain structurally sound for many years. A child needs a good academic and emotional foundation to develop independence and go out into the world as a happy and productive person. And an athlete must be anchored by a strong, scientifically based foundation of nutrition, training, and experience to stay in peak health and to perform successfully throughout life.

Part I is your introduction to your nutrition foundation. This section will translate the science of nutrition for strength training into the nuts and bolts of what you need to eat, day in and day out, to be a healthy, high-performing individual. Build a strong nutrition foundation, and muscular fitness, strength, and performance will follow.

1

Eating for Power

Think about how you'd like to look and feel. Imagine yourself with a body that's fit and firm with just the right amount of muscle. Imagine the joy of high strength and energy that give you the power to perform, day in and day out.

Keep those images in your mind's eye. This book will show you how to achieve them with a few nips and tucks in one of the most important fitness factors of all—nutrition. But we're not talking about just any type of nutrition. This is a book for people who strength train to stay in shape, compete in strength-training sports, or improve their athletic ability. In other words, you're a strength trainer if you lift weights a few times a week or train for competition. As a strength trainer, you have specific nutritional needs that depend on your type and level of activity.

So, what kind of strength trainer are you? Are you a bodybuilder, a power-lifter, an Olympic weightlifter, an athlete who strength trains for conditioning, or someone who works out with weights to stay in shape? All of these activities have different physical demands and different nutritional requirements, which is why you will find several individualized strength-training diets in chapters 12 through 15. But the common denominator is that all strength trainers, from competitors to recreational exercisers, are interested in the same thing: building lean muscle.

What Builds Muscle?

Most certainly, strength training builds muscle. But for this construction to take place, you have to supply the construction material: protein, carbohydrate, and fat. In a process called metabolism, the body breaks down these nutrients and uses the products to generate the energy required for growth and life.

During metabolism, proteins are broken down into amino acids. Cells use amino acids to make new proteins based on instructions supplied by DNA, our genetic management system. The DNA provides information on how amino acids are to be lined up and strung together. Once these instructions have been carried out, the cell has synthesized a new protein.

On the basis of this process, logic would tell you that the more protein you eat, the more muscle your body can construct. But it doesn't work that way. Excess protein is converted to carbohydrate to be used for energy or converted to fat for storage.

The way to make muscles grow is not by gorging on protein but by demanding more from it—that is, by making it work harder. The muscles will respond by taking up the nutrients they need, including amino acids from protein metabolism, so that they can grow. If you work your muscles hard, your muscle cells will synthesize the protein that the muscles need.

What Fuels Muscle?

To work your muscles hard, you have to provide the right kind of fuel. Muscle cells, like all cells, run on a high-energy compound known as adenosine triphosphate (ATP). ATP makes muscles contract, conducts nerve impulses, and promotes other cellular energy processes. Muscle cells make ATP by combining oxygen with nutrients from food, mainly carbohydrate. Fat is also used for fuel by muscles, but fat can be broken down only when oxygen is present. Muscle cells prefer to burn carbohydrate, store fat, and use protein for growth and repair.

Your cells generate ATP through any one of three energy systems: the phosphagen system, the glycolytic system, and the oxidative system.

The phosphagen system rebuilds ATP by supplying a compound called *creatine phosphate (CP)*. Once ATP is used up, it must be replenished from additional food and oxygen. During short, intense bursts of exercise such as weight training or sprinting, the working muscles exhaust the available oxygen. At that point, CP kicks in to supply energy for a few short seconds of work. CP can help create ATP when ATP is depleted. Any intense exercise lasting for 3 to 15 seconds will rapidly deplete ATP and CP in a muscle; they must then be replaced. Replenishing ATP and CP is the job of the other energy systems in the body.

The glycolytic system makes glucose available to the muscles, either from the breakdown of dietary carbohydrate during digestion or from the breakdown of muscle and liver glycogen, the stored form of carbohydrate. In a process called *glycolysis*, glycogen is disassembled into glucose in the muscles and, through a series of chemical reactions, ultimately converted into more ATP.

The glycogen reserve in your muscles can supply enough energy for about two to three minutes of short-burst exercise at a time. If sufficient oxygen is available, a lot of ATP will be made from glucose. If oxygen is absent or in short supply, the muscles produce a waste product from glucose called *lactic acid*. A buildup of lactic acid in a working muscle creates a burning sensation and causes the muscle to fatigue and stop contracting. Lactic acid exits the muscle when oxygen is available to replenish CP and ATP. A brief rest period gives the body time to deliver oxygen to the muscles, and you can continue exercising.

The third energy system is the oxidative system. This system helps fuel aerobic exercise and other endurance activities. Although the oxidative system can handle the energy needs of endurance exercise, all three energy systems kick in to some degree during endurance exercise. The phosphagen and glycolytic energy systems dominate during strength training.

Oxygen is not a direct source of energy for exercise; it is used as an ingredient to produce large amounts of ATP from other energy sources. The oxidative system works as follows: You breathe in oxygen, which the blood subsequently takes from your lungs. Your heart pumps oxygen-rich blood to tissues, including muscle. Hemoglobin, an iron-containing protein of the blood, carries oxygen to the cells to enable them to produce energy. Myoglobin, another type of iron-containing protein, carries oxygen primarily to muscle cells. Inside muscle cells, carbohydrate and fat are converted into energy through a series of energy-producing reactions.

Your body's ability to produce energy through any one of these three systems can be improved with the right training diet and exercise program. The result is a fat-burning, muscle-building metabolism.

Nutrition Principles for Strength Trainers

If you are serious about improving your physique and your strength-training performance, you'll do everything you can to achieve success. Unfortunately, advice given to strength trainers today is a hodgepodge of fact and fiction. What I'd like to do is separate one from the other by sharing several basic principles with you—principles that all strength trainers can follow to get in shape and achieve their personal best in performance. These principles are the same ones I have advocated for world-class athletes, Olympic contenders, and recreational strength trainers for more than 20 years. Let's review them here.

Eat Enough Calories

A key to feeling energized is to eat the right amount of calories to power your body for hard training. In the United States, the terms calorie and energy are often used interchangeably. Elsewhere, the joule is used as a measurement of energy. Although this book refers to calories, you can convert to kilojoules by multiplying the number of calories by 4.1868. A lack of calories will definitely make you feel like a wet dishrag by the end of your workout. A diet that provides fewer than 1,600 calories per day, for example, generally does not contain all the vitamins and minerals you need to stay healthy, prevent disease, and perform well. Very low-calorie diets followed for longer than two weeks can be hazardous to your health, and they do not provide the dietary reference intakes (DRIs) of enough of the nutrients needed for good health.

Historically, the recommended dietary allowances (RDAs) were the national standard for the amount of carbohydrate, protein, fat, vitamins, and minerals we need in our diets to avoid deficiency diseases and to maintain growth and health. The DRIs were established to update the RDAs based on more functional criteria rather than criteria based on deficiency diseases. Rather than focusing on avoiding disease, the DRIs focus on optimal performance both mentally and physically. But under certain conditions—stress, illness, malnutrition, and exercise—we may require a higher intake of certain nutrients. Studies have shown that athletes, in particular, may have to exceed the DRI of many nutrients. Some competitive bodybuilders have estimated their caloric intake to be greater than 6,000 calories a day during the off-season—roughly three times the DRI for the average person (2,000 calories a day for women and 2,700 calories a day for men).

How much you need of each nutrient depends on a number of factors, including your age and sex, how hard you train, and whether you are a competitive or recreational strength trainer, among other considerations. Generally, we find that strength trainers need to eat more protein, more of the right kinds of carbohydrate, and more of the right kinds of fat. What's more, they may be wise to supplement their diet with antioxidants and certain minerals. You'll learn more about these considerations as you read this book. If you are trying to gain muscle and lose body fat, eating enough calories and taking in enough nutrients will make the difference between success and failure.

Eat the Carbohydrate You Need

It's well known that most athletes, strength trainers included, don't eat enough carbohydrate, the primary fuel for the body. Most athletes eat diets in which only half of the total daily calories come from carbohydrate, but 6 to 7 grams of carbohydrate per kilogram of body weight should be consumed daily. That's more than half of an athlete's total calories, and this percentage should be as high as 60 percent for a heavyweight bodybuilder. Lots of bodybuilders prac-

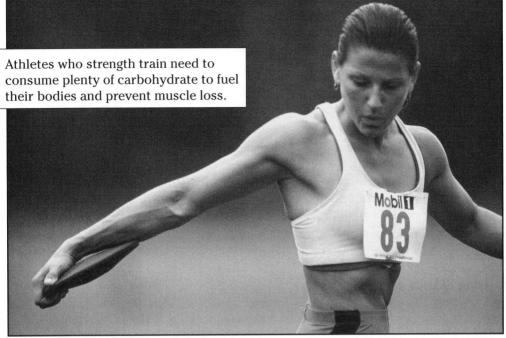

Athletes who strength train need to consume plenty of carbohydrate to fuel their bodies and prevent muscle loss.

© Rob Tringali / SportsChrome

tice low-carbohydrate dieting because they believe it promotes faster weight loss. The problem with these diets is that they deplete glycogen, the body's storage form of carbohydrate. Once glycogen stores are emptied, the body starts burning protein from tissues, including muscle tissue, to meet its energy demands. You lose hard-earned muscle as a result.

Many fitness-minded people shy away from foods high in carbohydrate, particularly breads and pasta. They think these foods will make them fat—a myth that is partially responsible for the unbalanced proportion of carbohydrate, fat, and protein in strength-training diets, which are typically too high in protein.

The real story on carbohydrate for weight control and muscle building is that you should select whole-food carbohydrate—natural, complex carbohydrate as close to its natural state as possible—instead of refined, processed carbohydrate. What's the difference? A blueberry is a whole-food carbohydrate; a blueberry toaster muffin is a processed carbohydrate.

One important reason why whole foods are better has to do with their high-fiber content. Fiber is the remnant of plant foods that remains undigested by the body. It's what keeps your bowel movements regular. Fiber is also a proven fat fighter. Research shows that people who eat healthy high-fiber diets have smaller waistlines, for example, and are able to better control their weight. The bottom line is that the right types of carbohydrate can help you manage your weight successfully. The only types of carbohydrate you should shy away from are sugars and highly processed foods. Even so, when used in a targeted way, sugars can be an athlete's best friend by providing the right fuel at the right time. But without a plan, they can be fattening.

You will learn more about carbohydrate in chapter 3, especially how to select the right types of carbohydrate in the right amounts at the right times so that you take in enough to fuel your muscles without gaining fat.

Vary Your Diet

You have probably admired the physiques of bodybuilders in magazines, and for good reason. They are muscular, well defined, and in near-perfect proportion—they look like the picture of health. But in many cases, bodybuilders eat incredibly unhealthy diets. The first study I ever conducted investigated the training diets of male competitive bodybuilders. What I found was that they ate a lot of calories, roughly 6,000 calories a day or more. The worrisome finding from this study was that they ate, on average, more than 200 grams of fat a day. That's almost as much fat as you'd find in two sticks of butter! In the short term, that's enough to make most people sick. Eaten habitually over time, such an enormous amount of fat may lead to heart disease.

Bodybuilding diets, especially precontest diets, tend to be monotonous, with the same foods showing up on the plate day after day. The worst example I've ever seen was a bodybuilder who ate chicken, pepper, vinegar, and rice for three days straight while preparing for competition. The problem with such a diet is that it lacks variety, and without a variety of foods, you miss out on nutrients essential for peak health.

Most bodybuilders don't eat much fruit, dairy products, and red meat. Fruit, of course, is packed with disease-fighting, health-building antioxidants and phytochemicals. Dairy products supply important nutrients like bone-building calcium. And red meat is an important source of vital minerals like iron and zinc.

When people limit or eliminate such foods from their diet, potentially serious deficiencies begin to show up. In studies conducted by myself and others, the most common deficiencies observed are those of calcium and zinc, particularly during the precompetition season. Many female bodybuilders have dangerous shortages of these minerals year round. A chronic short supply of calcium increases the risk of osteoporosis, a crippling bone-thinning disease. Although a woman's need for zinc is small (8 milligrams a day), adequate zinc is an impenetrable line of defense when it comes to protecting against disease and infection. In short, deficits of these minerals can harm health and performance. But the good news is that skim milk, red meat, and dark-meat poultry will help alleviate some of these problems. A 3-ounce (85-gram) portion of lean sirloin beef has about 6 milligrams of zinc; nonfat, 1 percent, or 2 percent milk has about 1 milligram of zinc in one 8-ounce (237-milliliter) glass; and 3 ounces (85 grams) of dark-meat turkey have about 4 milligrams of zinc.

Another nutritional problem among bodybuilders is fluid restriction. Just before a contest, bodybuilders don't drink much water, fearing it will inflate their physique to the point of blurring their muscular definition. Compounding the problem, many bodybuilders take diuretics and laxatives, a practice that flushes more water, as well as precious minerals called electrolytes, from the body. Generally, bodybuilders compete in a dehydrated state. At one contest, I saw two people pass out on stage—one because of severe dehydration, the other because of an electrolyte imbalance.

After a competition, bodybuilders tend to go hog wild with food. There's nothing wrong with this, as long as it's a temporary splurge for a few days or a week. But such dietary indulgence over a long time can lead to extra fat pounds.

Most bodybuilders, however, do a lot of things right, especially during the training season. For one thing, they eat several meals throughout the day—a practice that nutritionists recommend to the general public.

Time and Combine Your Food and Nutrients

To achieve superb shape and maximum performance, forgo the usual approach of three meals a day. Active people must fuel themselves throughout the day, eating small meals and snacks every two to three hours, preferably timed around their workout schedule. As we'll see, these meals don't include just any type of food.

When eating multiple meals, you always want to combine protein with carbohydrate and fat. Examples would be a turkey sandwich, a whole-wheat bagel with peanut butter, or an apple with nuts. Eating multiple meals also promotes variety in your diet and keeps your blood sugar levels even so that you avoid peaks and valleys throughout the day (a cycle that happens to promote fat storage).

By including small amounts of protein in meals and snacks, you can control your appetite, feed your muscles more efficiently, and maintain muscle when you're trying to lose fat. You also burn fat better because protein, as well as eating multiple small meals, has been shown to increase thermogenesis, the process by which your body converts ingested calories and stored fat into heat. Another advantage of multiple meals is mental performance. Regular, timed meals help you think and process information more effectively, increase your attention span, and boost your mood.

The bottom line is that small, frequent meals throughout the day are the best fat-burning, muscle-building strategy you can integrate into your lifestyle. Table 1.1 provides a look at how to time your meals properly and the benefits of doing so. The supplements listed in the table are discussed in detail elsewhere in this book.

Use a Food Plan

Any nutritional program aimed at losing body fat and building muscle should be based on a food plan that emphasizes lean protein, natural carbohydrate, and good fat. It should also include sample menus and recipes as well as information on how to make healthy selections that are personalized to your lifestyle. It should be neither so restrictive that it invites failure nor so unstructured as to be confusing. These are precisely the type of guidelines for food planning that you will find here.

Table 1.1   Timing Meals

Throughout the day

Fluids: 8-12 c (2-3 L) a day; at least 5 c (1 L) should be water.

Breakfast: Never skip this meal! It improves physical and mental performance and helps regulate weight.

Meals: Small, frequent protein–carbohydrate meals and snacks every 2-3 h.

Before exercise

Fluids: At least 8 oz (237 ml) before exercise.

Preexercise meal: At least 4 h before exercise so that the body properly assimilates carbohydrate for use by muscles.

Preexercise snack: 30-90 min before exercise. Snack should consist of 200-400 calories, including 30-50 g carbohydrate, 10-20 g protein, and 5-7 g fat. Snack can be food or meal-replacement supplement. This snack will provide additional energy for prolonged stamina and help decrease exercise-induced breakdown of muscle protein.

During exercise

Fluids: 7-10 oz (207-296 ml) every 10-20 min.

Glucose–electrolyte sport drinks: Sipping these during a workout has been shown to extend endurance. Use them during phases when you're trying to build muscle but not when you're trying to lose fat.

After exercise

Fluids: Replace each pound (.5 kg) of fluid lost with 16-24 oz (473-708 ml) of water or sport drink.

Carbohydrate: Consume .5 to 1 g/kg depending on what phase you're in.

Protein: Consume .5 g/kg protein with carbohydrate to encourage muscle growth. Postexercise snacks can be in the form of meal-replacement beverages with .5 to 1 g/kg of a high glycemic index and load carbohydrate and .5 g protein. Follow this within 2 h of exercise with a meal containing lots of carbohydrate and high-quality protein sources (e.g., fish, lean meats, low-fat dairy products, eggs).

Recovery supplements: Consume these with your meal replacement: creatine (2-5 g); glutamine (4-10 g); vitamin C (up to 500 mg); and zinc (up to 25 mg).

More specifically, if your goals are to develop lean muscle while reducing body fat, then your plan should take into consideration several factors, including balancing protein, carbohydrate, and fat; increasing your water intake; organizing your food into multiple meals; timing your intake; and incorporating certain dietary supplements into the mix.

You have to be exact about what you eat, and you need to make the right choices. Each calorie that you put into your mouth has to be results oriented. To drive your fat-burning machinery and lose weight, for example, you need to eat specific foods, such as dairy foods, whey protein, fish, soy, nuts, olives and olive oil, and green tea, to name a few. With the information you'll learn here, you can create a healthy diet that promotes fat loss and muscle gain.

Protein, Strength, and Muscle Building

For generations, athletes have believed that a high-protein diet will increase strength. This belief can be traced to a famous Greek athlete, Milo of Crotona, in the sixth century b.c.e. One of the strongest men in Greece, Milo was the wrestling victor in five Olympic Games and many other festivals. As the legend goes, he applied progressive resistance training by lifting a growing calf daily, and when the calf was four years old, he carried it the length of the Olympian stadium, killed it, roasted it, and ate it. It is written that his normal daily intake of meat was about 20 pounds (9 kilograms).

In the 1960s and 1970s, many people thought protein was a miracle food because muscle magazines hyped it so much. Bodybuilders and other athletes would follow diets made up mostly of meat, milk, and eggs. The raw-egg milkshake was particularly popular, thanks to Rocky Balboa. Why would anyone swill such a concoction? The answer is simple: misinformation. Articles and advertising from those days falsely communicated the notion that protein from raw foods, particularly eggs, is more available to the body for building muscle than protein from cooked foods is.

Not only is this notion absolutely untrue, it is dangerous. Eating raw eggs is a hazardous practice because eggs may be contaminated with the microorganisms that cause salmonella poisoning. Cooking eggs destroys bacteria, eliminating the risk of contracting this serious illness. Raw eggs should be avoided completely. If you want to add eggs to a supplemental drink, try pasteurized egg-white products instead of raw eggs, which is a safer practice. This form of egg whites can be cooked as well.

Cooking can also make protein more readily available to your body. A protein molecule is a string of amino acids connected together like a strand of pearls. If two strands of pearls were wound together and then twisted to double up on each other, they would resemble a protein molecule. Heating or cooking the protein molecule unwinds the string of amino acids, straightens it out, and separates it into smaller pieces. This is the process of heat denaturing, which is similar to the process of chemical denaturing, otherwise known as digestion. Cooking foods with protein can begin the digestive process and can actually decrease the net energy that the body must expend during digestion.

Protein is extremely vital in your diet, but by itself, it is not the magic bullet for muscle gain. Instead, protein and carbohydrate together are the magic bullet, especially in combination with the right kinds of fat. In other words, you must place equal emphasis on the right types of protein, carbohydrate, and fat in your diet. These nutrients work in concert to give you the edge on building body-firming muscle.

Power Profiles: Calorie Sources

Calories are certainly important in building muscle mass; however, the source of those calories is crucial if you want to maximize muscle and minimize body fat. A case in point is a professional rookie football player who wanted to lose weight to improve his speed on the field. Unless he trimmed down, his chance to be on the team was in jeopardy, so he needed a dramatic nutritional rescue.

This football player was eating slightly more than 7,000 calories a day. Broken down, those calories figured out to about 17 percent protein, 32 percent fat, and 49 percent carbohydrate. In daily fat grams, he was consuming a whopping 250 grams a day. The composition of his calories was an impediment to losing fat. I reconfigured his diet to 5,680 calories a day, with 15 percent of those calories coming from protein, 25 percent from fat, and 60 percent from carbohydrate. That mix slashed his fat grams to a healthier 142 grams a day.

He was eating a lot of unhealthy fat in foods like fried chicken, whole milk, and fast foods. For the high-fat foods, we substituted skinless chicken breasts, 1 percent milk, and fast-food choices such as salads and frozen yogurt that were lower in fat. In addition, we modified some of his favorite dishes such as sweet potato pie into healthier versions. He also began to load up on foods containing complex carbohydrate, like brown rice, whole wheat bread, fruits, and vegetables. Plus, he was using leaner protein sources with a wider variety of choices.

The upshot of these dietary changes was that he lost the weight, made the team, and had a great season. He is still a professional football player today.

The Scoop on Supplements

In the past several years, sales of dietary supplements have experienced explosive growth, surpassing $17 billion in sales a year and climbing. This growth has occurred despite the fact that some supplements have proven to be potentially harmful. Several years ago, for example, I would recommend that people take 400 IUs of vitamin E supplements, a fairly standard dosage. Today, however, I don't recommend anything higher than 100 to 200 IUs because of a study that found a slightly higher death rate (about 4 percent) in people who took 400 IUs of vitamin E or more than in those who took a placebo. That level of vitamin E amounted to an extra 48 deaths for every 10,000 people who were consuming it. With some supplements, there are just too many unknowns.

On the other hand, it appears that certain supplements are critical to good health. Omega-3 fatty acids are a good example. If you're not a fish eater, you should probably be taking omega-3 supplements because of their impressive list of health benefits. However, that's not to say that some day in the future research may surface that supplemental omega-3 fats aren't as beneficial as now thought.

Many of us tend to believe that certain supplements can cure disease. But in the case of vitamins and minerals, the only disease they will cure is one caused by a deficiency of that vitamin or mineral. It is always better to try to get your nutrients from whole foods, in which nutrients work synergistically to contribute to good health. But when you don't eat enough nutrients in your diet, supplementation with a daily multivitamin and mineral pill may be an important way to get what you need.

Beyond vitamin and mineral supplements, there is another class of nutrients called *nonessential supplements*. These are chemicals or compounds that don't cause classical signs of deficiency diseases if they are absent from the diet. Put another way, these supplements aren't required to maintain health or boost performance. We can certainly perform without nonessential supplements like medium-chain triglyceride (MCT) oil or creatine, but many strength trainers wouldn't be comfortable without them. Is it possible to reach new levels of performance by including nonessential supplements in our diets?

It's hard to say for sure, although the links between diet and performance are becoming clearer all the time. We have also come to realize that these links are more complex than we originally thought. Every day we read about new research discoveries relating to some factor in food that promises to boost energy or prevent disease. Sometimes these discoveries tell us that a factor previously considered nonessential may be important in improving health and energy.

Such information is all certain supplement manufacturers need to hear. Once one small piece of evidence surfaces—even in a single study—that a certain food factor may be helpful in preventing disease, building muscle, or enhancing performance, the next place you see that factor is in a supplement.

Unfortunately, supplement manufacturers don't have to follow the same rigorous review process that is required for new drugs. Supplements are legally considered food, not drugs. The U.S. Food and Drug Administration (FDA) expects the same kind of truth in labeling with supplements as it does with food. But in contrast to drugs, supplements do not have to be proven to work before they are placed on the market. Fortunately, though, a number of companies are conducting good research on their supplements. You can look at the manufacturer's website for supplements you use to see if the manufacturer has conducted research on the product. Ideally the research would be published in a scientific, peer-reviewed journal, meaning that other experts in the field have reviewed the research. This is the gold standard in scientific research, and it tells you the manufacturer has evidence to support its product claims.

Supplements have their place, and in chapters 8 and 9 I'll discuss targeted use of specific supplements by the right person, with the right goals, and under the right conditions. No supplement is beneficial unless you're following a healthy nutrition plan and training program and getting adequate rest.

Sport Nutrition Fact Versus Fiction:
Are Organic Foods Better for You?

Many strength trainers are opting to go organic to avoid the chemical fertilizers, pesticides, and additives used in many foods. Do you get an advantage in consuming organic foods?

In general, organically grown foods are grown in soil enriched with organic fertilizers rather than synthetic fertilizers and treated only with nonsynthetic pesticides. Organic farms use a soil-building program that promotes vibrant soil and healthy plants, usually including crop rotations and biological pest control.

We tend to think only of fruits and vegetables when we think of organic foods. However, organic meat, poultry, dairy, and egg products are also available. These foods come from farms that have been inspected to verify that they meet rigorous standards mandating the use of organic feed, that they prohibit the use of antibiotics, and that they require that animals have access to the outdoors, fresh air, and sunlight.

You can tell the difference between organically produced food and conventionally produced food by looking at package labels. The U.S. Department of Agriculture (USDA) has developed strict labeling rules to help consumers know the exact organic content of the food they buy. Look for the USDA Organic seal; it tells you that a product is at least 95 percent organic.

Organic foods do appear to have some advantages over conventionally produced foods. Here is what some of the latest research shows:

- Organic foods may be highly nutritious. Organic foods are higher in vitamin C and many minerals, antioxidants, and phytochemicals.

- Consuming organic foods appears to present fewer of the health hazards associated with pesticide contamination. In one study, children who ate organic produce and juice had only one-sixth the level of pesticide by-products in their urine compared with children who ate conventionally produced food. Thus, there are some important safety justifications for eating organic foods.

- One study found that farmworkers who apply pesticides as part of conventional farming have higher concentrations of pesticides in their bodies. Conceivably, if the trend continues toward organic farming, farmworkers may be protected from unhealthy exposure.

- Organic foods are not only good for you, they are good for the planet. Organic farming methods are less harmful to the environment than conventional methods. The use of natural products helps to improve the soil, and organic pest control generally relies on preventive measures such as crop rotation and biological controls. These methods place little to no stress on the earth and its wildlife inhabitants. According to one survey, now that organic agriculture is being embraced as environmentally sound and more sustainable than mainstream agriculture, consumers feel like they are contributing to a better future and an improved environment.

- Finally, I think that organic produce often tastes better. In Seattle, where I live, lots of organic food is grown locally. Consequently, the produce is very fresh because it doesn't have to be transported over thousands of miles.

Whether or not you decide to go organic, the most important move you can make for your health is to eat more fruits and vegetables. Much research shows that people can improve their health and quality of life by consuming more plant foods. Despite the use of pesticides, populations that eat large amounts of fruits and vegetables have lower rates of cancer and other life-threatening illnesses than populations that eat few fruits and vegetables.

In the end, the choice is yours. Purchasing organic foods is not just a nutritional issue but a political, social, and personal issue as well. If you want to treat the earth well and potentially protect workers from pesticide exposure, speak with your pocketbook: Buy organic.

You may pay more for organic produce, so if your pocketbook is light, buy fresh nonorganic produce and follow these guidelines for reducing pesticide residues in foods:

- Wash fresh produce in water. Use a scrub brush, and rinse the foods thoroughly under running water.

- Use a knife to peel an orange or grapefruit; do not bite into the peel.

- Discard the outer leaves of leafy vegetables such as cabbage and lettuce.

- Peel waxed fruit and vegetables; waxes don't wash off and can seal in pesticide residues.

- Peel vegetables such as carrots and fruits such as apples when appropriate. (Peeling removes pesticides that remain in or on the peel, but it also removes fiber, vitamins, and minerals.)

Where Do You Stand Now?

Analyze your present diet now to see exactly what you're eating, particularly in terms of the three energy nutrients. You should also analyze how much water you're drinking, because water is a critical nutrient. This analysis will make the following chapters more relevant and interesting. For example, when you're reading about protein, you may wonder how much protein you're eating now. With this analysis handy, you can find out quickly.

Using the form provided in appendix A on page 285, record everything you eat over the course of three days. Choose days that best represent your typical diet. Be as accurate as you can in terms of the amount of food you eat. Use the information in chapters 12 through 15 to help you figure out nutrients and calories.

2

Manufacturing Muscle

Inside your body, a marvelous process of self-repair takes place day in and day out, and it all has to do with protein, the nutrient responsible for building and maintaining body tissues.

Protein is present everywhere in the body—in muscles, bones, connective tissue, blood vessels, blood cells, skin, hair, and fingernails. This protein is constantly being lost or broken down as a result of normal physiological wear and tear and must be replaced. For example, about half of the total amount of protein in muscle tissue is broken down and replaced every 150 days.

The mechanism by which this repair occurs is really quite amazing. During digestion, protein in food is dismantled by other proteins (enzymes) into sub-units called *amino acids.* Amino acids then enter cells, and other enzymes, acting on instructions from DNA, put them back together as the new proteins needed to build and repair tissue. Virtually no other system in the world repairs itself so wonderfully. Every day, this process goes on and life continues.

Under any condition of growth—childhood, pregnancy, muscle building—the body manufactures more cells than are lost. From an energy source such as carbohydrate or fat, the body can manufacture many of the materials needed to make new cells. But to replace and build new protein, it must have protein from food. Unlike carbohydrate and fat, protein contains nitrogen, and nitrogen is required to synthesize new protein.

Protein, therefore, is absolutely necessary for the maintenance, replacement, and growth of body tissue. But protein has other uses, too. The body uses protein to regulate hormone secretion, maintain the body's water balance, protect against disease, transport nutrients in and out of cells, carry oxygen, and regulate blood clotting.

Protein and Muscle Building

Protein is a key player in the repair and construction of muscle tissue after exercise. By lifting weights, you force your muscles to lengthen when they want to contract. This action causes microscopic tears in your muscle fibers, which are the cause of the muscle soreness you feel a day or two after a workout. In response, your body makes muscle fibers bigger and stronger to protect against future tears.

The construction material for this process comes primarily from dietary protein, which is broken down in digestion into amino acids. As previously explained, amino acids enter the bloodstream and are transported to muscle cells to be synthesized into protein. There are two major types of muscle protein, actin and myosin. During muscular contraction, these muscle proteins slide over each other like two pieces of a telescope. When you build muscle, you're increasing the amount of actin and myosin in your muscles. This makes the muscle fibers increase in diameter, get stronger, and contract more powerfully.

Protein and Fat Burning

Studies have suggested that, compared with diets high in carbohydrate and low in fat, diets high in protein and low in fat promote greater weight loss. One reason is that lean protein helps stoke your fat-burning fires. Its thermogenic (heat-producing) effect may be as high as 22 percent, compared with as low as .8 percent for carbohydrate. In other words, you burn more calories by doing nothing more than eating slightly more protein and less carbohydrate.

A research article published in 2002 by Dr. Carol Johnston and colleagues from Arizona State University East in Mesa, Arizona, helps to explain the mechanism. Ten women aged 19 to 22 years consumed either a high-protein or high-carbohydrate diet, and then their energy production was measured two and a half hours after the meal. The study found that energy production was 100 percent higher on the high-protein diet than on the high-carbohydrate diet. Over the course of the day, postmeal energy production on the high-protein diet totaled 30 more calories at each test time. Johnston speculates that if this energy differential actually lasted for two to three hours after each meal (since each test point was two and a half hours after each meal), the added thermogenic effect of the high-protein diet may have been as high as 90 calories. What that means is that you can potentially burn more calories with extra protein in your diet. The high-protein diet contained 2 grams of protein per kilogram of body weight per day.

An increased sense of satiety is associated with the thermogenic effect of protein. Women placed on high-protein, moderate-carbohydrate meals have a greater sensation of fullness during meals that lasts for longer periods of time compared with low-protein meals. The difference is associated with the thermic effect of the meal. By following a high-protein, moderate-carbohydrate diet, you will feel more satisfied and have greater control over what and how much you eat.

To capitalize on the thermogenic effect of high-protein meals, you should consume protein in frequent meals and snacks throughout the day. This allows for the most efficient absorption and utilization of protein, and it helps to maintain higher levels of energy production to promote weight loss.

Protein and Strength-Training Performance

It would seem that the more construction material (protein) you supply your body, the more muscle you'll build. At least that's the train of thought strength athletes have followed for ages. But it doesn't quite work that way. Eating twice as much protein won't make your muscles twice as big. Furthermore, one problem with eating too much protein is that the excess can be stored as body fat.

To build muscle, you must maintain a positive nitrogen balance. Nitrogen leaves the body primarily in the urine and must be replaced by nitrogen taken in from food. Protein contains a fairly large concentration of nitrogen. Generally, healthy adults are in a state of nitrogen equilibrium, or zero balance—that is, their protein intake meets their protein requirement. A positive nitrogen balance means that the body is retaining dietary protein and using it to synthesize new tissue. If more nitrogen is excreted than consumed, the nitrogen balance is negative. The body has lost nitrogen—and therefore protein. A negative nitrogen balance over time is dangerous, leading to muscle wasting and disease.

Achieving a positive nitrogen balance doesn't necessarily mean you have to eat more protein. Muscle cells take up the exact amount of nutrients (including amino acids from dietary protein) they need for growth, and strength training helps them make better use of the protein that's available.

This fact was clearly demonstrated in 1995 by a group of Tufts University researchers led by Wayne W. Campbell. The researchers took a group of older men and women (aged 56 to 80 years) who had never lifted weights before, placed them on either a low-protein diet or a high-protein diet, and measured their nitrogen balance before and after participation in a 12-week strength-training program. The low-protein diet was actually based on the RDA for protein (.8 grams per kilogram of body weight daily). The high-protein diet was twice the RDA (1.6 grams per kilogram of body weight daily). The researchers wanted to see what effects each diet had on nitrogen balance during strength training.

What they discovered was interesting. Strength training enhanced nitrogen retention in both groups—protein was being retained and used to synthesize

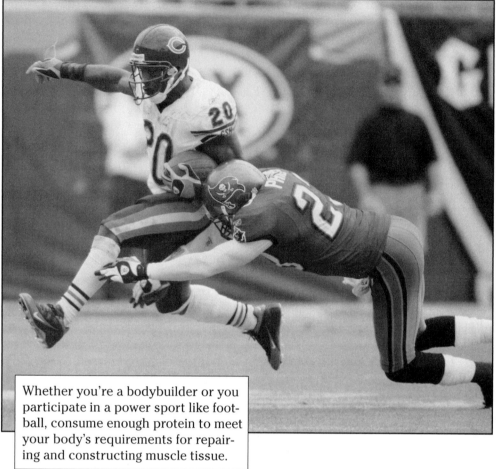

Whether you're a bodybuilder or you participate in a power sport like football, consume enough protein to meet your body's requirements for repairing and constructing muscle tissue.

© Tom DiPace / SportsChrome

new tissue. However, in the low-protein group, there was even better use of protein. Strength training caused the body to adapt and meet the demand for protein—even when the bare minimum requirement for protein was eaten each day. While this low level of protein intake may not be optimal for building muscle, this study shows how marvelously the body adjusts to what is available and how strength training makes muscle cells more efficient at using available protein to synthesize new tissue.

So, exactly how much protein should you eat for maximum performance and results? That question has been hotly debated in science for more than 100 years and by athletes since the time of the ancient Greeks. It has been difficult for nutrition scientists to reach a consensus on protein intake for several reasons. One reason has to do with the type and frequency of exercise you do. In endurance exercise, for example, protein can act as kind of a spare fuel tank, kicking in amino acids to supply fuel. If protein is in short supply, endurance athletes can peter out easily. In strength sports, additional dietary protein is needed to provide enough amino acids to synthesize protein in the muscles.

For generations, strength trainers have looked to protein as the nutritional panacea for muscle building. Is there any scientific basis to this belief?—New research shows that as a strength trainer, you may benefit from eating some extra protein.

Age and Protein Intake

It's no secret that as you age, you can lose muscle mass, strength, and function, partly because of inactivity. One way to reverse the downhill slide is by strength training. Study after study has shown that you can make significant muscle gains well into your 90s if you strength train.

Scientific research indicates that senior strength trainers can get a real boost from additional protein. At Tufts University, researchers gave supplemental protein to a group of elderly strength trainers, while a control group took no supplements. Based on CAT scans of muscle, the supplement group gained much more muscle mass than the control group did.

But what if you're not yet in your golden years? Can you get the same benefits from extra protein? Many studies say yes. Two groups of young bodybuilders following a four-week strength-training program ate the same diet, but with one exception. One group ate 2.3 grams of protein per kilogram of body weight (much more than the DRI), and the other group ate 1.3 grams of protein per kilogram of body weight. By the end of the study, both groups had gained muscle, but those eating the higher amount of protein had gained five times more!

Proper Protein Levels

At Kent State University, researchers divided strength trainers into three groups: (1) a low-protein group on a diet of .9 grams of protein per kilogram of body weight, which approximates the recommendation of .8 gram per kilogram for sedentary people; (2) a group on a diet of 1.4 grams of protein per kilogram of body weight; and (3) a group on a diet of 2.4 grams of protein per kilogram of body weight. Control groups with both sedentary subjects and strength-training subjects were also included.

Two exciting findings emerged. First, increasing protein intake to 1.4 grams triggered protein synthesis (an indicator of muscle growth) in strength trainers. There were no such changes in the low-protein group. Second, upping protein intake from 1.4 grams to 2.4 grams produced no further protein synthesis. This latter finding suggests that a plateau was reached, meaning that the subjects got more protein than they could use from 2.4 grams.

The research appears to indicate that if you strength train and eat more protein, you are going to enhance muscle development and preservation. But this doesn't necessarily mean you should start piling protein on your plate. Studies should always be interpreted with caution. Let's talk about how much protein you really need based on your activity level.

Your Individual Protein Requirements

As a strength trainer or bodybuilder, you need more protein than a less active person. Your requirement is higher than the current DRI of .8 gram of protein per kilogram of body weight a day, which is based on the needs of nonexercisers, but it's only slightly higher. (Don't forget, your body can work with a protein intake that meets the DRI.) Plus, individual protein requirements vary, depending on whether you're building muscle, doing aerobic exercise on a regular basis, or dieting for competition. Here's a closer look.

- **Muscle building.** With increases in training intensity, you need additional protein to support muscle growth and increases in certain blood compounds. On the basis of the latest research with strength trainers, I recommend that you eat 2.0 grams of protein per kilogram of body weight a day. Here's how you would figure that requirement if you weigh 150 pounds, or 68 kilograms (a kilogram equals 2.2 pounds):

$$2 \text{ g of protein} \times 68 \text{ kg} = 136 \text{ g of protein a day}$$

Strength trainers living in high altitudes need even more protein: 2.2 grams per kilogram of body weight daily. If you're a vegan, your protein needs are also 10 percent higher to make sure your diet is providing all the necessary amino acids:

$$2.2 \text{ g of protein} \times 68 \text{ kg} = 150 \text{ g of protein a day}$$

If you are new to strength training, you may need to eat more than a veteran strength trainer typically consumes—as much as 40 percent more.

- **Aerobic exercise.** On average, most strength trainers and bodybuilders perform an hour or two of intense weight training daily, plus five or more hours a week of aerobic exercise. If you are in this category, your protein needs are further elevated. Here's why.

During aerobic exercise lasting 60 to 90 minutes or more, certain amino acids—the branched-chain amino acids (BCAAs)—are used for energy in small amounts, particularly when the body is running low on carbohydrate, its preferred fuel source. One of the BCAAs, leucine, is broken down to make alanine, another amino acid, which is converted by the liver into blood sugar (glucose) for energy. This glucose is transported to the working muscles to be used for energy. The harder you work aerobically, the more leucine your body breaks down for extra fuel. In addition, studies show that obtaining amino acids such as leucine stimulates muscle repair, as well as muscular development, in the period following exercise.

Given this special use of amino acids as an energy and recovery source, you should increase your protein intake if your training program includes more than 5 hours a week of an endurance program. You may require as much as

2.2 grams of protein per kilogram of body weight. With the preceding example, you would calculate your requirements as follows:

$$2.2 \text{ g of protein} \times 68 \text{ kg} = 150 \text{ g of protein a day}$$

- **Competition dieting.** When cutting calories to get lean for looks or for competition, you risk losing body-firming muscle. Because muscle is the body's most metabolically active tissue, losing it compromises the ability of your body to burn fat. What's more, no bodybuilder wants to lose muscle before competition. One way to prevent diet-related muscle loss is to consume adequate protein while you're preparing for competition. Dieting bodybuilders need between 2.2 and 2.5 grams of protein per kilogram of body weight a day; I recommend 2.3 grams per day. Here is an example:

$$2.3 \text{ g of protein} \times 68 \text{ kg} = 156 \text{ g of protein a day}$$

Incidentally, the distribution of calories in this kind of plan will be 30 percent protein, 40 percent carbohydrate, and 30 percent fat (30–40–30). For more information on getting cut for competition, see chapter 15.

Proper Timing of Protein Intake

Let's say you've just finished an intense strength-training workout. If you could zoom in to the microscopic level of your muscles, you'd be astounded by the sight. There are tears in the tiny structures of your muscle fibers and leaks in your muscle cells. Over the next 24 to 48 hours, muscle protein will break down, and additional muscle glycogen will be used.

These are some of the chief metabolic events that occur in the aftermath of a hard workout. And although these events might look like havoc, they are actually a necessary part of recovery—the repair and growth of muscle tissue that take place after every workout. During recovery, the body replenishes muscle glycogen and synthesizes new muscle protein. In the process, muscle fibers are made bigger and stronger to protect themselves against future trauma.

You can do much to enhance the recovery process—including consuming protein before and after your workout. Having a small meal that includes protein and carbohydrate before your strength-training workout is very beneficial. In a review study (a study that looks at a bundle of research) of the role of protein in the athlete's diet, Dr. Peter W. Lemon, who has done cutting-edge research on protein, noted that protein meals consumed before exercise can result in greater gains in both muscle mass and strength than with training alone. The evidence here is too compelling to ignore, which is why I recommend small preexercise meals that include protein.

The next step is to eat a small meal immediately after exercise. Your body has already digested your preexercise protein, and it is working for you at the muscular level. Two or three hours later, as that effect wears off, your body begins to demand protein for the repair and recovery phase following a workout. According to research, you can jump-start the glycogen-making process by eating .5 gram of protein per kilogram of body weight, along with a high-glycemic carbohydrate, such as dextrose, maltodextrin, sucrose, or even honey, within 30 minutes of exercise. For example, if you weigh 150 pounds (68 kilograms), you should eat 34 grams of protein.

When protein is consumed along with carbohydrate, there's a surge in insulin. Insulin is like an acceleration pedal. It races the body's glycogen-making motor in two ways. First, it speeds up the movement of glucose and amino acids into cells, and second, it activates a special enzyme crucial to glycogen synthesis. Additional research shows that a carbohydrate and protein supplement ingested after exercise triggers the release of growth hormone in addition to insulin. Both are conducive to muscle growth and recovery.

Also, the availability of essential amino acids (see table 2.1) after exercise boosts the rate of muscle protein resynthesis in the body. On the basis of these findings, I recommend that you consume .5 to 1 gram per kilogram of body weight of a high-glycemic carbohydrate with .5 gram of a protein food or a quality protein supplement—preferably one that contains all the essential amino acids. (See table 3.2 on page 50 for a glycemic index of foods.)

High-Protein Diet Dangers

The high-protein, low-carbohydrate approach to weight control is a defeatist strategy if you are a strength trainer or bodybuilder. Not eating enough carbohydrate can lower your calorie intake, and when calories are restricted, your body will use protein from the diet to meet its energy demands. This leaves a reduced amount of protein available for the physiological functions that only protein can perform. Without enough protein, more muscle will be lost during weight loss, resulting in the undesirable effect of reduced metabolic rate. The bottom line is that you need carbohydrate along with protein to maintain muscle mass. Following a fat-loss diet that is 30 percent protein, which I recommended earlier in this chapter, is a win–win strategy. In this diet, you're lowering carbohydrate intake only slightly to make room for the extra protein, which will help drive fat burning.

The high-protein diets I object to are those that omit or drastically cut carbohydrate. Such diets promising quick weight loss continue to be the rage. These diets let you fill up on beef, chicken, fish, and eggs, with little emphasis on other foods like vegetables and grains.

What's wrong with such diets? To begin with, they're high in fat. The protein in animal foods is often coupled with large amounts of saturated fat and cholesterol. Excess dietary fat can make you gain body fat and can damage your heart. Most extreme protein diets are often low in fiber, too. Without enough bulk to

Table 2.1 Essential, Conditionally Essential, and Nonessential Amino Acids		
Essential	**Conditionally essential**	**Nonessential**
Isoleucine*	Arginine	Alanine
Leucine*	Cysteine (cystine)	Asparagine
Lysine	Glutamine	Aspartic acid
Methionine	Histidine	Citruline
Phenylalanine	Proline	Glutamic acid
Threonine	Taurine	Glycine
Tryptophan	Tyrosine	Serine
Valine*		

*Branched-chain amino acid.

Adapted from M.G. Di Pasquale. 2000, Proteins and amino acids in exercise and sport. In *Energy-Yielding Macronutrients and Energy Metabolism in Sports Nutrition*, edited by J.A. Driskell and I. Wolinsky (Philadelphia, PA: CRC Press), 119-162.

move things along, your whole digestive system slows down to a crawl, which can lead to constipation, diverticulosis, and other intestinal disorders.

In addition, most protein diets are dehydrating. Within the first week on a high-protein diet, you can lose a lot of weight, depending on your initial weight and body-fat percentage. You get on the scale, see an exhilarating weight loss, and feel wonderful, but most of this loss is water. You could be very dehydrated as a result, which spells trouble. If you weigh 150 pounds (68 kilograms), a mere 3-pound (1-kilogram) loss of water weight can make you feel draggy and hurt your exercise performance. The minute you go off this diet and eat some carbohydrate, water surges back into your tissues and you regain the lost water weight.

Clearly, your focus should not be on protein, but on a balance of nutrients. In chapters 12 through 15, you'll learn how to design your own personal eating plan, one that contains the right amount of protein, carbohydrate, and fat to help you build muscle and stay lean.

Fish Alert: Red Light or Green Light?

Fish is a food close to my heart. First of all, I love to eat it. Fish is such an incredibly healthy food that I tell my clients to eat five servings of fish each week as a protein source. But recent news about harmful pollutants in fish has put a note of caution into the praises being sung about fish.

Green Light

Fish is a quality source of protein that's low in fat and cholesterol. It's also a good source of niacin, vitamin B12, vitamin D, and omega-3 fatty acids. Studies have shown that people who include fish in their diet have better control of body weight. When fish is added to a weight-loss diet, more total fat and more abdominal fat are lost.

Omega-3 fats have been shown to decrease symptoms of inflammatory diseases like arthritis and colitis; reduce risks of heart disease, stroke, and certain types of cancers; and are linked with a lower risk of developing Alzheimer's disease. New research on omega-3 fats has established a strong link between dietary intake and mood, resulting in the use of omega-3 fats as part of an overall approach to managing and treating mild depression. For pregnant women, dietary omega-3 fats are important for fetal brain development, and they may reduce the risk of preterm births and slightly increase a child's cognitive abilities.

Red Light

Although fish is important in your diet, there can be some hazards associated with it. The damage we've done to the Earth's oceans has contaminated the environment where fish live and eat, leading to fish that may be contaminated with toxic chemicals.

Mercury

Concerns about mercury levels in several species of fish have been around for a long time, especially regarding the diets of pregnant women, nursing mothers, and young children. Mercury is a naturally occurring element in the environment and is also released into the air through industrial pollution. Mercury that falls from the air can accumulate in streams and oceans. Bacteria in the water cause chemical changes that transform mercury into methylmercury, and fish absorb the methylmercury as they feed in these waters. Methylmercury builds up more in some fish than others, depending on what they eat.

Methylmercury in the bloodstream of a fetus or young child can have adverse effects on the developing nervous system. Mercury is a potent neurotoxin, and prenatal exposure to even low levels can cause serious damage to the development of the brain, spinal cord, and nerves throughout the body.

Both the Environmental Protection Agency (EPA) and the FDA posted various advisories regarding the consumption of fish. These advisories often did not contain corresponding recommendations because the two organizations have different mandates: the EPA looks solely at health risks, whereas the FDA considers both safety and nutrition. Because these conflicting recommendations were not serving the public with useful information, the organizations drafted a joint consumer advisory in December 2004.

According to the advisory, pregnant women, women who might become pregnant, and nursing mothers should follow three rules:

1. Don't eat shark, swordfish, king mackerel, or tilefish because they contain high levels of mercury.
2. Mix up the types of fish and shellfish you eat since levels of mercury in fish can vary. Do not eat the same type of fish or shellfish more than once a week. You can safely eat up to 12 ounces (340 grams, or two to three meals) of other purchased fish and shellfish per week.
3. Check local advisories about the safety of fish caught by family and friends in local rivers and streams. If no advice is available, you can safely eat up to 6 ounces (170 grams, or one meal per week) of fish you catch from local waters, but don't consume any other fish during that week.

Follow the same rules when feeding fish and shellfish to young children, but the serving sizes should be smaller. The advisory also notes, "Tuna is one of the most frequently consumed fish in the United States. Mercury levels in tuna vary. Tuna steaks and canned albacore tuna generally contain higher levels of mercury than canned light tuna. You can safely include tuna as part of your weekly fish consumption."

From the U.S. Department of Health and Human Services and the U.S. Environmental Protection Agency, 2004. Available: http://www.cfsan.fda.gov/~dms/admehg3.html

Cancer-Causing Pollutants

The lead story in the News of the Week column published in the January 9, 2004, edition of the journal *Science* was about the dangers of eating farm-raised salmon. The concern is over the levels of cancer-causing pollutants found in farm-raised salmon, which are significantly higher than those in wild salmon.

Wild salmon are born in the cold rivers that run from Alaska to California. After hatching, they struggle to make their way to the ocean where they grow into a mature fish, returning to their natal rivers to spawn. Most wild salmon are caught in a short period during the late spring and summer when the fish migrate from the oceans to the rivers. This natural life process produces a lean, high-quality protein that is high in vitamins D and E and omega-3 fatty acids.

Contrary to the lives of wild salmon, farm-raised salmon are raised in an industrialized, contained habitat that allows for mass production. They are fed an artificial diet consisting of small fish that are ground up into fish meal. An artificial dye is added to the fish meal to give the salmon the pinkish hue that wild salmon get from their natural diet.

Pollutants get into farmed salmon through the small fish used in the fish meal. Pollutants such as factory runoff enter the habitat of small fish. The small fish absorb the pollutants, which are then highly concentrated in the fish meal. When the farmed salmon eat the fish meal, the pollutants are stored in the salmons' fat.

A study at Indiana University by Professor Ronald Hites and coworkers, published in the same January 9, 2004, edition of *Science*, analyzed 700 salmon from around the world for more than 50 contaminants. The greatest difference between farmed and wild salmon was in organochlorine compounds, particularly the cancer-causing polychlorinated biphenyls (PCBs), dieldrin, and toxaphene. Farmed salmon in Europe had the highest levels of these compounds, followed by those from North America. Farm-raised Chilean salmon were the cleanest.

The authors stated the possibility that eating more than one meal of farmed salmon per month may increase the risk of cancer. Then they got down to specifics. Table 2.2 shows the amount of salmon you can safely eat based on its origin.

Table 2.2 Safe Levels for Salmon Consumption	
Source of salmon	**Serving and frequency**
Scotland and Faroe Islands farm raised	2 oz (57 g) per month
Canada and Maine farm raised	4 oz (113 g) per month
Chile and Washington State farm raised	8 oz (227 g) per month
Wild salmon	64 oz (1,814 g) per month (1 lb or 454 g per week)

Adapted from Ronald A. Hites, et al. 2004, "Global assessment of organic contaminants in farmed salmon," *Science* 303: 226-229.

These recommendations are based on how much salmon is safe to eat for the average person. Advice for pregnant women is still under debate. Such pollutants can damage the developing endocrine system, immune system, and brain. The compounds build up in body fat and linger there for decades—where they can be passed to the fetus during pregnancy or to the baby through breast milk. The inclusion of farmed salmon in the diets of women of child-bearing age is a definite concern.

Yellow Light

Although the negative data look bleak, you should not eliminate fish from your diet, but you should proceed with caution. Based on studies examining the risk of developing heart disease, the American Heart Association (AHA) recommends that people with cardiovascular problems consume 6 to 12 ounces (170-340 grams) of fatty fish each week to raise their dietary intake of omega-3 fats. Because of the overwhelming health benefits of fish, I recommend five servings of fish a week to my clients.

Seafood choices that are generally low in contaminants include anchovies, sardines, oysters, crab, mussels, halibut, black cod, sole, turbot, and pollock. When you eat salmon, your best choice is wild salmon. If you choose farmed salmon, check where it was farmed; Washington State and Chile have the cleanest fish.

When it comes to tuna, there are some important points. While tuna steaks and canned albacore tuna tend to have higher levels of methylmercury, the size of the fish and where it is caught make an enormous difference. Fish become contaminated with mercury by eating smaller fish contaminated with mercury, and large fish eat more fish. The fish that they eat are more contaminated due to the volume of other fish that they consume, so the concentration of mercury rises with the weight of the fish. Conversely, the smaller the fish, the lower the concentration of mercury in its body.

Ocean waters vary in their level of mercury contamination. Tuna caught in cleaner waters have lower levels of mercury contamination. Fishing vessels that catch tuna for the large canneries whose products are most commonly found on supermarket shelves catch very large fish, 40 pounds (18 kilograms) in weight or higher. They want to catch fish in the most cost-effective manner, using nets, which often takes them to ocean waters with higher levels of mercury content. Tuna from these large canneries is generally high in mercury.

Privately owned boutique canneries in the Pacific Northwest catch smaller fish one at time by trolling rather than using a net. The fish weigh an average of 10 to 15 pounds (5-7 kilograms). These companies fish in cleaner waters because their smaller fishing vessels and different style of fishing allow them to be more flexible and maneuverable, leading to cleaner areas of ocean waters. These canned tuna are virtually free of mercury.

The canning process used by boutique canneries is also different, and it results in a superior product both in taste and nutritional content. Commercial canneries cook the fish twice, resulting in a substantial loss of natural oils and juices. Vegetable broth is then added along with additives such as pyrophosphate or hydrolyzed casein. This is the commercial canneries' water-pack method. The smaller canneries use a raw-pack method of canning, which cooks the fish one time only, in the can. All the natural juices and beneficial oils remain in the finished product. One cannery that has tested the levels of omega-3 fats in their tuna found 1.7 grams per serving, compared with .5 gram found in Starkist-brand tuna—four times the amount.

Like many other food concerns, fish safety comes down to becoming an informed consumer. Fish is far too healthy and delicious to eliminate from your diet, but you have to eat smart. Follow the guidelines and avoid unsafe fish while you are pregnant or nursing and when you feed young children. Choose the safe and clean varieties of salmon and tuna so that you can continue to enjoy them in your diet with confidence.

Red Meat

You may have shied away from red meat in the past because it tends to be high in fat and dietary cholesterol. Red meat, however, is a good source of protein, as well as iron, zinc, and other nutrients. Incidentally, so are dark-meat turkey and chicken.

Iron is necessary for manufacturing hemoglobin, which carries oxygen from the lungs to the tissues, and myoglobin, another transporter of oxygen found only in muscle tissue. The iron in red meat and other animal proteins is known as heme iron. The body absorbs heme iron better than it absorbs iron from plant foods, known as nonheme iron.

Zinc is a busy mineral. As one of the most widely distributed minerals in the body, zinc helps the body absorb vitamins, especially the B-complex vitamins. It is also involved in digestion and metabolism and is essential for growth. Like iron, zinc from animal protein is absorbed better than zinc from plant foods.

It may surprise you to learn that red meat can be very lean. In fact, 20 of the 29 lean beef cuts have, on average, only 1 more gram of saturated fat than a skinless chicken breast per 3-ounce (85-gram) serving (see table 2.3).

Table 2.3   The 20 Leanest Cuts of Beef

Cut	Saturated fat (g)	Total fat (g)
Eye of round roast and steak	1.4	4.0
Sirloin tip side steak	1.6	4.1
Top round roast and steak	1.6	4.6
Bottom round roast and steak	1.7	4.9
Top sirloin steak	1.9	4.9
Brisket, flat half	1.9	5.1
95% round beef	2.4	5.1
Round tip roast and steak	1.9	5.3
Round steak	1.9	5.3
Shank cross cuts	1.9	5.4
Chuck shoulder pot roast	1.8	5.7
Sirloin tip center roast and steak	2.1	5.8
Chuck shoulder steak	1.9	6.0
Bottom round steak	2.2	6.0
Top loin (strip) steak	2.3	6.0
Shoulder petite tender and medallions	2.4	6.1
Flank steak	2.6	6.3
Shoulder center (ranch) steak	2.4	6.5
Tri-tip roast and steak	2.6	7.1
Tenderloin roast and steak	2.7	7.1
T-bone steak	3.0	8.2

For comparative purposes, a 3-ounce (85-gram) serving of a skinless chicken breast has .9 gram of saturated fat and 3 grams of total fat.

Data from U.S. Department of Agriculture, Agricultural Research Service. 2005. USDA Nutrient Database for Standard Reference, Release 18. Nutrient Data Laboratory Home Page, http://www.ars.usda.gov/ba/bhnrc/ndl.

Beef Safety Tips

Consumer confidence in beef is fairly high despite concerns around the globe regarding mad cow disease. Even so, you should take precautions to protect yourself against any meat-related disease, including foodborne illnesses. Here's what you can do to take charge of beef safety:

- Choose beef cuts that are likely to be free of bone tissue and nervous-system tissue (the brain, spinal cord, and nerve endings). These tissues are the most infectious part of a cow with mad cow disease. Safer beef cuts include boneless cuts such as boneless steaks, chops, and roasts, as well as beef products from grass-fed and organic cattle. T-bone steaks, porterhouse steaks, prime ribs with bone, beef tips, and bone-in roasts carry miniscule risk.

- Avoid ground beef as much as possible; it may contain bone and nervous-system tissue. If you do eat ground beef, use a food thermometer to make sure that it is cooked to 160 degrees Fahrenheit (66 degrees Celsius), eliminating any foodborne bacteria in the meat. Wash the thermometer immediately after using it. If you order ground beef in a restaurant, ask your server if it has been cooked to at least 155 degrees Fahrenheit (71 degrees Celsius) for 15 seconds (a safe option for restaurants).

- Be wary of products that contain beef extracted by advanced meat recovery (AMR) machines that squeeze out as much meat as possible from cow carcasses. AMR meat may be used in hot dogs, taco fillings, pizza toppings, sausages, and beef jerky made from ground or chopped meat. Unfortunately, manufacturers are not yet required to identify AMR beef on food labels.

Red meat clearly has some nutritional pluses. The key is to control the amount of fat you get from meat. Here's how.

1. **Serving size.** Keep the serving size moderate, because about 3 ounces (85 grams) of lean beef contains just 8.4 grams of total fat and 21 grams of total protein and is about the size of a deck of cards or the palm of a woman's hand. To get 3 ounces (85 grams) of cooked meat, start with 4 ounces (113 grams) of uncooked, boneless meat.

2. **Grade.** Beef is graded according to fat marbling: prime, choice, and select. Select is the leanest grade. When choosing beef, look for lean cuts closely trimmed of fat, or trim them yourself at home before cooking them. Pork is also a leaner meat than it used to be. The leanest cuts of pork come from the loin and leg areas, and a 3-ounce (85-gram) cooked and trimmed portion of any of these cuts contains fewer than 9 grams of fat and 180

calories. Lamb and veal are also lower in fat than beef. Follow the same guidelines for selecting lean cuts.

3. **Preparation.** To keep a lean cut tasty after cooking, you must handle and prepare it properly. Because leaner cuts have less fat to keep them moist and juicy, the method of preparation is important. More tender cuts, like loin cuts, can be broiled or grilled and served immediately. Avoid overcooking. Beef can also be marinated to tenderize it. Because it is the acid in the marinade (vinegar, citrus juice, or wine) that tenderizes the meat, oil can be replaced with water without diminishing the tenderizing effect. To improve the tenderness of roasts, carve them into thin slices on the diagonal and across the grain when possible.

Going Meatless, Staying Muscular

Can you be a vegetarian and still build muscle? Absolutely—as long as you plan your diet properly. The key is to mix and match foods so that you get the right balance of amino acids.

You can think of amino acids as a construction crew building a house. Each crew member has a specific function, from framing to wiring. If just one crew member calls off, then the construction job doesn't get finished. It's the same with amino acids. There are 22 amino acids, all of which combine together to construct proteins required for growth and tissue repair. For your body to build protein, all of these amino acids must be on the job. If just one amino acid is missing or even if the concentration of an amino acid is low, protein construction comes to a halt.

Of the 22 amino acids, 8 cannot be made by the body; they must be supplied by the food you eat. These 8 amino acids are called the *essential amino acids.* Seven of the 22 amino acids are termed *conditionally essential amino acids.* This means that they are made by the body but, under certain conditions, are required in greater amounts. The remaining 7, which can be manufactured by the body, are known as the nonessential amino acids. Your body makes nonessential amino acids from carbohydrate and nitrogen and by chemically re-sorting essential and nonessential amino acids. (The essential, conditionally essential, and nonessential amino acids are listed in table 2.1 on page 25)

Foods that contain all the essential amino acids in the amounts required for health and growth are called *complete proteins.* Proteins found in dairy products, eggs, meat, poultry, fish, and other animal sources are complete proteins. Various plant foods typically provide incomplete proteins that either completely lack or are low in a particular essential amino acid. The essential amino acid that is missing or in short supply is called the *limiting amino acid.*

To get enough essential amino acids from a vegetarian diet, select foods that complement one another's limiting amino acids. In other words, mix and match foods during the day so that foods low in one essential amino acid are balanced by those that are higher in the same amino acid. It's not necessary to combine these proteins at one meal; you can simply eat a variety of protein sources throughout the day. For example, grains contain a limited amount of lysine but a higher amount of methionine. Legumes such as navy beans, kidney beans, and black beans are high in lysine but low in methionine. Thus, by combining grains and legumes, you create a complete protein meal. Soybeans are an exception and are considered a complete protein. Other fully nutritious protein combinations include the following:

- Rice and beans
- Corn and beans
- Corn and lima beans
- Corn tortillas and refried beans
- Pasta and bean soup

If you are a vegetarian who chooses to eat milk and eggs, you needn't worry about combining foods. The protein in milk, eggs, cheeses, and other dairy products contains all the essential amino acids you need for tissue growth, repair, and maintenance. A word of caution, though: Dairy products can be high in fat, so be sure to choose low-fat or nonfat dairy foods such as milk, cheese, and yogurt. As for eggs, limit yourself to one egg yolk a day. Most of the protein is found in the egg white anyway.

Whether you choose to include or exclude meat in your diet is a matter of personal choice. If you decide to go meatless, plan your diet carefully to avoid certain nutritional danger zones—namely, iron, zinc, and B12 deficiencies. These deficiencies can hurt exercise performance. Here are some tips for avoiding deficiencies if you're a vegetarian strength trainer.

- **Get enough protein.** A challenge for vegetarian strength trainers is to obtain the 2 grams of high-quality protein per kilogram of body weight required daily to support muscle growth. You can do this by including plenty of low-fat dairy products and protein-rich plant sources in your diet. If you are a pure vegan (you eat no animal foods at all), increase your daily protein intake to 2.2 grams of protein per kilogram of body weight.

- **Include some sources of heme iron.** As noted, all types of animal protein contain the more easily absorbed form of iron, heme iron. If you're a semivegetarian—that is, still eating fish or chicken but no red meat—you're in luck, because chicken and fish contain heme iron. If you avoid animal proteins, you won't be consuming heme iron. That means you have to work harder to get all the iron that you need. No easy absorption tactics will be available to you.

Power Profiles: Vegetarianism

I once worked with a professional basketball player who, for philosophical reasons, was a lacto-ovovegetarian. A lacto-ovovegetarian eats no animal foods except for dairy and egg products. He was determined to stick to his vegetarian game plan both on the road and at home.

Unexpectedly, this player's biggest problem was not protein. He was getting plenty of protein from dairy products. But he wasn't getting enough iron, selenium, and zinc—minerals that are plentiful in meat. In addition, his diet was high in fat because he was eating a lot of cheese-laden vegetable lasagna.

To solve the mineral problem, he began taking a mineral supplement containing the RDA of the minerals he was lacking. After basketball practice, he started drinking one or two meal-replacement beverages, which contain extra nutrients and fit perfectly into a lacto-ovovegetarian diet.

With my help, he discovered several new low-fat recipes, like vegetarian chili, that he could pack for road trips as long as he had a microwave oven in his hotel room. He took dried fruit on the road, too, which can be eaten anywhere and is loaded with minerals and energy-packed calories.

At home, he began to vary his diet using vegetarian staples such as beans, tofu, rice, and peanut butter. By varying his diet, he was also getting plenty of quality calories to fuel both training and competition. Equally important, he learned that he didn't have to sacrifice his beliefs for athletic performance.

- **Watch the meat, fish, and poultry factor.** Meat, fish, and poultry (MFP) contain a special quality called the *MFP factor* that helps your body absorb more nonheme iron. When meat and vegetables are eaten together at the same meal, more nonheme iron is absorbed from the vegetables than if the vegetables had been eaten alone. If you're a semivegetarian, your slightly lower iron intake will signal your body to absorb extra iron from vegetables.

- **Include vitamin C sources.** Fruits, vegetables, and other foods that contain vitamin C help the body absorb nonheme iron. For example, if you eat citrus fruits with an iron-fortified cereal, your body will absorb more iron from the cereal than if it had been eaten alone.

- **Guard against a B_{12} deficiency.** Vitamin B_{12} is one of the most significant nutrients typically missing from the diets of vegans. That's because vitamin B_{12} is available only from animal products. Fortunately, the body needs only tiny daily amounts of this vitamin (the DRI is 2.4 micrograms for adults), which is used in the manufacture of red blood cells and nerves. Even so, a deficiency is serious, potentially causing irreversible nerve damage.

Fermented foods, such as the soybean products miso and tempeh, supply some vitamin B_{12} from the bacterial culture that causes fermentation, but generally not enough. Vegans should eat foods fortified with B_{12} or take supplements to ensure a healthy diet.

- **Watch iron and zinc blockers.** Some foods contain phytates, oxalates, or other substances that block the absorption of iron and zinc in the intestine. Coffee and tea (regular and decaffeinated), whole grains, bran, legumes, and spinach are a few examples of foods containing blockers. These foods are best eaten with sources of heme iron or vitamin C to help your body absorb more iron and zinc.

- **Consider iron and zinc supplements.** Our bodies don't absorb the iron that comes from vegetables as easily as the iron that comes from animal foods. Nonmeat eaters, especially active people or menstruating women, must pay attention to their dietary iron needs. Animal flesh is the major source of zinc in most diets, so all vegetarians may be at greater risk of having low intakes of this mineral.

Although dietary supplements are not replacements for food, it may be a good idea to supplement if iron and zinc are in short supply in your diet. Daily supplementation of iron and zinc at 100 percent of the DRI is insurance against harmful deficiencies.

Protein Quality and Types

As an exerciser or athlete, you should be concerned about the quality as well as the type of protein you eat. The bottom line is that you need either high-quality protein or a variety of protein sources to ensure adequate intake of all eight essential amino acids—particularly after exercise.

Protein is rated on its quality, or content of essential amino acids. To rate the quality of the protein in foods, scientists have developed a number of measurement methods. Here's a rundown of the three most common methods:

- **Protein digestibility corrected amino acid score (PDCAAS).** The protein values you read on food labels are calculated using the PDCAAS. It describes the proportion of amino acids in a protein source, as well as its digestibility, or how well a protein is used by the body. In calculating the PDCAAS, the food is first assigned a score based on its amino acid composition. The score is then adjusted to reflect its digestibility.

Digestibility, which varies from food to food, is important. Generally, more than 90 percent of the protein in animal foods is digested and absorbed, whereas about 80 percent of the protein in legumes is used. Between 60 and 90 percent of the protein in fruits, vegetables, and grains is digested and absorbed.

With the PDCAAS, the highest possible score is 100. For reference, egg whites, ground beef, milk powder, and tuna have scores of 100; soy protein has a score of 94.

• **Protein efficiency rating (PER).** The PER reflects a particular protein's ability to support weight gain in test animals and gives researchers a good indication of which foods best promote growth. The yardstick for comparison is the growth produced by the complete protein found in egg whites or milk. Egg protein, in particular, is considered the perfect protein, because it contains all eight essential amino acids in the ideal proportions and is the reservoir of nutrients to grow a bird.

• **Biological value (BV).** The BV represents the percentage of protein absorbed from a particular food that your body can use for growth and repair rather than for energy production. As with the PER, the BV of egg whites serves as the yardstick by which other protein sources are compared. Complete proteins tend to have high biological values, whereas incomplete proteins have lower values. Lower BV foods are used mainly for fuel rather than for growth and repair.

To bump up the protein in your diet, consider eating additional sources of protein besides lean fish, poultry, or meat, such as low-fat dairy and soy protein. I am a major proponent of milk in the diets of athletes, for two important reasons. First, when taken after strength training, milk protein has been shown to influence the development of muscle. Specifically, milk protein stimulates the uptake of amino acids by the muscle, a process that leads to the building of muscle. The two proteins found in milk are whey and casein; both are beneficial in producing muscle gains (see the following discussion). Also, research hints that lactose, a sugar found in milk, may also be instrumental in stimulating muscle development. This is probably because lactose slightly elevates insulin, and insulin is necessary for pushing protein into muscle cells for energy, growth, and development.

The second reason I advocate milk is because milk is naturally high in tryptophan. This amino acid elevates brain levels of serotonin, a natural chemical that makes you feel good mentally and emotionally. This result indirectly affects muscle growth—when you're in a good mood, you feel more motivated to work out and achieve your fitness goals.

Here's a rundown on the benefits of various types of protein to consider as additions to your diet.

• Whey is a natural, complete protein derived from cow's milk and available in protein supplements, and it provides numerous benefits to those who strength train. Whey is considered a fast protein because it is digested and absorbed quickly, making amino acids readily available for muscle repair. Whey is thus ideal to consume immediately after exercise because of its rapid uptake. It appears to work even better for muscle building when taken with a carbohydrate. Another intriguing fact about whey is that animal studies suggest that it stimulates fat-burning mechanisms in the liver and muscle, as well as making more fat available for fuel during exercise. Whey is also rich in leucine, a BCAA that helps burn body fat while preserving lean muscle tissue.

- Casein is another milk-derived protein, also available in protein supplements. It is considered a slow protein because it generally forms into a solid in the stomach and is delivered to the muscles more slowly, in a time-released fashion. Consuming casein before working out is a good move because of this sustained action in feeding your muscles. Both whey and casein are high in glutamine, an amino acid that assists in muscle building and in fortifying the immune system.

- Soy protein is a complete protein extracted from soybeans that provides the essential amino acids to meet basic protein needs. However, a diet that is 100 percent dependent on soy protein may not be adequate to meet the needs of a person trying to gain muscle and strength. Soy is a good source of protein if you are a vegan or are sensitive to milk. Soy protein also contains isoflavones, which have a number of potential health benefits.

Soy milk, however, does not work as well as cow's milk in stimulating muscle gains. In a study of young men who completed five days of resistance training for 12 weeks, they had greater muscular gains when they consumed cow's milk versus soy milk. The researchers speculate that protein found in cow's milk works more effectively to trigger the muscle-making process.

- Egg (ovalbumin) protein was once considered the best source of protein, especially in supplements. But because egg protein is fairly expensive compared with other forms of quality protein, its popularity has decreased. As we get further into the book, I will talk about supplemental protein and how to use it to your advantage when building lean muscle.

The Bottom Line on Protein

Protein is definitely a key to manufacturing muscle, and the latest research shows that strength trainers who are building muscle, are vegetarians, or cross-train require slightly elevated amounts of protein. You don't have to go overboard, though, because your body will extract exactly what it needs. By following the recommendations here, you'll get the optimal amount of protein to build muscle and maintain strength.

Sport Nutrition Fact Versus Fiction:

Do Supplemental Amino Acids Build Muscle?

For a long time, a debate has raged as to whether exercisers and athletes should take amino acid supplements as a natural way to enhance the muscle-building process. Today, the talk focuses more on the timing and type of protein and amino acid intake relative to muscle growth and performance. There is a mound of research validating the need to take protein before and after exercise in order to activate the repair and growth of lean muscle mass. Table 2.4 covers good sources of protein that you can get from food.

As for amino acids in particular, a study at the University of Texas tested the hypothesis that 6 grams of essential amino acids taken orally stimulates the manufacture of lean muscle when taken one to two hours after strength training. The two amino acids used in the study were leucine and phenylalanine. When volunteers took a drink containing these amino acids following strength training, there was a positive increase in net muscle protein in their muscles—an indication that new muscle was being manufactured.

Another amino acid, arginine, has been shown to initiate recovery following exercise. In one study, exercisers consumed either a carbohydrate supplement or a carbohydrate–arginine supplement one, two, and three hours after exercise. The supplements were formulated with either 1 gram of carbohydrate per kilogram of body weight or 1 gram of carbohydrate plus .08 gram of arginine per kilogram of body weight. During the four-hour recovery period, the increase in muscle glycogen was more rapid in those who had consumed the carbohydrate–arginine formula.

The researchers attributed this response to arginine's ability to increase the availability of glucose for muscle glycogen storage during recovery. There were some untoward side effects associated with the carbohydrate–arginine supplement, however, including bitter taste and diarrhea.

As for the BCAAs (leucine, isoleucine, and valine), they make up about one-third of your muscle protein. They work together to rebuild muscle protein, which is dismantled by exercise, and act as fuel for exercise. The harder you work out, the more leucine your body will use. After aerobic exercise, plasma leucine levels drop 11 to 33 percent; after strength-training exercise they drop 30 percent. Furthermore, high-intensity aerobic exercise drains skeletal muscle stores of leucine.

Supplementing your diet with leucine (50 milligrams per kilogram of body weight a day) along with consuming 1.26 grams of protein per kilogram of body weight each day can prevent a decrease in leucine during five weeks of speed and strength training, according to one study. Other research indicates that consuming BCAAs (30 to 35 percent leucine) before or during endurance training may decrease, and even prevent, the rate of protein degradation in the muscle, plus spare muscle glycogen.

Should you supplement with BCAAs? Consider these facts: Your body starts drawing on BCAAs for fuel during exercise only if you're not taking in sufficient carbohydrate (carbohydrate keeps the body from burning too much of its BCAA supply). In other words, you should be able to get all the BCAAs you need from food. That's easy to do. Each of the following foods contains all the BCAAs you need to prevent protein breakdown during aerobic exercise:

- 3 ounces (85 grams) of water-packed tuna
- 3 ounces (85 grams) of chicken

- 1 cup (245 grams) of nonfat yogurt
- 1 cup (180 grams) of cooked legumes

In addition, a great way to replace BCAAs lost during exercise is to consume dairy products or whey protein after your workouts.

Table 2.4 Good Sources of Protein

Food	Amount	Protein (g)	Calories
Animal foods			
Beef, lean, sirloin, broiled	3 oz (85 g)	26	172
Roasted chicken breast (boneless, no skin)	3 oz (85 g)	26	140
Sole or flounder, baked or broiled	3 oz (85 g)	21	100
Turkey	3 oz (85 g)	25	145
Dairy products			
Cheese	1 oz (28 g)	8	107
Cottage cheese, 2%	½ c (105 g)	16	101
Egg, boiled	1 large	6	78
Egg white, cooked	1 large	4	78
Milk, dried nonfat, instant	½ c (34 g)	12	122
Milk, low-fat, 1%	1 c (237 ml)	8	102
Milk, nonfat	1 c (237 ml)	8	86
Yogurt, low-fat, plain	8 oz (227 g)	13	155
Yogurt, low-fat, fruit	8 oz (227 g)	11	250
Nuts, seeds, and nut products			
Peanuts, dry roasted	1 oz (28g)	7	166
Peanut butter	2 tbsp (32 g)	8	190
Pumpkin seeds, dry roasted	½ c (114 g)	6	143
Sunflower seeds, dry roasted, hulled	2 tbsp (32 g)	3	93
Soy products			
Soybeans, cooked	½ c (90 g)	15	149
Soy milk	1 c (237 ml)	8	79
Tofu	½ c (126 g)	10	94
Vegetables, high protein			
Black beans, boiled	½ c (86 g)	8	114
Chickpeas (garbanzos), boiled	½ c (82 g)	7	135
Lentils, boiled	½ c (99 g)	9	115
Pinto beans	½ c (86 g)	7	117

Although the research into amino acid supplements is compelling, I am still not a proponent of these supplements. I would rather see you get your amino acids naturally—from food. And just as important, time your protein intake by having a small mixed meal of protein, carbohydrate, and some fat both before and after your strength-training sessions.

Food remains the best protein source for your body. One of the main reasons has to do with absorption. All nutrients are absorbed better when they come from real food. There are substances in foods, which scientists have termed *food factors,* that help the body absorb and use nutrients. We don't even know what many of these food factors are, but we do know that they aren't found in food supplements.

As for protein, it is one of the best-absorbed foods, particularly animal protein. Scientific research has found that 95 to 99 percent of animal protein is absorbed and used by the body. Even protein from plant sources is well absorbed: More than 80 percent of the protein from high-protein plants is put to use by the body.

If you eat a variety of protein, you don't need to take protein or amino acid supplements. Just 1 ounce (28 grams) of chicken contains 7,000 milligrams of amino acids. To get that much, you might pay $20 for an entire bottle of amino acid supplements!

3

Fueling Workouts

From the oatmeal you eat for breakfast to the baked potato you eat for dinner, carbohydrate is the leading nutrient fuel for your body. During digestion, carbohydrate is broken down into glucose. Glucose circulates in the blood, where it is known as blood sugar, to be used by the brain and nervous system for energy. If your brain cells are deprived of glucose, your mental power will suffer, and because your brain controls your muscles, you might even feel weak and shaky.

Glucose from the breakdown of carbohydrate is also converted to glycogen for storage in either liver or muscle. Two-thirds of your body's glycogen is stored in the muscles, and about one-third is stored in the liver. When muscles use glycogen, they break it back down into glucose through a series of energy-producing steps.

It is no surprise that pastas, cereals, grains, fruits, vegetables, sport drinks, energy bars, and other types of carbohydrate are the foods of choice for endurance athletes, who load up on carbohydrate to improve their performance in competition. But carbohydrate is just as necessary for strength trainers as it is for endurance athletes—in the right amounts, and combined with protein and fat. The glycogen provided by carbohydrate is the major source of fuel for working muscles. When carbohydrate is in short supply, your muscles get tired and heavy. Carbohydrate, particularly in combination with protein and fat, is a vital nutrient that keeps your mind and muscles powered for hard training and muscle building.

The Force Behind Muscle Building and Fat Burning

Among the nutrients, carbohydrate is the most powerful in affecting energy levels. But it also affects muscle-building and fat-burning power. It takes about 2,500 calories to build just 1 pound (.5 kilogram) of muscle. That's a lot of energy! The best source of that energy is carbohydrate. It provides the cleanest, most immediate source of energy for body cells, and the body prefers to burn carbohydrate over fat or protein. Carbohydrate spares protein from being used as energy, and leaves protein free to do its main job—build and repair body tissue, including muscle.

Carbohydrate is a must for efficient fat burning, too. Your body burns fat for energy in a series of complex chemical reactions that take place inside cells. Think of fat as a log on a hearth waiting to be ignited. Carbohydrate is the match that ignites fat at the cellular level. Unless enough carbohydrate is available in key stages of the energy-producing process, fat will just smolder—in other words, it will not burn as cleanly or completely.

Increase Carbohydrate Calories

The single most important nutritional factor affecting muscle gain is calories, specifically calories from carbohydrate. Building muscle requires a rigorous strength-training program. A tremendous amount of energy is required to fuel this type of exercise—energy that is best supplied by carbohydrate. A carbohydrate-dense diet allows for the greatest recovery of muscle glycogen stores on a daily basis. This ongoing replenishment lets your muscles work equally hard on successive days. Studies continue to show that carbohydrate-dense diets give strength-trained athletes an edge in their workouts, and the bottom line is, the harder you train, the more muscle you can build.

To build a pound (.5 kilogram) of muscle, add 2,500 calories a week. This means introducing extra calories into your diet. Ideally, women must increase their calorie intake by 300 a day and men must increase their intake by 400. This is the optimal increase to begin building muscle without gaining fat, as research has shown.

You should increase your calorie consumption gradually so that you don't gain too much fat. What I suggest to strength trainers in a building phase is to start by introducing only 300 to 350 calories more per day. Then after a week or two, add another 300 to 400 calories a day. As long as you're not gaining fat, start introducing extra calories into your diet weekly, again at the same

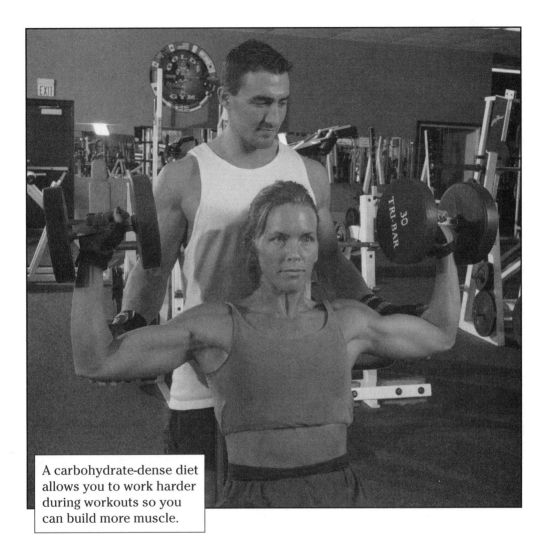

A carbohydrate-dense diet allows you to work harder during workouts so you can build more muscle.

rate of 300 to 400 calories. (Incidentally, for losing fat, you can drop calories by the same amount—300 calories a day for women and 400 calories a day for men.)

But back to increasing calories: Most of these additional calories should come from carbohydrate in the form of food and liquid carbohydrate supplements. An example of 300 to 400 calories worth of carbohydrate from food is 1/2 cup (70 grams) of pasta, half of a bagel, and one banana. It just doesn't take that much additional food to increase your carbohydrate intake. Later in the book, I'll show you how to time your carbohydrate intake properly and how to combine the additional carbohydrate with the right foods in order to enhance muscle building.

When I'm working with someone, I make sure their protein and fat needs are taken care of; then I look at their carbohydrate intake. That's how I will adjust calories, by increasing or decreasing carbohydrate calories. Carbohydrate calories are the fuel, so if someone wants to gain weight, carbohydrate calories go up; to lose fat, carbohydrate calories go down. Remember, carbohydrate should always be eaten in combination with the right amount of protein and the right amount of fat; it should not be consumed alone except perhaps in a sport drink when you just can't eat any additional solid food. (Sport drinks, however, should be consumed during training, not as a beverage during the day.)

To be really exact, you can match your carbohydrate intake to your weight. A strength trainer who wants to build muscle should take in about 7 grams of carbohydrate per kilogram of body weight a day. An athlete who cross-trains with strength training, wants to build, and does any type of endurance activity needs about 8 to 9 grams per kilogram of body weight a day.

Supplementing with liquid carbohydrate, including smoothies, is an excellent way to increase those calories, boost carbohydrate and protein consumption, and take in nutrients conveniently. It's also a great way to consume nutrients when you don't feel like eating, particularly after a heavy weight-training session. In addition, liquid nutrition is absorbed faster than nutrition from solid foods is. Liquid supplementation also appears to support muscle growth. In a landmark experiment, competitive weightlifters took a liquid high-calorie supplement for 15 weeks. The goal of the study was to see how the supplement affected the athletes' weight gain, body composition, and strength. The weightlifters were divided into three groups: those using the supplement and no anabolic steroids, those using the supplement plus anabolic steroids, and a control group taking no supplements or steroids but participating in exercise. The supplement contained 540 calories and 70.5 grams of carbohydrate, plus other nutrients.

All the participants followed their usual diets. The steroid group and the control group ate most of their calories from fat rather than carbohydrate (45 percent fat, 37 percent carbohydrate). The supplement group ate more carbohydrate and less fat (34 percent fat, 47 percent carbohydrate). What's more, the supplement group ate about 830 more calories a day than the control group and 1,300 more calories a day than the steroid group.

Here's what happened: The weight gain in both supplemented groups was significantly greater than in the control group. Those in the supplement-only group gained an average of 7 pounds (3 kilograms); those in the supplement and steroid group, 10 pounds (4.5 kilograms); those in the control group, 3.5 pounds (1.5 kilograms). Lean mass in both the supplement and steroid groups more than doubled compared with the control group. The supplement group lost .91 percent body fat, whereas the steroid group gained .5 percent body fat. Both the supplement and steroid groups gained strength—equally.

These results are amazing. They prove that ample calories and carbohydrate are essential for a successful strength-training and muscle-building program. Even more astounding is the fact that you can potentially attain the same results with diet alone as you can with drugs. That's powerful news for drug-free strength trainers everywhere. In chapter 12, you'll learn how to plan your own carbohydrate-dense diet to support muscle growth.

Choose the Right Carbohydrate

Not just any type of carbohydrate is appropriate for building lean mass and developing a fit, streamlined physique. The right types of carbohydrate come from unrefined, whole foods such as fruits, vegetables, legumes, and whole grains. There is also some carbohydrate in milk due to lactose, the milk sugar. By contrast, the wrong types of carbohydrate come from processed foods, including sugar, high-fructose corn syrup, white flour, white rice, commercial baked goods, many packaged foods, and alcohol. Processed foods have been stripped of their important nutritional factors, including fiber. Because they lack fiber, it is easy to eat huge quantities of calories without feeling full. Foods with processed carbohydrate are the ones you should mostly avoid.

Sport Nutrition Fact Versus Fiction:

Does Carbohydrate Make You Fat?

Recently, several books hit the bookstores claiming that carbohydrate-dense diets make you fat and are therefore bad. The authors based this theory on the fact that some people (about 25 percent of the population) are insulin resistant, a condition in which the pancreas oversecretes insulin to maintain normal blood levels of glucose after a carbohydrate-dense meal. This oversecretion theoretically causes carbohydrate to be converted to stored body fat.

While this may be true for a sedentary population, it's just not the same case with athletes and other active people. In fact, for bodybuilders, insulin is an anabolic hormone that helps build muscle mass by fueling the muscles.

As someone who's active, you're already keeping your insulin levels in line. Though the exact mechanism isn't clear, exercise makes muscle cells more sensitive to insulin. For glucose to enter muscle cells, it has to have help from insulin. Once insulin gets to the outer surface of the cell, it acts like a key and unlocks tiny receptors surrounding the cell. The cell opens and lets glucose in for use as fuel. Maintaining muscle tissue through strength training helps normalize the flow of glucose from the blood into muscle cells where it can be properly used for energy.

Should you be worried about eating pasta and bread? No! But you should be eating a variety of whole-carbohydrate foods like beans, whole grains, fruits, and vegetables in addition to bread and pasta. Even in the unlikely event you are insulin resistant, the variety minimizes the effects, along with mixing carbohydrate with protein and fat. Also, staying active helps control body weight and builds muscle tissue, which helps regulate the body's use of glucose.

Insulin and carbohydrate are not the bad guys when it comes to fat—calories and poor diet planning are. You gain body fat when you make poor choices and eat more calories than you burn. It's just that simple.

Not surprisingly, people who eat the right types of carbohydrate tend to have lower body weights and better control of blood lipids and carbohydrate metabolism when compared with those who eat predominantly simple sugars. Increased whole-grain intake in particular is associated with decreased risks of obesity, coronary heart disease, type 2 diabetes, insulin resistance, and many causes of illness. Thus, by replacing bad types of carbohydrate with good ones, you gain better control over most of the physiological and metabolic risk factors associated with the development of obesity and chronic disease.

High in Fiber

The right carbohydrate is high in fiber, which is found only in plant foods, primarily whole foods and largely unprocessed foods. It is a structural and storage form of carbohydrate and is not digested as it passes through the human digestive system. Fiber is classified by its ability to dissolve in water, and there are two types: water soluble and water insoluble. Soluble fibers, which come primarily from beans, fruits, and whole grains, can be dissolved in water and include plant material such as gums, mucilages, pectin, and some hemicelluloses. Insoluble fibers, which come primarily from vegetables, beans, whole wheat, and fruit skins, do not dissolve in water and include lignins, cellulose, and some hemicelluloses. The two types of fiber both improve the work of the intestines, although in different ways. Water-soluble fiber is generally sticky and viscous and slows down the movement of food through the digestive tract. Water-insoluble fiber acts like a stool softener and bulk former and keeps things moving through the system.

Want to know an easy way to stay lean and healthy? Add 5 more grams of fiber to your diet every day. Just 5 more grams a day will reduce your chances of experiencing an expanding waistline and becoming overweight. The latest research out of France has shown that a 5-gram increase in total dietary fiber can reduce the risk of becoming overweight by almost 11 percent and reduce the risk of an expanding waistline by almost 15 percent. This relationship was particularly strong with insoluble fiber from fruit, dried fruit, nuts, and seeds.

Another study published by a research group from Harvard showed that women who increased fiber intake by about 8 grams per day ate 150 fewer calories per day than those who decreased their fiber intake by 3 grams per day during the study. During the 12 years of the study, the women with the highest fiber consumption lost about 8 pounds (3.5 kilograms), compared with a nearly 20-pound (9-kilogram) weight gain for those who cut their fiber intake during those years.

How does fiber work its weight-controlling wonders? First, high-fiber foods take longer to eat, resulting in a full, satisfied feeling. Second, they lower levels of insulin, a hormone that stimulates appetite. Third, more energy (calories) is used up during the digestion and absorption of high-fiber foods. Fourth, high-fiber diets are lower in calories and help you naturally manage your weight. In addition, studies have substantiated that one of the primary reasons people succeed at keeping weight off is that they stick to a high-fiber diet over time. One more important point: By avoiding obesity through a high-fiber diet, you lower your risks for the development and progression of cardiovascular disease, cancer, hypertension, and diabetes. Table 3.1 provides a list of the best high-fiber foods for strength trainers, bodybuilders, exercisers, and other athletes.

Here's a question a lot of my clients ask me when I advise upping their fiber intake: How do you get a lot of fiber in your diet without feeling bloated or being in the bathroom all the time? The answer is to stick to your regimen of smaller multiple meals that include carbohydrate, protein, and fat. These small, frequent meals give you time-released energy while lowering the total volume of fiber you take in at any one time. You'll also experience less gas with smaller, more frequent meals. That's because the friendly bacteria in your gut feeds off fiber. A by-product of bacterial digestion can be gas, but if you take in fiber in smaller amounts, less gas is produced. If you have trouble with bloating, the following list includes the high-fiber foods that form the least gas:

- Fresh fruits with skin, dried fruits, and fruit juices with pulp
- Potatoes, sweet potatoes, and yams with skin
- Peas
- Carrots
- Winter squash
- Tomatoes
- Romaine, leaf, Boston, and Bibb lettuces
- Whole grains and cereals

Low Glycemic Ratings

In addition to being high in fiber, the right types of carbohydrate are also low on the glycemic index, and when portion sizes are controlled, they have low glycemic loads. The glycemic index is a measure of how quickly sugar is released into the bloodstream after eating a food containing 50 grams of digestible carbohydrate. Foods high on the index raise blood sugar levels rapidly; foods lower on the index cause a slower response. Highly refined foods are generally digested more quickly compared with whole foods and raise blood sugar levels more rapidly. However, this is not always the case. The volume of carbohydrate consumed is also a big factor. While the creators of the glycemic index understood that and kept the volume constant to 50 grams, many of the normal portion sizes contain less than 50 grams of carbohydrate.

The concept of glycemic load was created in order to more specifically understand the metabolic response to carbohydrate. While the glycemic index uses a constant 50-gram portion of digestible carbohydrate, all foods do not contain equal volumes of digestible and indigestible (fiber) carbohydrate. The

Table 3.1 Food Sources of Dietary Fiber Ranked by Amount of Fiber

Food, standard amount	Dietary fiber (g)	Calories
Navy beans, cooked, 1/2 c (91 g)	9.5	128
Bran ready-to-eat cereal (100%), 1/2 c (30 g)	8.8	78
Kidney beans, canned, 1/2 c (89 g)	8.2	109
Split peas, cooked, 1/2 c (98 g)	8.1	116
Lentils, cooked, 1/2 c (99 g)	7.8	115
Black beans, cooked, 1/2 c (86 g)	7.5	114
Pinto beans, cooked, 1/2 c (86 g)	7.7	122
Lima beans, cooked, 1/2 c (85 g)	6.6	108
Artichoke, globe, cooked, 1 each	6.5	60
White beans, canned, 1/2 c (90 g)	6.3	154
Chickpeas, cooked, 1/2 c (82 g)	6.2	135
Great northern beans, cooked, 1/2 c (89 g)	6.2	105
Cowpeas, cooked, 1/2 c (83 g)	5.6	100
Soybeans, mature, cooked, 1/2 c (90 g)	5.2	149
Bran ready-to-eat cereals, various, ~1 oz (~28 g)	2.6-5.0	90-108
Crackers, rye wafers, plain, 2 wafers	5.0	74
Sweet potato, baked, with peel, 1 medium	4.8	131
Asian pear, raw, 1 small	4.4	51
Green peas, cooked, 1/2 c (80 g)	4.4	67
Whole-wheat English muffin	4.4	134
Pear, raw, 1 small	4.3	81
Bulgur, cooked, 1/2 c (91 g)	4.1	76
Mixed vegetables, cooked, 1/2 c (82 g)	4.0	59
Raspberries, raw, 1/2 c (62 g)	4.0	32
Sweet potato, boiled, no peel, 1 medium	3.9	119
Blackberries, raw, 1/2 c (72 g)	3.8	31
Potato, baked, with skin, 1 medium	3.8	161
Soybeans, green, cooked, 1/2 c (90 g)	3.8	127
Stewed prunes, 1/2 c (124 g)	3.8	133
Figs, dried, 1/4 c (37 g)	3.7	93
Dates, 1/4 c (45 g)	3.6	126
Oat bran, raw, 1/4 c (18 g)	3.6	58
Pumpkin, canned, 1/2 c (123 g)	3.6	42
Spinach, frozen, cooked, 1/2 c (95 g)	3.5	30
Shredded wheat ready-to-eat cereals, various, ~1 oz (~28 g)	2.8-3.4	96

Food, standard amount	Dietary fiber (g)	Calories
Almonds, 1 oz (28 g)	3.3	164
Apple with skin, raw, 1 medium	3.3	72
Brussels sprouts, frozen, cooked, 1/2 c (78 g)	3.2	33
Whole-wheat spaghetti, cooked, 1/2 c (70 g)	3.1	87
Banana, 1 medium	3.1	105
Orange, raw, 1 medium	3.1	62
Oat bran muffin, 1 small	3.0	178
Guava, 1 medium	3.0	37
Pearled barley, cooked, 1/2 c (79 g)	3.0	97
Sauerkraut, canned, solids and liquids, 1/2 c (71 g)	3.0	23
Tomato paste, 1/4 c (131 g)	2.9	54
Winter squash, cooked, 1/2 c (103 g)	2.9	38
Broccoli, cooked, 1/2 c (78 g)	2.8	26
Parsnips, cooked, chopped, 1/2 c (78 g)	2.8	55
Turnip greens, cooked, 1/2 c (72 g)	2.5	15
Collards, cooked, 1/2 c (95 g)	2.7	25
Okra, frozen, cooked, 1/2 c (92 g)	2.6	26
Peas, edible pod, cooked, 1/2 c (80 g)	2.5	42

From the U.S. Department of Health and Human Services and the U.S. Department of Agriculture, 2005, *Dietary guidelines for Americans 2005*. Available: http://www.health.gov/dietaryguidelines/dga2005/document/html/appendixB.htm.

volume of food that a subject eats to get the right amount of digestible carbohydrate varies from food to food, making portion sizes and the index measure inconsistent with what the average person might actually eat. Glycemic load combines the glycemic index with the amount of food typically eaten, or the load, and it has been shown to be physiologically relevant to increases in blood sugar and insulin levels. Table 3.2 provides the glycemic index and load for common foods.

Nibbling, or eating smaller meals more frequently, allows you to eat smaller portions and reduces the amount of carbohydrate that you eat at one time, or the load. Choosing foods lower on the glycemic index that are less processed, like whole fruit instead of fruit juice or beans instead of bread, will give you that timed-release response to digestion that keeps your blood sugar levels more even. Since carbohydrate is digested more rapidly than protein or fat, when you eat combinations of foods like an apple with peanut butter or bread with cheese, you mimic the whole-food response and slow digestion down, while still getting that slow release of sugar into the bloodstream and preventing weight gain. Rather than having to eat a diet devoid of carbohydrate, you can still enjoy carbohydrate and get the same weight-loss benefit.

Table 3.2 Glycemic Index by Glycemic Load

Foods	Glycemic load	Glycemic index
Low glycemic load breads, cereals, and grains		
All-Bran cereal	8	42
Whole-meal rye bread	8	58
Hamburger bun	9	61
Cinnamon, raisin, pecan bread	9	63
Barley flour bread	9	67
Gluten-free bread	9	69
White bread	10	70
Whole-wheat bread	9	71
Popcorn	8	72
Waffles	10	76
Low glycemic load fruits		
Apples	6	38
Pears	4	38
Strawberries	1	40
Oranges	5	42
Peaches	5	42
Grapes	8	46
Raw apricots	5	57
Pineapple	7	59
Cantaloupe	4	65
Watermelon	4	72
Low glycemic load vegetables		
Peanuts	1	14
Chickpeas	8	28
Pinto beans	10	39
Carrots	3	47
Sweet corn	9	54
Beets	5	64
Pumpkin	3	75
Low glycemic load miscellaneous foods		
Fat-free milk	4	32
Reduced-fat chocolate milk	9	34
Honey	10	55
Sucrose (table sugar)	7	68
Popcorn, plain	8	72

Foods	Glycemic load	Glycemic index
Medium glycemic load breads, cereals, and grains		
Fettucine	18	40
Sourdough wheat bread	15	54
Buckwheat	16	54
Wild rice	18	57
Raisin Bran cereal	12	61
RyCrisp crackers	11	63
Puffed wheat cereal	13	67
Cheerios	15	74
Shredded Wheat	15	75
Medium glycemic load fruits		
Apple juice	12	40
Orange juice	12	50
Bananas	12	52
Apricots, canned in light syrup	12	64
Lychee, canned in syrup	16	79
Medium glycemic load vegetables		
New potatoes	12	57
Sweet potatoes	17	61
Parsnips	12	97
Medium glycemic load miscellaneous foods		
Vegetarian pizza, thin crust	12	49
Cheese pizza	16	60
Gatorade	12	78
High glycemic load breads, cereals, and grains		
Spaghetti	20	42
Macaroni	23	47
Linguine	23	52
White rice	23	64
Couscous	23	65
Oatmeal, quick-cooking	24	69
Plain white bagel	25	72
White rice, instant	31	74
Cornflakes	21	81
High glycemic load vegetables		
Baked russet potatoes	26	85

While you may never memorize the list of foods with the lowest glycemic load, there are a few pointers that you can use to give you a general sense of which foods are lower on the scale:

- Whole, unprocessed foods in their natural state are lower on the glycemic-load scale compared with processed foods.
- Raw, uncooked foods are lower than cooked.
- Solid foods are lower than liquid foods.
- Foods higher in fiber, fat, and protein are lower on the glycemic-load scale.
- A smaller portion will give a lower load compared with a larger portion.
- Exact glycemic index and load numbers are available at www.glycemicindex.com.

Carbohydrate: How Much, How Often?

Clearly, there are plenty of reasons to fill up on carbohydrate, particularly the whole, unrefined kind. First, though, you have to understand that there is a ceiling on how much carbohydrate your body will stock. Think of a gas tank; there are only so many gallons it will hold. Try to fill it with more, and it will only overflow. Once your carbohydrate stores fill up in the form of glycogen, the liver turns the overflow into fat, which is then stored under the skin and in other areas of the body.

The amount of muscle glycogen you can store depends on your degree of muscle mass. Just as some gas tanks are larger, so are some people's muscles. The more muscular you are, the more glycogen you can store.

To make sure you get the right amount of carbohydrate and not too much, figure your daily carbohydrate intake as follows: To build muscle, consume 7 grams of carbohydrate per kilogram of body weight daily. Divide your body weight in pounds by 2.2 in order to get your body weight in kilograms, then multiply by 7. If you want to maintain, lose fat, or cut, you can find your customized carbohydrate needs in chapters 12, 14, and 15.

Once you increase your carbohydrate to the right level, you should start making additional strength gains. Ample amounts of carbohydrate will give you the energy to push harder and longer for better results in your workout.

Bread, Cereal, Rice, and Pasta

Bread, cereal, rice, and pasta—all foods from grains—are among the types of carbohydrate you need each day to maintain health and prevent disease. But according to most surveys, Americans eat very little of these precious foods (21 percent of total calories) compared with the rest of the world. One serving of a grain product is equal to one slice of bread, 1 ounce (28 grams) of ready-to-eat cereal, or 1/2 cup (70-79 grams) of cooked cereal, rice, or pasta.

Along with many fruits and vegetables, the grain group of foods contains complex carbohydrate, which you know best as starch. Starch is to the plant what glycogen is to your body, a storage form of glucose that supplies energy to help the plant grow. At the molecular level, starch is actually a chain of dozens of glucose units. The links holding the starch chain together are broken apart by enzymes during digestion into single glucose units that are circulated to the body's cells.

Although primitive humans probably gnawed on whole kernels, today we grind or mill grains to ease their preparation and improve their palatability—hence the term *refined grains*. Milling subdivides the grain into smaller particles. For example, the wheat kernel can be milled to form cracked wheat, fine granular wheat, or even finer whole-wheat flour. Refining processes also remove the germ or seed, as well as the bran, a covering that protects the germ and other inner parts of the grain.

When the endosperm, a starch layer that protects the germ, is separated from a corn kernel, you get such products as grits or cornmeal. Another processing technique is abrasion, in which the bran of rice or barley is removed and the remaining portion is polished. The result is white rice or pearled barley.

As parts of the kernel such as the germ or bran are removed, so are the nutrients they contain—fiber, unsaturated fat, protein, iron, and several B-complex vitamins. These are replaced in cereal products in a process known as enrichment. However, enriched cereals are not nearly as nutritious as the original grains, so you should minimize your consumption of them. Furthermore, they lack the fiber found in whole grains.

I recommend that most of the starchy foods in your diet be whole grains. First, they are higher in fiber. Second, unlike refined foods, whole grains are less likely to cause insulin resistance, when elevated blood sugar circulates in the blood because body cells respond abnormally to the action of insulin. High intakes of refined foods can lead to insulin resistance.

As a strength trainer, you're probably used to eating a lot of oatmeal, rice, and other common grains. For variety, you might experiment with grains that are less well known but are now widely available in supermarkets. For instance, tabbouleh, a Middle Eastern dish, is a delicious cold salad made from bulgur wheat. The Russians traditionally use kasha, or roasted buckwheat groats, to make both warm and cold dishes and stuffings. Barley makes a hearty soup, and pearled whole-wheat semolina is the traditional variety for making couscous, a Moroccan dish.

Fruits and Vegetables

You've heard it since grade school: Eat your fruits and vegetables, and you'll be healthy. Somewhere between then and now, you may have become skeptical of that advice. It seems too simplistic. After all, human health and nutrition science must be more complicated than that! But science has put grade school advice to the test and turned up some provocative findings. In a nutshell, the advice you heard as a kid is not only sound, it may be life saving.

Thanks to continuing research, there are now more reasons than ever to eat lots of fruits and vegetables. In addition to their high vitamin, mineral, and fiber content, fruits and vegetables are full of other nutritional treasures like the following:

- **Antioxidants.** Vitamins and minerals such as vitamin A, beta-carotene, vitamins C and E, and selenium fight disease-causing substances in the body called *free radicals.* Antioxidants have some real benefits for strength trainers; see chapter 7 for more details.

- **Phytochemicals.** These plant chemicals protect against cancer, heart disease, and other illnesses. Table 3.3 lists some of the important phytochemicals found in various types of carbohydrate.

- **Phytoestrogens.** These are special phytochemicals found in tofu and other soy foods that may protect against some cancers, lower dangerous levels of cholesterol, and promote bone building. Phytoestrogens are also listed in table 3.3.

There are lots of reasons why we should be piling more fruits and vegetables on our plates. First, plant foods provide significant protection against many types of cancer. People who eat greater amounts of fruits and vegetables have about half the risk of getting cancer and less risk of dying of cancer.

For example, tomatoes may protect against prostate cancer. In a study sponsored by the National Cancer Institute, researchers identified lycopene as the only carotenoid associated with a lower risk of prostate cancer. Cooked tomato products are concentrated sources of lycopene. Thus, tomato sauce, stewed tomatoes, tomato paste, tomato juice, pizza sauce, and spaghetti sauce are rich in lycopene. People who consumed more than 10 servings of these combined foods per week had a significantly decreased risk of developing prostate cancer compared with those who ate fewer than one and a half servings per week.

Here's more proof of the cancer-fighting power of fruits and vegetables: A study of 2,400 Greek women showed that women with the highest intake of fruit (six servings a day) had a 35 percent lower risk of breast cancer compared with women who had the lowest fruit intake (fewer than two servings a day).

The number of fruits and vegetables in your daily diet makes a difference in cardiovascular health, too. Researchers tracked 832 men aged 45 to 65 as part of the famous Framingham Heart Study, which has followed the health of residents of a Boston suburb since 1948. For every increase of three servings of fruits and vegetables that the men ate per day, there was approximately a 20 percent decrease in their risk of stroke. A previous study reported a similar finding among women. Those who ate lots of spinach, carrots, and other

Table 3.3   Phytochemicals for Fitness

Phytochemical	Food source	Protective action
Allyl sulfides	Garlic, onions, shallots, leeks, chives	Lower risk of stomach and colon cancers
Sulforafanes, indoles, isothiocyanates	Broccoli, cabbage, Brussels sprouts, cauliflower, kohlrabi, watercress, turnips, Chinese cabbage	Lower risk of breast, stomach, and lung cancers
Carotenes	Carrots, dried apricots and peaches, cantaloupe (rock melon), green leafy vegetables, sweet potatoes, yams	Lower risk of lung and other cancers
Lycopene, *p*-coumaric acid, chlorogenic acid	Tomatoes	Lower risk of prostate and stomach cancers
Alpha-linolenic acid, vitamin E	Vegetable oils	Lower risk of inflammation and heart disease
Monoterpenes	Cherries, orange-peel oil, citrus-peel oil, caraway, dill, spearmint, lemongrass	Lower risk of breast, skin, liver, lung, stomach, and pancreatic cancers
Polyphenols	Green tea	Lower risk of skin, lung, and stomach cancers
Phytoestrogens	Soy foods, including tofu, miso, tempeh, soybeans, soy milk, isolated soy protein	Lower risk of breast and prostate cancers, decrease in symptoms of menopause

vegetables and fruits rich in antioxidants had a 54 percent lower risk of stroke than other women.

There's more: In the United States, men with low vitamin C intakes have significantly higher risk of cardiovascular disease and death compared with men who eat the highest levels of vitamin C. Risk of heart disease appears to be the lowest in people who eat an average of at least 11 pounds (5 kilograms) of citrus fruit per year.

Want to better control your blood pressure? Eat more fruit. It's loaded with potassium and magnesium—two minerals that have been credited with possibly lowering blood pressure. Research shows that people who follow the dietary patterns of various ethnic backgrounds tend to have lower blood pressure than those who follow the typical American diet. The reason is that people who maintain their traditional diet patterns eat twice as many servings of fruits and vegetables as people who transition to the average American diet. Other research indicates that high blood pressure can be lowered—without medication—if you eat a diet packed with fruits and vegetables.

Fruit, in particular, is important for weight control and weight loss. Case in point: Researchers in Spain wanted to identify the differences between the diets of overweight or obese elderly people and the diets of normal-weight elderly people. Amazingly, here's what they learned: There was no difference in calorie intake between the two groups. However, the overweight and obese group ate more of their calories from protein and less from carbohydrate compared with the normal-weight group. In addition, the overweight or obese subjects ate less fruit than the normal-weight subjects did. This goes to show that the composition of your diet can have a huge impact on whether you gain body fat.

Can you get the same health benefits from popping supplements as from food? Not exactly. New research has discovered that food factors like antioxidants and phytochemicals work best to fight disease when you get them from food rather than when they are isolated as supplements. In other words, a vitamin and mineral supplement, or any other kind of nutritional supplement, can't match the power of food.

To get the disease-fighting benefits of fruits and vegetables, you should eat a minimum of three to five servings of vegetables and two to four servings of fruit every day. One serving of a vegetable is equal to 1/2 cup (91 grams) cooked or chopped raw vegetables; 1 cup (38 grams) raw, leafy vegetables; 1/2 cup (90 grams) cooked legumes; or 3/4 cup (178 milliliters) vegetable juice. One serving of a fruit is equal to one medium piece of raw fruit, half of a grapefruit, one melon wedge, 1/2 cup (62 grams) berries, 1/4 cup (37 grams) dried fruit, or 3/4 cup (178 milliliters) of fruit juice.

Energy Bars

Energy bars, which are a convenient, ready-to-eat source of carbohydrate, have come a long way since I first ate a PowerBar close to 20 years ago. There was no question then that food was a better choice, but it was hard to eat a cheese sandwich and an apple while cycling along the rugged coast of Maine. A PowerBar was desirable because I could wrap it around my handlebars, peel it off, and eat it as I rode. Bars have now become specialized to boost energy for activity, to add protein for dieting or building muscle, or to generally replace a small meal or snack.

For the most part, energy bars come in three varieties: those containing lots of carbohydrate and little fat; those formulated with a more equal combination of carbohydrate, protein, and fat; and those that emphasize protein.

For strength trainers, the carbohydrate in energy bars is a fast way to replace glycogen stores, which are lost during heavy exercise, to help the body recover. If you need to add fiber to your diet, look for bars that contain fiber-rich whole foods like oats, nuts, and fruit, whose carbohydrate provide a steady release of energy. Some of these often contain as many as 5 grams of fiber. You'd be wise to check the calorie counts of these products, however.

They can contain anywhere from 200 to 400 calories per bar. If you're trying to shed body fat, you could unwittingly sabotage your diet by eating bars instead of whole foods such as fruits and vegetables.

Table 3.4 includes food sources of carbohydrate that are important in a strength-training diet. Now, let's look at how you can plan your meals to include enough carbohydrate to train at peak levels.

Table 3.4 Good Food Sources of Carbohydrate			
Food	**Amount**	**Carbohydrate (g)**	**Calories**
Fruits			
Apple	1 medium	21	81
Orange	1 medium	15	62
Banana	1 medium	28	109
Raisins	1/4 c (36 g)	29	109
Apricots, dried	1/4 c (33 g)	25	107
Vegetables			
Corn, canned	1/2 c (82 g)	15	66
Winter squash	1/2 c (103 g)	10	47
Peas	1/2 c (80 g)	13	67
Carrot	1 medium	7	31
Breads			
Whole wheat	2 slices	26	138
Bagel, plain	1 whole (3.5-in. or 9-cm diameter)	38	195
Whole-wheat English muffin	1 whole	27	134
Pita pocket, whole wheat	1 whole (6.5-in. or 16-cm diameter)	35	170
Bran muffin, home-made	1 small	24	164
Matzo	1 sheet	24	112
Granola bar, hard	1 bar	16	115
Granola bar, soft	1 bar	19	126
Low-fat granola bar, Kelloggs	1 bar	29	144
PowerBar Original	1 bar	45	240
PowerBar Pria	1 bar	16	110

(continued)

Table 3.4, continued

Food	Amount	Carbohydrate (g)	Calories
Grains and cereals			
Grape Nuts	¼ c (29 g)	22	97
Raisin Bran	½ c (31 g)	21	86
Granola, low-fat	¼ c (26 g)	19	91
Oatmeal, plain, instant	1 packet	18	104
Oatmeal, cinnamon spice, instant	1 packet	35	177
Shredded Wheat (spoon sized)	½ c (25 g)	20	83
Kashi puffed cereal	1 c (12 g)	20	99
Sport drinks			
6% glucose-electrolyte solution	8 oz (237 ml)	14	50
High-carbohydrate replacer	12 oz (355 ml)	70	280
Meal replacer	11 oz (325 ml)	59	360
Pasta and starches			
Baked potato, with skin	1 large	46	201
Baked sweet potato	1 c (200 g)	49	206
Whole-wheat spaghetti, cooked	1 c (140 g)	37	174
Brown rice, cooked	1 c (195 g)	46	218
Legumes			
Baked beans, vegetarian, canned	1 c (254 g)	52	236
Navy beans, canned	1 c (182 g)	54	296
Black beans	1 c (172 g)	34	200
Baby lima beans, frozen, cooked	1 c (182 g)	35	189
Lentils, cooked	1 c (198 g)	40	230

Carbohydrate Before and During Your Workout

Preworkout carbohydrate: Is it a good idea? It depends. If you're in a mass-building phase and want to push it to the max, fuel yourself with carbohydrate before and during your workout. In this phase, the best timing recommendation for eating before exercise is to eat a small meal of carbohydrate and protein one and a half to two hours before working out. This meal should contain about 50 grams of carbohydrate (200 calories) and 14 grams of protein (56 calories). These amounts can vary based on your individual calorie needs as well as the amount of food you can tolerate before exercise.

If you are trying to lose fat, you want to minimize the carbohydrate you take in before your workout since you are training to burn fat. I suggest cutting your carbohydrate–protein meal in half. Thus, your meal would contain about 25 grams of carbohydrate and 14 to 15 grams of protein.

And, of course, you should make sure you are always well hydrated. Drink 2 cups (473 milliliters) of fluid within two hours of working out and another cup (237 milliliters) 15 minutes before exercise. Following this pattern will ensure that you gain the greatest energy advantage from your preexercise meal without feeling full while you exercise.

If you want a little extra boost, try drinking a liquid carbohydrate just before your workout. In a study of strength trainers, one group consumed a carbohydrate drink just before training and between exercise sets. Another group was given a placebo. For exercise, both groups did leg extensions at about 80 percent of their strength capacity, performing repeated sets of 10 repetitions with rest between sets. The researchers found that the carbohydrate-fed group outlasted the placebo group, performing many more sets and repetitions.

Another study turned up a similar finding. Exercisers drank either a placebo or a 10 percent carbohydrate beverage immediately before and between the 5th, 10th, and 15th sets of a strength-training workout. They performed repeated sets of 10 repetitions, with three minutes of rest between each set. When fueled by the carbohydrate drink (1 gram per kilogram of body weight), they could do more total repetitions (149 versus 129) and more total sets (17.1 versus 14.4) than when they drank the placebo. All this goes to show that carbohydrate gives you an energy edge when consumed before and during a workout. The harder you can work out, the more you can stimulate your muscles to grow.

If you sip a carbohydrate drink over the course of a long workout, be aware that you can take in too many calories. When counseling clients, I recommend that they alternate between drinking a carbohydrate beverage and drinking water during training, especially if their workouts last more than an hour. That way, they don't consume too many calories from the carbohydrate drink.

The key is to figure out how many grams of carbohydrate you need daily. If you supplement with a sport drink, be sure to count the carbohydrate in the drink as well. Consider your goals—mass building or fat burning—and listen to your body for signs of fatigue. Adjust your carbohydrate intake accordingly, depending on your goals and energy level.

During strength training, glycogen is pulled from storage to replace ATP, the energy compound inside cells that powers muscular contractions. The ATP is broken down in the cells through a series of chemical reactions. The energy released from this breakdown enables the muscle cells to do their work. As you train, the glycogen in your muscles progressively decreases. You can deplete as much as 26 percent of your muscle glycogen during high-intensity strength training.

Some people might argue that a 26 percent decrease isn't enough to affect strength-training performance. After all, endurance athletes lose as much as 40 percent or more of their glycogen stores during a competitive event. What's the big deal? Well, research has shown that glycogen depletion is localized to the muscles you work. Let's say you train your legs today. During your workout, glycogen depletion occurs mostly in your leg muscles, but not much in your arms, chest, or elsewhere in your body. If scientists measured your glycogen levels after exercise, they might find a 26 percent depletion overall. But your leg muscles could be totally emptied. Hard training depletes glycogen from the individual muscles worked.

Recovery Nutrition

After working out, you want your muscles to recover. Recovery is the process of replenishing muscle glycogen. The better your recovery, the harder you'll be able to train during your next workout. There are three critical periods in which you must feed your muscles with carbohydrate, as explained in the following discussion.

1. **Immediately after your workout.** Your muscles are most receptive to producing new glycogen within the first few hours after your workout. That's when blood flow to muscles is much greater, a condition that makes muscle cells practically sop up glucose like a sponge. Muscle cells are also more sensitive to the effects of insulin during this time, and insulin promotes glycogen synthesis. You should therefore take in some carbohydrate along with protein immediately after you work out. (Remember that protein helps jump-start the manufacture of glycogen.) The best type of carbohydrate for refueling is carbohydrate with a high-glycemic index because it will be rapidly absorbed.

If you are in a building phase, I suggest that you consume 1 to 1.5 grams of carbohydrate per kilogram of body weight as soon as possible after exercise. If you are losing fat, consume .5 to 1 gram per kilogram as soon as possible after exercise—the higher amount if you are a man, the lower amount if you are a woman. Think of it this way: Have a meal consisting of a 3-to-1 ratio of carbohydrate to protein as soon as possible after exercise. Protein is the key to building muscle after exercise; carbohydrate is more about refueling. My Muscle Formula Plus smoothie recipe on page 265 contains the proper ratio of carbohydrate, protein, and fat for refueling.

Honey, particularly in the form of a carbohydrate gel, is also a good post-workout choice because honey is a high-glycemic carbohydrate. A research study found that combining honey with a protein supplement may boost postworkout recovery and help prevent drops in blood sugar after exercise. In this particular study, honey outperformed maltodextrin—a starch that has been the standard among the various types of recovery carbohydrate.

If you're not hungry for food at this time (most of us aren't), polishing off a sport drink is a convenient alternative. It's a great way to refuel with carbohydrate calories as well as rehydrate your body. A sport drink containing glucose, sucrose, or a glucose polymer (all high on the glycemic index) is a rapid and efficient restorer of glycogen. Some of these drinks may also contain fructose, which isn't as fast at replenishing muscle glycogen as either glucose or sucrose. Try to avoid fructose (excluding fruit, because fruit always contains a mixture of fructose and glucose) as the sole source of carbohydrate in the period immediately after your workout. Stick to choices high on the glycemic index that contain primarily glucose, sucrose, and maltodextrins.

2. **Every two hours after your workout**. Continue to take in carbohydrate every two hours after your workout until you have consumed at least 100 grams within four hours after exercise and a total of 600 grams within 24 hours after your workout. That equates to roughly 40 to 60 grams of carbohydrate an hour during the 24-hour recovery period. (Many women may not need this much. Follow the menu plans in chapters 12 through 15 for customized postworkout meals.)

A word of caution: There is a drawback to foods high on the glycemic index. They may produce a fast, undesirable surge of blood sugar. When this happens, the pancreas responds by oversecreting insulin to remove sugar from the blood. Blood sugar then drops too low, and you can feel weak or dizzy.

Foods low on the glycemic index, on the other hand, provide a more constant release of energy and are unlikely to lead to these reactions. By mixing and matching low- and high-glycemic foods in your diet, you can keep your blood sugar levels stable from meal to meal. The watchword here is moderation. Don't overdose on high-glycemic foods or beverages.

3. **Throughout the week.** To keep carbohydrate replenishment on track, stay on a carbohydrate-dense diet from week to week. An excellent study of hockey players, whose sport requires both muscular strength and aerobic endurance, found that during a three-day period between games, a high-carbohydrate diet caused a 45 percent higher glycogen refill than a diet lower in carbohydrate. By consistently fueling yourself with carbohydrate, you can keep your muscles well stocked with glycogen.

You can also supercharge your energy levels. In another study, athletes filled up on carbohydrate for three straight days. They then pedaled at a super-high level of intensity—104 percent of their $\dot{V}O_2$max, which describes the ability of the body to take in, transport, and use oxygen. The athletes were able to perform this ride for 6.6 minutes straight, compared with only 3.3 minutes after eating a very low-carbohydrate diet (2.6 percent carbohydrate). As this illustrates, carbohydrate is pure gas for high-intensity exercise.

Should You Practice Carbohydrate Loading?

Endurance athletes practice a type of nutritional jump-start known as carbohydrate loading, which involves increasing the amount of glycogen stored in the muscle just before an endurance competition. With more glycogen available, the athlete can run, cycle, or swim longer before fatigue sets in, thus gaining a competitive edge. When done properly, carbohydrate loading works wonders for endurance athletes.

Among strength athletes, bodybuilders have experimented the most with carbohydrate loading. Their goal is not endurance, but bigger muscles. In general, about seven days before the contest, the bodybuilder cuts back on carbohydrate. This is the depletion stage. Then, a few days before the contest, the bodybuilder starts increasing carbohydrate intake. This is the loading stage. The depletion stage theoretically prepares the muscles to hold more glycogen once more carbohydrate is eaten just before competition. With more glycogen, the muscles supposedly look fuller.

But does this actually happen? Not really, says one study. Researchers put nine men, all bodybuilders, on a carbohydrate-loading diet. The diet involved three days of heavy weight training (designed to deplete muscle glycogen) and a low-carbohydrate diet (10 percent of the calories were from carbohydrate, 57 percent from fat, and 33 percent from protein). This was followed by three days of lighter weight training (to minimize glycogen loss) and a diet of 80 percent carbohydrate, 5 percent fat, and 15 percent protein. A control group followed the same strength-training program but ate a standard diet. At the end of the study, the researchers measured the muscle girth of all the participants. The results? Carbohydrate loading did not increase muscle girth in any of the bodybuilders.

There are enough data available in the sport nutrition literature to conclude that strength athletes derive no real benefit from carbohydrate loading. Your diet should contain ample carbohydrate on a daily basis, but this is not carbohydrate loading. Keep in mind, too, that carbohydrate depletion can actually result in the loss of hard-earned muscle.

Mental Muscle

The amount of carbohydrate in your diet can affect your mental performance. Not only is carbohydrate fuel for muscles, it's also fuel for your brain. On a diet very low in carbohydrate, you can feel quite out of sorts—anxious, easily upset, irritable, or depressed. These are all signs of hypoglycemia, too little glucose in the blood.

At Auburn University, researchers put seven female cyclists on three different diets: a low-carbohydrate diet (13 percent of calories from carbohydrate); a moderate-carbohydrate diet (54 percent of calories from carbohydrate); and a high-carbohydrate diet (72 percent of calories from carbohydrate). The cyclists followed each of the three diets for one week at a time. While on the low-carbohydrate diet, the cyclists felt tired, tense, and depressed and were more likely to get angry.

Mounds of research have shown that carbohydrate does have a positive effect on state of mind. In a very real sense, sufficient carbohydrate is a natural mood elevator.

Sport Nutrition Fact Versus Fiction:

What's the Story on High-Fructose Corn Syrup?

Used as an inexpensive sweetener in many processed foods, high-fructose corn syrup (HFCS) is corn syrup containing a high proportion of glucose, which is then treated with an enzyme that converts part of the glucose to the much sweeter fructose. This process results in an inexpensive replacement for cane sugar. HFCS can contain up to 90 percent fructose, but most of the HFCS found in beverages contains approximately 55 percent fructose.

The major sources of HFCS in the diet are soft drinks, and soft-drink consumption continues to rise. A 1998 study on soft-drink consumption titled "Liquid Candy," published by the nonprofit Center for Science in the Public Interest (CSPI), reported that Americans are drinking twice as much soda as they did 25 years ago. In 1998, the average male aged 12 to 19 years old consumed more than two cans of soda per day. That's 50 grams or 200 calories of fructose, or about 10% of the average person's energy need, without even considering other dietary sources of fructose.

Fructose consumption takes up a significant amount of calories every day, and the increase in fructose consumption has coincided with a remarkable increase in obesity during the same two decades. Is this just a coincidence, or is something else going on?

Researchers from the Department of Nutrition at the University of California, Davis; the USDA Western Human Nutrition Research Center at Davis, California;

the Monell Chemical Sense Institute; and the University of Pennsylvania, Philadelphia, have recently published a landmark review of the scientific literature on fructose, weight gain, and insulin resistance syndrome, popularly called syndrome X or metabolic syndrome. They have proposed the theory that fructose in the form of HFCS may be primarily responsible for the epidemic of obesity and abnormalities seen as part of syndrome X, including insulin resistance, impaired glucose tolerance, hyperinsulinemia, hypertriacylglycerolemia, and hypertension.

It has been understood for several years that fructose is metabolized differently in the body than glucose is. While the body prefers to metabolize glucose into energy or store it as glycogen to fuel muscle cells, fructose is metabolically processed in the liver and preferentially turned into fat rather than used as energy. Studies have shown that fructose ingestion increases rates of fat production in humans, but ingesting the same number of calories as glucose does not cause the same response.

Not only does fructose turn into fat, it shuts down the mechanisms that keep the body from turning into a fat-making machine by letting the body know when it's consumed enough energy. According to numerous studies, fructose does not stimulate the production of two key hormones, insulin and leptin, which are involved in the long-term regulation of energy balance. Unlike glucose, fructose does not stimulate the secretion of insulin from the pancreas. While at low levels of fructose intake this may be desirable for type 2 diabetics and others, it is far from desirable for anyone trying to lose body fat. Insulin influences the regulation of body fat by inhibiting food intake and increasing energy expenditure. After a meal, insulin is secreted in response to the carbohydrate that has been eaten. Along with its job of ushering glucose into cells, insulin acts as a signal for how much food has been eaten and when it is time to stop eating. If insulin is not secreted, then there is no mechanism to turn off energy intake, and weight gain and obesity may develop.

Leptin is a protein manufactured in fat cells that functions as a circulating signal to limit fat stores and fat production by inhibiting food intake and increasing energy expenditure. Insulin stimulates leptin production, thus playing a key role in the regulation of fat stores. When carbohydrate is consumed as part of a meal, it is digested to glucose, insulin is secreted and stimulates leptin production, hunger is abated, and energy expenditure is increased. Body weight stays in balance. When HFCS is consumed, this cascade of events is by-passed, crippling the internal mechanisms for calorie control and energy balance.

In addition to its pivotal role in the development of obesity, the research group from California and Pennsylvania proposes a chief role for fructose in the development of insulin resistance, impaired glucose tolerance, hyperinsulinemia, abnormal lipid profiles, and high blood pressure.

Thus, there is mounting evidence that fructose, in the form of HFCS or sucrose, is an undesirable ingredient in the diet. While small amounts are not harmful and do not interfere with energy metabolism, the large amounts found in soft drinks and many processed foods may be at the root of the body's inability to maintain energy balance and control body weight.

Managing Fat

After about an hour of intense exercise, your glycogen supply can dwindle to nothing. But not so with your fat stores—another energy source for muscles. Compared with the limited but ready-to-use glycogen stores, fat stores are practically unlimited. In fact, it's been estimated that the average adult man carries enough fat (about a gallon, or 4 liters) to ride a bike from Chicago to Los Angeles, a distance of roughly 2,000 miles (3,219 kilometers).

If fat stores are nearly inexhaustible, why worry about carbohydrate intake and glycogen replenishment? And why not supplement your diet with fat as an extra source of energy? True, there is a large enough tank of fat on your body to fuel plenty of exercise. (That's one reason there's no need to supplement with extra fat.) But the problem is that fat can be broken down only as long as oxygen is available. Oxygen must be present for your body to burn fat for energy, but not to burn glycogen. In the initial stages of exercise, oxygen is not yet available. It can take 20 to 40 minutes of exercise before fat is maximally available to the muscles as fuel. The glucose in your blood and glycogen in your muscles are pressed into service first.

That's not to say fat is hard to burn. It isn't. But how efficiently your body burns fat depends on your level of conditioning. One of the advantages of strength training and aerobic exercise is that your body improves its ability to burn fat as fuel in two major ways.

First, exercise (particularly aerobic exercise) enhances the development of capillaries to the muscles, thus improving blood flow where it's needed. In addition, exercise increases myoglobin, a protein that transports oxygen from the blood into muscle cells. With better blood flow and greater oxygen to the muscles, the body becomes more efficient at burning fat, which is why you should not neglect the aerobic portion of your training.

Second, exercise stimulates the activity of hormone-sensitive lipase, an enzyme that promotes the breakdown of fat for energy. The more fat you can break down and burn, the more defined you will look.

Fat is definitely an exercise fuel, but it is a second-string source of energy for strength trainers. During strength training, your body still prefers to burn carbohydrate for energy, either from glucose in the blood or glycogen in the muscles. Fat is certainly one of the more controversial topics in nutrition. It is crucial in your diet, but it also has a bad reputation. Let's try to clear up the confusion once and for all.

Fat Facts

There are three major types of fatty material in the body: triglycerides, cholesterol, and phospholipids. Triglycerides, true fats, are stored in fat tissue and in muscle. A small percentage of fatty material is found in the blood, circulating as free fatty acids, which have been chemically released from the triglycerides. Of the three types of fatty material, triglycerides are the most involved in energy production, and research with bodybuilders has found that triglycerides, including the fat found in muscle, serve as a significant energy source during intense strength training. Not only will strength training help you build muscle, it will also help you burn body fat.

Cholesterol is a waxy, light-colored solid that comes in two different forms. You might call the first kind "the cholesterol in the blood," and the second, "the cholesterol in food." Required for good health, blood cholesterol is a constituent of cell membranes and is involved in the formation of hormones, vitamin D, and bile (a substance necessary for the digestion of fat). Because your body can make cholesterol from fat, carbohydrate, or protein, you don't need to supply any cholesterol from food.

When you eat a food that contains cholesterol, that cholesterol is broken into smaller components that are used to make various fats, proteins, and other substances that your body requires. The cholesterol you eat doesn't become the cholesterol in your blood. Although it is important to reduce your intake of high-cholesterol foods, it is even more important to lower your intake of saturated fat (the kind found mostly in animal foods). That's because the liver manufactures blood cholesterol from saturated fat. The more saturated fat you eat, the more cholesterol your liver makes.

If your liver produces large amounts of cholesterol, the excess circulating in the bloodstream can collect on the inner walls of the arteries. This accumulation is called *plaque*. Trouble starts when plaque builds up in an artery, narrowing the passageway and choking blood flow. A heart attack can occur when blood flow to the heart muscle is cut off for a long period of time and part of the heart muscle begins to die. High blood cholesterol is therefore a major risk factor for heart disease, but it is one that in many cases can be controlled with exercise and a healthy diet.

Cholesterol may be present in blood as a constituent of low-density lipoprotein (LDL) or of high-density lipoprotein (HDL). LDL and HDL affect your risk of heart disease differently. LDL contains the greater amount of cholesterol and may be responsible for depositing cholesterol on the artery walls. LDL is known as bad cholesterol; the lower your blood value of LDL, the better.

HDL contains less cholesterol than LDL. Its job is to remove cholesterol from the cells in the artery wall and transport it back to the liver for reprocessing or excretion from the body as waste. HDL is the good cholesterol; the higher the amount in your blood, the better.

A total cholesterol reading of greater than 200 milligrams per deciliter may be a danger sign. Generally, your HDL should be greater than 35 and your LDL should be less than 130. High levels of triglycerides in your blood can reflect an excess of alcohol or saturated fat in your diet and can increase your risk of heart disease. It is advisable to have your cholesterol and triglycerides checked annually. Table 4.1 shows what your cholesterol numbers mean.

Table 4.1 Cholesterol Numbers

Total cholesterol	
<200 mg/dL	Desirable
200-239 mg/dL	Borderline high
>240 mg/dL	High
LDL cholesterol	
<100 mg/dL	Optimal
100-129 mg/dL	Near optimal/above optimal
130-159 mg/dL	Borderline high
160-189 mg/dL	High
>190 mg/dL	Very high
HDL cholesterol	
<40 mg/dL	Low
>60 mg/dL	High
Triglycerides	
<150 mg/dL	Desirable
150-199 mg/dL	Borderline high
200-499 mg/dL	High
>500 mg/dL	Very high

Source: American Heart Association. www.americanheart.org.

The third type of fatty material, phospholipids, is involved primarily in the regulation of blood clotting. Along with cholesterol, phospholipids form part of the structure of all cell membranes and are critical in the cell membranes of brain cells and nervous-system cells.

Fat in Foods

As an exerciser, strength trainer, or bodybuilder concerned with your appearance, you may be confused by mixed messages concerning dietary fat. What is the real story? The latest word is that fat is actually good for you and good for weight control, as long as you eat the right kinds. Sure, too many fat calories, just like too many carbohydrate calories or too many protein calories, can turn into body fat. But the right kinds of fat calories actually help you lose fat and keep you healthy in body and mind. You'll need help figuring out how much fat and what kind of fat to eat to stay healthy. Here's a closer look.

Fatty acids from food, the tiny building blocks of fat, are classified into three groups according to their hydrogen content: saturated, polyunsaturated, and monounsaturated. Saturated fatty acids are usually solid at room temperature and, with the exception of tropical oils, come from animal sources. Beef fat and butter fat are high in saturated fatty acids. Butter fat is found in milk, cheese, cream, ice cream, and other products made from milk or cream. Low-fat or skimmed-milk products are much lower in saturated fat. Tropical oils high in saturated fat include coconut oil, palm kernel oil, and palm oil and also include the cocoa fat found in chocolate. They are generally found in commercial baked goods and other processed foods.

Polyunsaturated and monounsaturated fats are usually liquid at room temperature and come from nut, vegetable, or seed sources. Polyunsaturated fats like vegetable shortening and margarines are solid because they have been hydrogenated—a process that changes the chemical makeup of the fat to harden it. The resulting fat is composed of substances known as trans-fatty acids, which recent studies have shown to raise blood cholesterol. Trans-fatty acids are more harmful than saturated fats when it comes to your heart; no levels of trans fat are safe, and they should be avoided altogether. Fortunately, food manufacturers are now required to label the existence of trans fats on their products if their packaged foods enter interstate commerce in the United States. You should be able to look at the Nutrition Facts label and see how many grams of trans fats are in your food.

Monounsaturated fatty acids are found in large amounts in olive oil, canola oil, peanut oil, and other nut oils. Monounsaturated fats appear to have a protective effect on blood cholesterol levels. They help lower the bad cholesterol (LDL) and maintain the higher levels of good cholesterol (HDL).

Essential Fats

Of all dietary fat, certain types of polyunsaturated fat are considered essential. Two of these are linoleic acid and alpha-linolenic acid (ALA). The chemical structure of linoleic acid is referred to as an *omega-6* fat, and the chemical structure of linolenic acid is an *omega-3* fat. While these fats are essential, they are not needed in very large amounts. Your body can't make them; you have to get them from food. They are required for normal growth, maintenance of cell membranes, and healthy arteries and nerves. As well, essential fats keep your skin smooth and lubricated and protect your joints. They also assist in the breakdown and metabolism of cholesterol. Vegetable fats such as corn, soybean, safflower, and walnut oils are all high in essential fats, as are nuts and seeds. The total amount required for good health is 6 to 10 percent of total fat intake, or a total of 5 to 10 grams a day.

In addition to linolenic acid, there are two other omega-3 fats that are considered essential and are found virtually only in fish: eicosapentaenoic acid (EPA) and docosahexaenoic acid (DHA). EPA and DHA are found predominantly in marine oils while ALA is found mostly in plant foods. All three are important and are not interchangeable in amounts that will support health and performance.

Unfortunately, most people's intake of omega-3 fats is pitifully low. One reason is that we are eating more omega-6 fats, displacing omega-3 fats and creating an unhealthy imbalance. Sources of omega-6 fats include all the types of oils used in commercial cooking, baking, and food processing, including safflower, sunflower, soybean, corn, and cottonseed oils. Nutrition experts now recommend that we eat omega-6 fats and omega-3 fats in a healthier ratio, increasing our intake of omega-3 oils and decreasing our intake of omega-6 oils. You should substitute olive oil and canola oil, which are lower in omega-6 fats and higher in monounsaturated fats, for the other oils in your diet. Then increase the amount of fish that you eat to increase your omega-3 intake. Some have suggested a 1:1 or 2:1 ratio of omega-6 fats to omega-3 fats; others advocate a 4:1 ratio. These ratios have been associated with lower incidence of heart disease and cancer in populations where the consumption of omega-3 fats is traditionally higher.

Evidence is emerging that when this ratio is out of whack—when there is a high intake of omega-6 fat and a low intake of omega-3 fat—the fatty acid metabolism is altered in the body. The brain releases hormones and neurotransmitters (brain chemicals involved in sending messages) that tell the body to hold on to fat and to not burn it. It appears, then, that by raising levels of omega-3 fats in your diet, you create a better fat-burning effect. You really do need to eat the right kind of fat to feed your brain and burn body fat.

Omega-3 fatty acids, in particular, have far-reaching benefits for health and the management of chronic disease. Current research shows that they lower blood levels of triglycerides and a heart-damaging form of cholesterol called very low-density lipoproteins (VLDL). In addition, omega-3 fats lower blood pressure in people with high blood pressure and may reduce the risk of sudden cardiac death. Omega-3 fats are also required for the development of the retina. Lack of omega-3 fat in the diets of pregnant women may adversely affect the eyesight of newborns.

There is emerging evidence, too, that omega-3 fats may bolster the immune system through their strong anti-inflammatory influence. In recent years, scientists have discovered that the development of many diseases is influenced by chronic inflammation in the body. Inflammation is an essential part of the body's healing process, brought on when the immune system tries to battle disease-causing germs and repair injured tissue. When that battle is over, the army of inflammation-triggering substances is supposed to withdraw, but in many cases it does not. Chronic inflammation is the result, and it has been implicated in heart disease, diabetes, arthritis, multiple sclerosis, cancer, and even Alzheimer's disease. Omega-3 fats appear to help circumvent chronic inflammation.

Omega-3 Fatty Acids and Brain Health

Treatment of depression, anxiety, and stress with omega-3 fatty acids is garnering a lot of attention in medical circles. About 60 percent of the brain is composed of fat, and the primary fat in the brain is omega-3 fat. When omega-3 fats are in short supply in the diet, other fats get involved in brain building, and as a result, the health of brain cells is impaired. The membrane of each brain cell, for example, becomes rigid, and it takes longer for electrical impulses to travel from one cell to another. This means messages are not being carried rapidly from brain cell to brain cell. Consequently, you don't think clearly, and your memory may become foggy. Depression and anxiety can also set in. Increasing levels of omega-3 fats in the diet has been shown to help alleviate these problems.

Based on these health benefits, the AHA now recommends that you eat two to three fish meals a week. The best fish sources of omega-3 fatty acids are wild salmon, mackerel, black cod, cod, halibut, rainbow trout, shellfish, sardines, herring, and tuna. (Refer to table 4.2 for nutritional information on seafood.) Omega-3 fats are also found in green leafy vegetables, nuts, canola oil, tofu, and flaxseed. However, it is not the same omega-3 fat as that which is found in fish oil. It is ALA, the third kind of omega-3 fat besides EPA and DHA. ALA must be converted to EPA and DHA in the body in order to be useful. On the best of days, when you eat flax or get ALA from any of the other sources, only 5 percent of it is changed into EPA and DHA. Furthermore, you must be well nourished and very healthy to get that 5 percent exchange rate. Most people don't have the capability to fully reach 5 percent. While flaxseed and other sources of omega-3 fats other than fish have benefits, they are not a good substitute for EPA and DHA. I recommend to my clients that they eat five fish meals a week, and when they are on the road and can't get fish, I recommend that they supplement their diet with fish oil capsules.

Table 4.2   Alaska Seafood Nutrition Information[1]

	Calories	Protein (g)	Fat (g)	Saturated fat (g)	Sodium (mg)	Cholesterol (mg)	Omega-3 (g)
Alaska salmon							
King chinook	231	25.7	13.4	3.2	60	85	1.7
Sockeye (red)	216	27.3	11.0	1.9	66	87	1.2
Coho (silver)	139	23.5	4.3	1.1	58	55	1.1
Keta (chum)	154	25.8	4.8	1.1	64	95	0.8
Pink	149	25.6	4.4	0.7	86	67	1.3
Alaska whitefish							
Halibut	140	26.7	2.9	0.4	69	41	0.5
Cod	105	23.0	0.8	0.1	91	47	0.3
Pollock	113	23.5	1.1	0.2	116	96	0.5
Rockfish	121	24.0	2.0	0.5	77	44	0.4
Flounder	117	24.2	1.5	0.4	105	68	0.5
Sablefish	250	17.2	19.6	4.0	72	63	1.8
Alaska shellfish[2]							
King crab	97	19.4	1.5	0.1	1072	53	0.4
Snow crab	115	23.7	1.5	0.2	691	71	0.5
Dungeness crab	110	22.3	1.2	0.2	378	76	0.4
Pacific oysters	163	18.9	4.6	1.0	212	100	1.4
Shrimp	99	20.9	1.1	0.3	224	195	0.3
Alaska canned salmon							
Sockeye (red)	153	20.5	7.3	1.6	538 (75)[3]	44	1.2
Pink	139	19.8	6.0	1.5	554 (75)[3]	55	1.7

[1]Source: Values from USDA National Nutrient Database (www.nal.usda.gov/fnic/foodcomp), released August 9, 2004. Values for 100 g edible portion, cooked dry heat unless otherwise noted. Omega-3 values represent the sum of eicosapentaenoic acid (EPA) and docosahexaenoic acid (DHA).

[2]Values for 100 g edible portion, cooked moist heat.

[3]Values for 100 g edible portion, without salt, drained solids with bone.

Courtesy of the Alaska Seafood Marketing Institute. www.alaskaseafood.org

Omega-3 Supplementation

It is a good idea to supplement your diet with fish oil. Enough research justifies its use; however, you need to choose wisely. The product you choose should be a good source of EPA and DHA, with at least 500 milligrams of fish oil.

I prefer an enteric-coated product, meaning that it's not digested until it reaches your intestines. That means you won't have fishy burps or a fishy aftertaste in your mouth. It is more expensive, however. The product I take when I'm traveling and don't eat enough fish is Fisol, but there are many good products available. You want to make sure that the product you buy sells quickly and does not sit on the shelf forever, so watch the expiration date on the label. If you are a vegetarian who does not eat fish, then supplementing with oils from marine algae may be helpful.

If you don't like swallowing large pills, there is a product you can purchase through the Internet at www.omega3brainbooster.com. It is an omega-3 product in powder form that you can add to juice or to yogurt. In 1 teaspoon (5 ml), you get 500 milligrams of fish oil and very little fishy taste or smell.

A word of caution: If you are eating five fish meals a week, you don't need to supplement. If you eat less fish and choose to take supplements, don't overdo it. If a little is good, a lot is not better. Take the recommended doses, because overdosing can have negative health consequences. An excess of these oils can cause internal or external bleeding. As a fat, they're also high in calories and can promote weight gain when too many are taken.

Essential Fat Needs

If you slash fat to miniscule levels or cut it out altogether, you risk developing an essential fat deficiency. This is not a widespread problem, because Americans get their fill of fat. Even so, I have seen many athletes, bodybuilders in particular, go to extremes in cutting fat. When this happens, the body has trouble absorbing the fat-soluble vitamins A, D, E, and K. Furthermore, the health of cell membranes is jeopardized because low-fat diets are low in vitamin E. Vitamin E is an antioxidant that prevents disease-causing free radicals from puncturing cell membranes, and it also helps in the muscle repair process that takes place after exercise. Men who go on a low-fat diet put their bodies in hormonal jeopardy, since fat is required to make the male hormone testosterone. Women who slash their fat will feel terrible in general, and will even start to crave processed carbohydrate.

You can also go overboard on fat. Too much dietary fat causes weight gain and gradually leads to obesity and related health problems. Excessive saturated fat in the diet can also elevate cholesterol, particularly the dangerous type (LDL). On the other hand, polyunsaturated and monounsaturated fats have been shown to cut cholesterol levels. However, polyunsaturated fat may also lower the protective type of cholesterol (HDL). Very high intakes of polyunsaturated fat have been linked to higher risks of cancer.

So where's the happy medium between too much fat and too little? According to the AHA, the maximum amount of fat considered healthy in your daily diet is 30 percent or less, based on the number of calories you eat over several days (such as a week). Saturated fat should be 7 to 10 percent or less of total daily calories; polyunsaturated fat should also be at 10 percent or less; and monounsaturated fat should make up to 15 percent of total calories. To help manage depression, anxiety, and stress, a diet that contains these amounts is considered a good target. Dietary cholesterol should be kept to a daily maximum of 300 milligrams, according to the AHA. To get more specific, here are some recommendations:

DRIs for Essential Fats

Linoleic acid: 12 grams daily for women; 17 grams daily for men

Linolenic acid: 1.1 grams daily for women; 1.6 grams daily for men

EPA and DHA combined: 2 grams daily, based on a 2,000 calorie diet (This is a United Kingdom recommendation because there is no EPA and DHA DRI for the United States.)

Fat Recommendations for Active People

If you're an exerciser, bodybuilder, or strength trainer trying to stay lean, you should control your total fat intake in order to control your total calorie intake. Keep your fat intake at 25 to 30 percent of calories each day. Your diet should contain much more unsaturated than saturated fat: 5 percent saturated, 10 to 15 percent monounsaturated, and 7 to 10 percent polyunsaturated.

One way to monitor your fat intake is by counting the grams of fat in your diet each day. You can calculate your own suggested daily fat intake by using the following formulas:

Total fat:

$$\frac{\text{Total calories} \times 30\% = \text{daily calories from fat}}{9} = \text{g total fat.}$$

$$\text{Example: } \frac{2{,}000 \text{ calories} \times .3 = 600}{9} = 67 \text{ g total fat.}$$

Saturated fatty acids (SFA):

$$\frac{\text{Total calories} \times 5\% = \text{daily calories from SFA}}{9} = \text{g SFA}.$$

$$\text{Example:}\quad \frac{2{,}000 \text{ calories} \times .05 = 100}{9} = 11 \text{ g SFA}.$$

Following the Power Eating plan, first determine your protein and carbohydrate needs. All of your leftover calories are fat calories—most of which should be monounsaturated and polyunsaturated fats. Be sure to read food labels for the fat content per serving of the foods you buy in the supermarket. The grams of fat are listed on any food package that provides a nutrition label.

Fat Substitutes and Fat Replacers

Many low-fat foods replace the fat with starch, fiber, protein, and other forms of fat. But why even bother with fat substitutes and fat replacers when you need the right kinds of fat in your diet? Go ahead and continue to enjoy healthy fat in foods such as olive oil, nuts, avocadoes, and nut and seed oils. Your body needs and deserves them.

What's more, we don't yet know what effect artificial fat has on health. There's a concern among nutritionists and other health advocates that consumers may get so carried away with eating fat-free foods that they'll not obtain enough of the healthy fat that our bodies truly need.

Reducing Bad Fat in Your Diet

Saturated fat, trans fat, and cholesterol in your diet can lead to high cholesterol in the blood, which in turn clogs blood vessels, contributing to heart disease and stroke. You should be vigilant about reducing these fats in your diet. When there is no nutrition information available about a particular food, remember these helpful hints about the sources of saturated fat, trans fat, and cholesterol in foods.

- The major sources of saturated fat are meats and whole-milk dairy products. Choose lean cuts of select meat like round, sirloin, and flank, and eat portions that are no larger than the palm of your hand. Chicken, turkey, and fish are always leaner meat choices.

- When preparing and eating meat, make sure to trim all visible fat and skin. Use cooking racks to bake, broil, grill, steam, or microwave the meat in order to avoid melting the fat back into the meat.

- When eating lunch meat, select low-fat chicken or turkey breast rather than high-fat bologna or salami.

- Dairy foods are very important in your diet, including for weight control. To cut the fat in dairy foods, choose low-fat products rather than whole-milk products, and include them in your diet two to three times each day.

- Cholesterol is found only in animal products, and egg yolk is a concentrated source. Substitute two egg whites for one yolk, or use an egg substitute. Limit your intake to one egg yolk per day.

- Processed and prepared foods, especially snack foods, can be concentrated sources of fat. Hydrogenated vegetable fat contains trans-fatty acids that promote heart disease, so pay the most attention to the types and total amounts of fat in the food. Read labels carefully, even if the packaging says the product is light, to determine whether products really are lower in fat.

All the accumulated sport nutrition information tells us that the right kinds of dietary fat have profound effects on weight management, mood, and overall health. If we cut out all the fat in our diets, we eliminate not only the bad saturated fat, but also the good unsaturated fat. In today's world, the effective message is that the wrong fat can hurt, and the right fat can help. As long as you balance your calories, a diet high in lean protein, good carbohydrate, and good fat will leave little room for unhealthy foods to creep in. Keep your sight on all the good foods you need to eat every day and then the bad foods won't get you down.

Sport Nutrition Fact Versus Fiction:

Is Chocolate Healthful or Harmful?

Answer: Healthful! Chocolate is a healthy choice in prudent amounts. First, when you're feeling low or run down, a bit of chocolate not only is a way to pamper ourselves, but it actually works with our brain chemistry to lift our mood and make us feel better. The combination of sugar and fat in chocolate elevates two key neurotransmitters, serotonin and endorphins. Low levels of these brain chemicals are linked with depression and anxiety. By raising them you feel calmer, more relaxed, and happier. Not bad for a few hundred calories!

Second, eating chocolate may actually make us healthier. This finding originated with the research on dietary saturated fat and its association with an increased risk of developing heart disease. Over a decade ago, the discovery that stearic acid, the predominant saturated fat in chocolate, actually has a neutral effect on blood cholesterol levels exonerated chocolate from the list of foods that are bad for your heart. Even feeding subjects one whole chocolate bar a day didn't change levels of blood cholesterol.

What's more, scientists have discovered that chocolate is full of antioxidants, including flavonols and flavonoids. These compounds appear to have cardioprotective effects, including antioxidant properties, the ability to reduce the stickiness of blood cells, and the ability to help the lining of blood vessels remain dilated, allowing blood to pass more freely and keep blood pressure at normal levels.

The richest source of flavonols is cocoa powder. It is also the healthiest source since it is devoid of sugar and very low in fat and calories. Next on the list is baking chocolate and dark chocolate. Dark chocolate has twice the amount of flavonols as milk chocolate.

Curious about the antioxidant content of cocoa compared with wine and tea, Dr. Chang Yong Lee of Cornell University tested the antioxidant content of the following beverages: one cup (237 ml) of hot water containing 2 tablespoons (30 ml) of pure cocoa powder, one cup (237 ml) of water containing a standard-size bag of green tea, one cup (237 ml) of black tea, and a 5-ounce (148-ml) glass of California merlot (red wine). On a per-serving basis, the antioxidant concentration in cocoa was the highest. Its concentration was almost two times stronger than in red wine, two to three times stronger than in green tea, and four to five times stronger than in black tea. Dr. Lee also found that hot cocoa triggers the release of more antioxidants than cold cocoa.

A study published by Dr. Mary Engler and colleagues at the University of California, San Francisco, investigated the effects of a flavonoid-rich dark chocolate on endothelial function (the function of the cells lining blood vessels), oxidative stress, blood lipids, and blood pressure in 21 healthy adult subjects. The subjects were assigned to eat either a daily high-flavonoid or low-flavonoid dark chocolate bar for two weeks. There were no obvious differences between the two bars. The subjects were instructed to keep their diets the same as usual, except to eliminate all other foods and beverages high in flavonoids, alcohol, vitamin supplements, and nonsteroidal anti-inflammatory drugs. The results showed that endothelial function improved with the consumption of the high-flavonoid chocolate bars. Blood vessels were more dilated and blood flow was freer. Other biochemical measures indicated a strong association with the intake of flavonoids. No differences in oxidative stress or lipid profiles were seen between the two groups.

Deciding which side of the line chocolate falls on goes back to two major tenets of nutrition: variety and moderation. To be sure, chocolate bars, whether they contain dark or milk chocolate, are high in calories, sugar, and fat. When searching for sources of antioxidants in your diet, remember that fruits, vegetables, fish, nuts, seeds, and tea are rich sources of many important nutrients and antioxidants. Flavonol-rich cocoa is available in candy bars, cocoa powder, and even desserts. On a regular basis it is probably best to get your flavonols from a cup of cocoa that is lighter in fat and calories. Then, when you can really enjoy it, savor your piece of dark chocolate like you would sip from a glass of fine wine.

5

Burning Fat

Why do you want to lose body fat? To compete in a lower weight class? Get ready for a bodybuilding contest? Improve your performance? Look better in your clothes? All are admirable goals for fat loss, and there are umpteen ways to reach them. Two of the most widely used and unhealthy methods are crash dieting and fad dieting.

Crash dieting involves a drastic reduction in calories, usually to about 800 calories or fewer a day, and results in equally drastic consequences, such as the following:

- **Muscle and fluid losses along with fat loss.** If you lost 20 pounds (9 kilograms) in 20 days, the first 6 to 10 pounds (2.5-4.5 kilograms) would be fluid and the rest, fat and muscle. You are not gaining anything by dropping a lot of weight in a short period of time.

- **Loss of aerobic power.** Your body's capacity to take in and process oxygen, or $\dot{V}O_2$max, will decline significantly. As a result, less oxygen will be available to help your muscle cells combust fat for fuel.

- **Loss of strength.** This is a major handicap if you need strength and power for competition or to get through a workout without fizzling out.

- **Metabolic slowdown.** Crash dieting slows your metabolic rate to a crawl. Your metabolic rate is the speed at which your body processes food into energy and bodily structures. It is made up of two interrelated factors: basal metabolic rate (BMR) and resting metabolic rate (RMR). Your BMR represents the energy it takes just to exist; it is the energy required to keep your heart beating, your lungs breathing, and your other vital internal functions going strong. Basal metabolic needs must be met. If you're a woman, for example, you spend as many as 1,200 to 1,400 calories a day just fueling the basic work of your body's cells. Imagine the harm you are doing to life processes by subsisting on a diet of 800 calories a day!

RMR includes your BMR plus additional energy expenditures required for the light activities of waking up, getting dressed, sitting up, and walking around. Your RMR accounts for about 60 percent of the energy you expend daily. The higher this rate, the more efficient your body is at burning fat.

Specifically, it is your RMR that slows down when you restrict calories. In a one-year study of overweight men, those who cut calories to lose weight (as opposed to those who exercised) experienced a significant drop in their RMR. One reason was that they lost muscle tissue, and RMR is closely linked to how much muscle you have. The moral of the story is that following restrictive diets for an extended period will decelerate your RMR, and you can kiss good-bye the muscle you worked so hard to build.

Crash dieting is a losing proposition all the way around. There is nothing to be gained—except more weight! About 95 to 99 percent of all people who go on such diets are likely to regain their weight plus interest within a year.

Fad diets—eating plans that eliminate certain foods and emphasize others—are just as bad as crash diets. A major problem with fad diets is that they are nutritionally unbalanced, and you could be missing out on some of the key nutrients you need for good health. An analysis of 11 popular diets revealed deficiencies in one or more essential nutrients, several of the B-complex vitamins, calcium, iron, and zinc. One diet derived 70 percent of its calories from fat. Such dangerously high levels of fat can lead to heart disease.

But there are other problems, too. Take the mostly protein diet (with hardly any carbohydrate), one of the most popular fad diets among strength trainers. And no wonder it's popular! At first, it works great. You get on the scale, see a huge weight loss, and feel wonderful—until you go off the diet. Then the weight comes back as fast as it left. That is because mostly protein diets are dehydrating; they flush water right out of your system to help the body get rid of excess nitrogen. Dehydration is dangerous, too, potentially causing fatigue, lack of coordination, heat illnesses such as heat stress and heatstroke, and in extreme cases (a loss of 6 percent or more of body fluid), death. Even with a mere 2 percent drop in body weight as fluid, your performance will diminish. That is the equivalent of 3 pounds (1 kilogram) of water loss in a 150-pound (68-kilogram) person. Even though very low-carbohydrate diets do help you lose more pounds faster, the research is clear that the diet is incredibly monotonous, and virtually everyone goes off the diet and gains the weight right back and then some—not much of a solution for a lifetime, or even the next year.

Enough said about what doesn't work. There are antifat exercise and diet strategies that do work, namely a fat-burning training program and an individualized, nutritionally balanced eating plan that emphasizes a balanced combination of carbohydrate, protein, and the right kinds of fat. Before beginning, though, you should set some physique goals.

Go for Your Goal

Whether you realize it or not, you already know what your goal is. Just ask yourself: At what weight, or body-fat percentage, do I look, feel, or perform the best? The answer to that question is your goal.

The first step is to figure out how close to the mark you are. There are lots of ways to figure this out, including height and weight charts, body mass index (BMI) calculations, and bathroom scales. But the problem with most of these is that they are not very accurate for people who strength train. None of these methods takes into account the amount of muscle you have on your body; they might even indicate that you are overweight!

Bathroom scales tempt you to step on them every morning. That can be a downer, because your weight goes up and down daily as a result of normal fluid fluctuations. It can be easy to get obsessed with the numbers you see on the scale, especially because when you begin a program to lose fat, following the proper diet, exercising, and drinking enough water, you may often gain weight before you lose it. Here's why: For every molecule of glycogen stored in your muscles, you store an additional three molecules of water inside your muscles, which lie there ready to assist in metabolism. When you step on the scale, you may experience a gain that is water weight.

A better measurement technique is body-composition testing, which determines how much of your weight is muscle and how much is fat. Several methods are in use. One is underwater weighing, considered the gold standard and very accurate if done properly with the right equipment. But it is not convenient—I certainly don't have a water tank in my office—and it can be rather expensive.

Another method that is rapidly improving in reliability and validity is bioelectrical impedance analysis (BIA), which involves passing a painless electrical current through the body by means of electrodes placed on the hands and feet. Fat tissue won't conduct the current, but fat-free tissue (namely water found in muscle) will. Thus, the faster the current passes through the body, the less body fat there is. Readings obtained from the test are plugged into formulas adjusted for height, gender, and age to calculate body-fat and fat-free mass percentages.

You can now purchase bathroom scales on which you can weigh yourself while measuring your body composition with BIA at the same time. These scales are not necessarily accurate, but as long as you follow the weigh-in instructions, you can see trends in your body composition changes. You should be well hydrated, because if you are dehydrated even a little, as most people are, you won't get an accurate reading. Also, don't eat within three to four hours of weighing, and don't drink any alcohol within 12 hours of weighing. When instructions are followed, these scales are fairly reliable in showing whether your body fat percentage is increasing or decreasing. If you want to keep tabs on your body composition, it is a good idea to check it only once every few weeks since it takes time for this change to occur.

Another accurate method of checking body composition is the skinfold technique, which measures fat just under the skin and uses those measurements to calculate body composition, including body-fat percentage. One of the keys to getting accurate and reliable measurements with the skinfold method is to use the same technician, time after time, month after month. That way, you don't get as much variability in the measurements.

I use another strategy with strength trainers and athletes, one that can be a real motivator as you progress toward your goal. I have them take circumference measurements (with a cloth tape measure) of selected widths on the upper arm, chest, waist, hips, thighs, and calves. Take these measurements every four to six weeks to see the evidence of the positive changes that strength training, combined with the right diet, makes in your body.

Your Optimal Body-Fat Percentage

Exactly what is optimal in terms of body fat? Healthy ranges of body fat are 20 to 25 percent for women and 15 to 20 percent for men. But if you are a strength trainer or bodybuilder, it is desirable to have even lower percentages: 10 to 18 percent for women and 5 to 15 percent for men.

The Female Athlete Triad

Many elite female athletes have less than 10 percent body fat. Female competitive runners, for example, may have as little as 5 or 6 percent body fat, according to some studies. A low percentage of body fat may be perfectly normal and desirable for some female athletes because it enhances sport performance. As long as you don't consciously restrict calories while training for a sport, there is nothing unhealthy about having a naturally lean figure. However, calorie restriction combined with overexercising depletes body-fat stores to unhealthy levels, which elevates the risk of a syndrome known as the female athlete triad.

The female athlete triad refers to three interrelated health problems seen in women: disrupted eating habits, menstrual irregularities, and weak bones. If you have the female athlete triad, you may suffer from an eating disorder such as anorexia or bulimia, or you may have reduced energy availability due to cutting your food intake too low for your exercise level. Your menstrual periods have ceased. You may also have the beginnings of osteoporosis, a disease that makes your bones thin and weak.

You are at the highest risk for the female athlete triad if you

- are a competitive athlete;
- are involved in sports such as gymnastics or bodybuilding that require you to check your weight often;
- exercise more than you need to, without taking in enough calories;

- constantly diet for performance, appearance, or both;
- have perfectionist personality traits;
- have stopped eating with your family and friends; and
- have the attitude that amenorrhea (loss of your period), excessive exercise, and weight loss are positive attributes in athletics.

Some symptoms of the female athlete triad are weight loss, absent or irregular periods, fatigue and stress fractures, and increase in illness due to a weakened immune system. I have occasionally encountered the female athlete triad in my practice. For example, I once worked with a woman who was an ultraendurance athlete and did an extreme amount of exercise. She had begun to experience bone fractures all over her body, along with various illnesses. Her period had become very irregular. Once we talked, it was apparent that she was consuming fewer calories than her body required to carry out all its activity. We corrected this situation through a higher-calorie diet with the correct percentages of protein, carbohydrate, and fat. Ultimately, she had to cut back on her exercise to regain her health. Once she was healthy she was able to return to her sport in much better shape than she left it.

What typically happens is that women deliberately try to lose weight in an effort to improve their performance or appearance, and so body fat is drastically reduced. In response, the ovaries cut back production of estrogen. When estrogen is reduced, menstrual periods become irregular or cease altogether. With poor diet and low calcium intake along with low estrogen levels, osteoporosis becomes a serious concern that can result in fracture risk.

To prevent the female athlete triad, as well as treat it,

- follow a healthy, energy-rich diet adequate for the demands of your sport;
- increase your caloric intake, including getting adequate calcium and vitamin D to help guard against osteoporosis;
- cut back on your training intensity; and
- get under the medical supervision of a sports medicine physician, who may prescribe hormone replacement therapy temporarily to replace lost estrogen and to stop your body from losing any more bone strength.
- For more information and resources on the female athlete triad, visit www.femaleathletetriad.org.

Body Dysmorphia in Men

Women aren't the only ones who obsess about their weight and appearance; men can be just as preoccupied. Body dissatisfaction in men has nearly tripled over the last three decades. An obsessive dissatisfaction with one's body is termed *body dysmorphia,* which is seen largely in men, and tends to manifest in athletes. Whereas women tend to think their bodies are bigger than in reality, men with this disorder tend to falsely believe that their body or their muscles are too small. They may have a poor body image and an obsessive desire to build muscle and avoid gaining fat.

Some of the signs of body dysmorphia include the following:

- Excessive strength training (spending countless hours in the gym) and other compulsive exercising that interferes with work and life
- Body checking (looking in mirrors and other reflections) or avoiding mirrors altogether
- Obsessive weighing
- Lack of time spent with family or friends
- Use of anabolic steroids

If you find you're training excessively and you're worried about it interfering with daily life, and if your joy in life has diminished at the same time, then seek counseling, since this disorder is psychiatric in nature. It does not respond to aesthetically oriented interventions such as exercise programs, diets, or plastic surgery to correct perceived bodily flaws. Some research indicates that antidepressants may help. See a qualified psychologist if you or someone you love may be suffering from this disorder.

Your Weight-Loss Goal Formula

Once you have determined your body composition through an appropriate method, you can figure out how many pounds you need to lose to reach a lower body-fat percentage with the following formula:

1. Present body weight × present body-fat % = fat weight
2. Present body weight – fat weight = fat-free weight
3. Fat-free weight / desired % of fat-free mass = goal weight
4. Present body weight – goal weight = weight-loss goal

As an illustration, let's say you weigh 140 pounds (63.5 kilograms), with a present body-fat percentage of 12 percent. Your goal is to achieve 7 percent body fat. Your goal weight will be composed of 7 percent fat and 93 percent fat-free mass. How many pounds do you need to lose? Here's the calculation:

$$140 \text{ lb } (63.5 \text{ kg}) \times .12 = 16.8 \text{ lb } (7.6 \text{ kg}) \text{ fat weight.}$$

$$140 \text{ lb } (63.5 \text{ kg}) - 16.8 \text{ lb } (7.6 \text{ kg}) = 123.2 \text{ lb } (55.9 \text{ kg}) \text{ fat-free weight.}$$

$$\frac{123.2 \text{ lb } (55.9 \text{ kg})}{.93} = 132.5 \text{ lb } (60.1 \text{ kg}).$$

140 lb (63.5 kg) – 132.5 lb (60.1 kg) = 7.5 lb (3.4 kg).

To arrive at 7 percent body fat, you need to lose 7.5 pounds (3.4 kilograms). Naturally, you want those 7-plus pounds to be fat pounds. Here's a look at how to maximize fat loss and minimize muscle loss.

Exercise and Fat Loss

Your objective is to lose body fat without losing muscle mass. You don't want to lose strength or endurance, either, and you don't want your performance to suffer. So how can you keep on the losing track? Forget about diet for a moment; the other key is exercise.

When it comes to burning fat, exercise is your best friend in three ways:

1. **The more exercise you do, the less you have to worry about calories.** By burning 300 to 400 calories a day through exercise, you enhance the rate of fat burning. As I noted previously, these caloric deficits have been tested in research and proven accurate.

2. **Exercise hikes your RMR.** After you exercise, your RMR stays elevated for several hours, and you burn extra calories even at rest. If you strength train, you get even more of a metabolic boost: The muscle you develop is calorie-burning, metabolically active tissue. Having more muscle tissue cranks your metabolic rate even higher.

At Colorado State University, researchers recruited 10 men, aged 22 to 35, to see what effect strength training had on metabolism. At various times in the study, the men participated in strength training, aerobic exercise, or a control condition of quiet sitting. During the experiment, the subjects were fed controlled diets with a composition of 65 percent carbohydrate, 15 percent protein, and 20 percent fat.

In the strength-training portion of the experiment, the men performed a fairly standard, yet strenuous, routine: five sets of 10 different upper- and lower-body exercises for a total of 50 sets. They worked out for about 100 minutes. For aerobic exercise, the men cycled at moderate intensities for about an hour.

The researchers reported these findings: Strength training produced a higher rate of oxygen use than either aerobic exercise or quiet sitting, meaning that it was a better elevator of RMR. The men's RMR stayed elevated for about 15 hours after working out. Clearly, strength training stood out as a metabolic booster and a calorie burner. With strength training, it is easy to keep fat off and control your weight.

3. **Exercise preserves muscle.** If you lose 10 pounds (4.5 kilograms) of body weight, you may be lighter, but if 5 pounds (2 kilograms) of that loss are muscle, you sure won't be stronger, and your performance can suffer. Appearance-wise, you can still look flabby when muscle tissue is lost. Exercise is one of the best

ways to make sure you are shedding weight from fat stores rather than from muscle stores.

Researchers have put this principle to the test. In a study of 10 overweight women, half of the women were placed in a diet-plus-exercise group and half of the women in an exercise-only group. The women in the first group followed a diet that reduced their calories by 50 percent of what it took to maintain their weight, and they worked out aerobically six times a week. The women in the exercise-only group followed the same aerobic exercise program but followed a diet designed to stabilize their weight.

After 14 weeks, it was time to check the results. Here is what happened: Both groups lost weight. But the composition of that loss was vastly different between the groups. In the group that dieted and exercised, the weight lost was 67 percent fat and 33 percent lean mass. In the group that only exercised, the women lost much more fat—86 percent fat and only 14 percent lean mass! Not only that, RMR declined by 9 percent among the dieters, whereas it was maintained in the exercisers.

What does all this tell us? Sure, you can lose weight by low-calorie dieting. But you risk losing muscle. Not only that, your metabolic rate can plummet, sabotaging your attempts at successful weight control. With exercise and a nonrestrictive diet, you preserve calorie-burning muscle and keep your metabolism in gear.

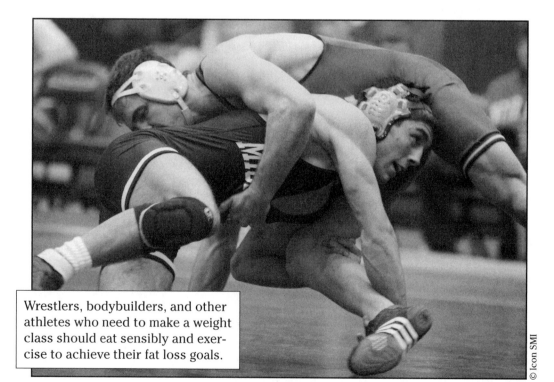

Wrestlers, bodybuilders, and other athletes who need to make a weight class should eat sensibly and exercise to achieve their fat loss goals.

© Icon SMI

Exercise Intensity Counts

The term *intensity* has several different meanings depending on the type of exercise you do, but it basically describes how hard you work out. With aerobic exercise, intensity can be measured by heart rate, which indicates the amount of work your heart does to keep up with the demands of various activities, including exercise.

For optimal fat burning, you should exercise at a level hard enough to raise your heart rate to 70 to 85 percent of your maximum heart rate, which is expressed as 220 minus your age. At low-intensity exercise—20 minutes or longer at around 50 percent of your maximum heart rate—fat supplies as much as 90 percent of your fuel requirements. High-intensity aerobic exercise at roughly 75 percent of your maximum heart rate burns a smaller percentage of fat (around 60 percent) but results in more total calories burned overall, including more fat calories.

To illustrate this concept, here's a comparison based on studies of aerobic intensity. At 50 percent of your maximum heart rate, you burn 7 calories a minute, 90 percent of which come from fat. At 75 percent of your maximum heart rate, you burn 14 calories a minute, 60 percent from fat. So at 50 percent intensity, where 90 percent of the calories are from fat, you are burning only 6.3 fat calories per minute (.9 × 7 calories per minute), but at 75 percent intensity, where only 60 percent of the calories are from fat, you are burning as much as 8.4 fat calories per minute (.6 × 14 calories per minute). In short, you burn more total fat calories at higher intensities.

If it is difficult for you to exercise at a high intensity, try increasing your duration—how long you exercise. You can burn just as much fat at a lower intensity by working out longer as you can by exercising at a higher intensity for a shorter duration.

To increase your rate of fat loss, gradually increase your aerobic exercise sessions from 30 to 60 minutes or strive for longer distances. For example, jogging a mile (1.5 kilometers) expends about 100 calories. Jog 5 miles (8 kilometers), and you will burn 500 calories.

Another option related to duration is frequency—working out more times a week to obtain a greater caloric expenditure. Perhaps you could add spinning, cardiovascular step class, kickboxing, or aerobic dance to your aerobic program for some variety as well as for some extra calorie burning.

Intensity in strength training refers to how much weight you lift. For your muscles to respond—that is, get stronger and better developed—you have to challenge them to handle heavier weights. That means continually putting more demands on them than they're used to, progressively increasing the weight you lift from workout to workout. The more muscle you can develop, the more efficient your body becomes at fat burning, because muscle is the most metabolically active tissue in the body.

Competitive Strategy of a Professional Bodybuilder

Years ago, a group of researchers at Arizona State University studied the diet and exercise strategies of Mike Ashley, known in bodybuilding circles as "Natural Wonder," because he does not use anabolic steroids. During an eight-week precontest period, Mike did the following:

- Consumed roughly 5,000 calories daily—3,674 calories from food plus a carbohydrate-rich sport drink—and an amino acid supplement.

- Took in an additional 1,278 calories a day from supplemental MCT oil (see page 174 for more about MCTs). This meant that 25.5 percent of his calories came from a fat source, not including food intake. However, MCTs are not metabolized like conventional fat; the body uses them immediately for energy rather than storing them as fat. (Although MCTs represent a more compact source of energy—9 calories per gram versus 4 calories per gram for carbohydrate—this approach is not recommended for everyone. The nutrition plan outlined in chapter 13 has wider application and will work for more people.)

- Trained on a stair-climbing machine for a full hour, six days a week.

- Weight trained six days a week, dividing his routine into two or three workouts a day. In total, Mike worked out five to six hours a day at a high level of intensity.

With these strategies—lots of quality calories and lots of intense exercise—Mike was able to reduce his body fat from 9 percent to a contest-sharp 6.9 percent, without sacrificing muscle.

You don't have to start working out five hours a day (unless perhaps you are a professional bodybuilder training for a contest). But there is a connection between exercise and diet to burn body fat. You don't necessarily have to cut calories; you can actually keep them high. Exercising at moderate to high levels of intensity will take care of the fat.

Antifat Diet Strategies

The old-fashioned way of figuring out how many calories you should eat to lose weight is to just chop off 500 to 1,000 calories from your current diet. One pound (.5 kilogram) of fat is equivalent to 3,500 calories. According to the laws of thermodynamics, if you feed yourself 500 calories fewer than you need each day for seven days, theoretically you should lose 1 pound (.5 kilogram) at the end of the week. Double that amount and you should lose 2 pounds (1 kilogram). But dietitians have known for years that it never works this way, and this strategy becomes more frustrating as the weeks of dieting wear on.

At Georgia State University, Dr. Dan Benardot wondered why these seemingly clear laws of physics don't hold true within the human body. His research has shown that once food enters the biological system of the body, there are more variables at work than the simple number of calories that are given off by a pound of fat when measured directly in a science lab. The human body is a living organism, and the drive for survival allows the rules of the system to change based on thousands of years of adaptation to the environment. Dr. Benardot tested two groups of female gymnasts and runners: One group ate a diet of 500 fewer calories than they needed to maintain their weight each day, and the other group ate 300 fewer calories. What he found was astounding: The group that ate 300 fewer calories had a lower percentage of body fat than the group that actually ate less food. His theory is that when too few calories are eaten, resting energy expenditure (REE) slows down to meet the energy available to the body.

The ability of the body to slow metabolic rate to meet available energy has long been understood by scientists. Called *starvation adaptation,* it is induced in extreme circumstances of famine to allow the body to survive far longer than would be predicted based on normal metabolic rates of energy use. Dr. Benardot is proposing for the first time that even under mild states of energy deficit, energy use slows down. There is no benefit to eating far fewer calories than your body needs. In fact, he calls a 300-calorie deficit the ideal metabolic window for women to lose the most amount of fat in the shortest amount of time.

So forget low-calorie dieting. When you reduce your caloric intake by 300 calories (women) or 400 calories (men), you can keep your metabolic rate high enough to continue to burn fat at a good clip. Additionally, you want to have enough energy to perform at peak levels both physically and mentally. Here's how to eat to give yourself the best chance at losing fat and saving muscle.

- **Don't starve yourself.** Because you strength train and probably do aerobics as well, you actually need more food, not less. Researchers at Tufts University found that when older men and women began a strength-training program, they needed 15 percent more calories just to maintain their body weight. This finding is not so surprising, really. With strength training, the exercisers began to expend more calories. Plus, their RMR increased because they had built more muscle.

You can figure out exactly how many calories you need to lose fat. Based on my research with competitive bodybuilders, I have concluded that an intake of 35 to 38 calories per kilogram of body weight a day is reasonable for fat loss and muscle preservation. The minimum is 29 to 32 calories per kilogram for a rapid cut. Anything less than that is too restrictive, and you won't be well nourished.

Let's say you weigh 180 pounds (82 kilograms). Here's how to figure your calorie requirements to lose fat: 82 kg × 35 calories / kg = 2,870 calories. For maintaining body weight, you should eat up to 44 calories per kilogram of body weight a day, or 3,608 calories a day. If you want to build muscle and you increase your exercise intensity, duration, or frequency, go even higher—to 54 calories per kilogram of body weight, or 4,428 calories a day.

If you still need a calorie deficit to continue losing fat or to break a plateau, get that deficit by increasing your activity level and modifying your calories slightly. For example, restrict your calories by about 300 to 400 calories a day and increase your aerobic exercise. This deficit, again, is the ideal metabolic window for weight loss.

- **Correct your dietary fat.** Be sure to include the right kinds of fat in your diet, including omega-3 fats from fish and monounsaturated fat from olive oil, avocadoes, nuts and seeds, and nut and seed oils. A recent Australian study showed that when premenopausal women ate diets rich in monounsaturated fat, the diet helped them preserve muscle while losing weight. Diets high in omega-3 fats may actually protect against obesity; many studies have observed the fat-burning effect of omega-3 fats. Include up to five fish meals in your diet each week. The more muscle you maintain while losing fat, the greater your chance of keeping the weight off for good.

- **Preserve muscle with protein.** To lose mostly fat and keep your metabolism running in high gear with muscle mass preserved, you must have adequate protein in your diet. Protein also helps control your appetite. If you go on a diet that is too low in calories, there is a good chance that your dietary protein will not be used to build tissue but instead will be broken down and used for energy much like carbohydrate and fat are. As a reminder, for losing body fat the nutrient profile of your diet should be 30 percent protein, 40 percent carbohydrate, and 30 percent fat.

- **Concentrate on the right kinds of carbohydrate.** These include high-fiber foods and foods with a low-glycemic load (see chapter 3), which promote fat loss. Regardless of what you hear or read, the right kinds of carbohydrate are critical to fat loss for reasons that bear repeating. First, carbohydrate is required in the cellular reactions involved in burning fat. Second, it spares protein from being used as fuel. Third, carbohydrate restocks the body with glycogen, which helps power the muscles during exercise. Fourth, when your body is digesting carbohydrate, your metabolic rate goes higher than it does when metabolizing fat. Finally, complex carbohydrate is loaded with fiber, which has its own set of fat-burning benefits.

If you are strength training and doing aerobics as part of your fat-loss program, you need to eat 4 to 5 grams of carbohydrate per kilogram of body weight daily for men and 3 grams per kilogram of body weight daily for women. This amount will keep you well fueled for high-intensity exercise while still allowing enough room for your extra protein needs.

- **Monitor added sugar in your diet.** Added sugar in your diet promotes fat gain by reducing the sensitivity of your cells to insulin so that insulin cannot shuttle sugar into your muscle. It then heads to the liver, which turns the sugar into fat. When you eat low glycemic-load foods, you avoid this situation entirely.

Case in point: Researchers at Indiana University in Bloomington, Indiana, analyzed the diets of four groups of people: lean men (average body fat of 15 percent), lean women (average body fat of 20 percent), obese men (average body fat of 25 percent), and obese women (average body fat of 35 percent). The obese men and women ate more of their calories from fat (as high as 36 percent of total calories) and refined sugars, such as candy, doughnuts, and ice cream, which are also high in fat, than the lean men and women. In other words, there was a link between high-fat, high-sugar diets and obesity.

The lesson is this: Change the composition of your diet to keep the fat off. This means cutting down on high-fat, sugary foods. If you have a sweet tooth, choose dark chocolate or combine the sweet food with a protein and a healthy fat so that you slowly absorb the food and slowly release sugar and, ultimately, insulin into your bloodstream. Stay away from beverages and foods sweetened with high-fructose corn syrup, which has been linked to the incidence of obesity.

You may have thought about using artificially sweetened foods, but proceed with caution. See the section on artificial sweeteners on page 90 for more on the controversy over their use.

- **Don't skip breakfast.** Skipping breakfast is not a good way to lose body fat; in fact, it could even make you fatter! Most people who skip breakfast make up those calories, with interest, throughout the day. In Madrid, Spain, researchers found that overweight and obese people spent less time eating breakfast and ate smaller quantities and less varied types of food at breakfast compared with normal-weight people. Eating breakfast stokes your metabolic fires for the day. By contrast, going hungry in the morning is just another form of fasting, which slows down your metabolism. Plus, your physical and mental performance will suffer when you are running on empty.

If you're like me, you're rushed in the morning, with barely enough time to shower and dress, let alone eat breakfast. If that is the case, eat what you can. Something is better than nothing. A study done in England found that because ready-to-eat cereals are high in vitamins and minerals and low in fat, they make a great choice for breakfast. When choosing cereals, whole grains, low sugar, and high fiber are the best bets.

The best breakfasts include a combination of carbohydrate, protein, and fat. If you are always on the go, you need some nutritious breakfasts that take minutes to fix. There are several breakfast recipes in chapter 16 to help you. Some of these can even go on the road with you—so there is no excuse to skip breakfast!

Power Eating Fact Versus Fiction:

Do Artificial Sweeteners Have a Place in a Fat-Loss Program?

Artificial sweeteners have always been controversial. As a strength trainer, be aware of the controversies because you most likely eat a lot of food, some of which you may sweeten with these products. Here's some history on the oldest artificial sweeteners and an update on some of the newer sweeteners on the market.

The oldest artificial sweetener on the market is saccharin. A zero-calorie sweetener, saccharin was originally developed in 1900 to help people with diabetes and improve the taste of medically supervised diets. Though it is still on the market, commonly found as the product *Sweet 'N Low,* many nutrition experts and consumer advocate groups consider saccharin to be unsafe, because studies show that it causes cancer in rats.

In 1981, the FDA approved the use of aspartame. Commercially available as Equal, aspartame is an artificially synthesized compound of two natural ingredients, the amino acids phenylalanine and aspartic acid. Aspartame is virtually calorie free and 200 times sweeter than sugar.

Aspartame's natural ingredients and superior taste catapulted it to popularity. But no sooner had the FDA approved the use of aspartame than its safety came into question. It was already well known that eating aspartame could be dangerous for people with phenylketonuria (PKU), an inability to metabolize phenylalanine. All products containing aspartame must be labeled with a warning for people who have PKU. The most sensationalized concern around aspartame is reports of headaches by some consumers after using aspartame. Although there are many anecdotal reports, no confirmation of any specific dangers in using aspartame exist. In general, aspartame is considered probably safe by nutrition experts.

In 1988, another sweetener was approved—acesulfame-K. It is 200 times sweeter than sugar, yet has a bitter taste. The K in its name stands for potassium. Acesulfame-K is not metabolized by the body. You can cook and bake with it. Marketed under the names *Sunette* and *Sweet One,* this sweetener has not been adequately tested, according to some nutrition experts and consumer advocate groups.

Sucralose is 600 times sweeter than sugar and is made from a process that begins with regular sugar. Marketed under the name *Splenda,* sucralose has been approved for use in many products, including baked goods, baking mixes, nonalcoholic beverages, chewing gum, desserts, fruit juices, confections, toppings, and syrups. You can cook with sucralose and add it directly to food. The FDA reviewed more than 100 animal and human studies and concluded that sucralose was safe.

Neotame was approved by the FDA in 2002 and is supposedly sweeter than other artificial sweeteners on the market. It is made from phenylalanine and aspartic acid. Unlike aspartame, people with PKU can consume it. Consumer advocate groups consider Neotame to be safe.

Tagatose is a low-calorie natural sugar that has been approved by the FDA for use in foods, beverages, and other products. Manufactured from lactose, a simple sugar found in milk, tagatose looks like sugar, tastes like sugar, and best of all, cooks like sugar. The major difference between tagatose and sugar is that tagatose has roughly 6 calories per teaspoon compared with 16 calories for sugar. Tagatose has a low glycemic response, meaning that it won't push blood sugar and insulin to unhealthy levels. Tagatose has been shown in research to help with weight control. It is also a probiotic, promoting healthy bacteria in the intestines for better digestion. Tagatose is sold under the name *Naturlose*.

Sugar alcohols are used as artificial sweeteners in many foods, particularly low-carbohydrate products, and include erythritol, sorbitol, maltitol, mannitol, xylitol, lactitol, and isomalt. They are derived from fruit or produced from a sugar called dextrose. Most sugar alcohols contain .2 to .4 calorie per gram (sugar provides 4 calories per gram). Sugar alcohols are not digested in the small intestine the way regular sugar is. Instead, they pass straight through to the large intestine, where they are broken down by fermentation. As a result, they do not raise blood sugar as much as regular sugar does. For this reason, sugar alcohols are thought to be better than sugar for people with diabetes. A downside of sugar alcohols is that, if eaten in excess, they have a laxative effect.

Another sweetener used in many low-carbohydrate products is glycerine, a common food additive with a syrupy consistency and sweet taste. Even though glycerine is metabolized in the body like a carbohydrate, it does not turn into blood sugar or have the same effect on insulin activity that regular carbohydrate does. Glycerine is typically used in packaged foods to keep them from drying out. This is one reason you find it as an ingredient in many protein bars.

Stevia is a sweetener you can find mainly in health food stores. It is not allowed to be added to food but is sold as a supplement because it is technically an herb. The main ingredient in stevia is stevioside; it is virtually calorie free and hundreds of times sweeter than sugar. Stevia has not been widely tested, but in some animal studies it has been shown to adversely affect the male reproductive system, cause mutations in the genetic material of cells, and interfere with the absorption of carbohydrate. Most nutrition experts say that it is fine to use a little stevia once or twice a day in a cup of tea or other food. More studies are needed on this herb to fully determine its safety profile.

My advice on all artificial sweeteners is to use them sparingly. Don't forget that they show up in foods such as flavored yogurts, diet supplements, beverages, and many low-calorie and low-carbohydrate foods, so you might be ingesting more than is safe or necessary. Keep tabs on what you're eating and read labels.

Individualize Your Diet

Making dietary changes doesn't mean giving up your favorite foods or completely altering your lifestyle. Simply moderate how much of your favorite foods you eat by having them less often, and then learn how to make healthier substitutions. Making dietary changes also involves putting together the right proportions of protein, carbohydrate, and fat—and making sure your calories are sufficient to fuel your activities. I have included sample diets in chapter 14 as examples of how to eat to lose fat and develop muscle. These should help you plan your own menus. As further help along those lines, let me give you a case study of a young man I recently worked with who exemplifies exactly what can happen when you follow my Power Eating recommendations.

Mark is 35 years old and owns his own business. When we met at the end of April 2005, he weighed 187 pounds (85 kilograms), with 19 percent body fat; his height is 6 feet (183 centimeters). At the time, he was eating 2,900 calories a day, which broke down to 159 grams of protein, 286 grams of carbohydrate, 115 grams of fat, and 15 grams of alcohol. His protein intake was 22 percent of his total calories, carbohydrate was 39 percent, fat was 36 percent, and alcohol was 3 percent. Mark's goals were to lose fat and gain muscle to support his training and enhance his performance in the sports he enjoyed. He worked out with weights five times a week, did stationary cycling almost every day for about an hour, and took yoga once a week for an hour. We decided that he needed to see a personal trainer who could set up a healthier, more balanced exercise program, because it appeared to me that he might be overtraining. After he did that, we got down to nutrition business.

I started by lowering Mark's intake to 2,600 calories a day. He needed to increase his protein intake. His carbohydrate consumption was just about right, but he had to increase low glycemic-load foods. His total fat intake was slightly higher than what his body needed, and like carbohydrate, he needed to select healthier fat. At the start of his program, he began at 2,635 calories. The breakdown was as follows: 185 grams of protein (2.2 grams per kilogram of body weight); 204 grams of carbohydrate (3.3 grams per kilogram); and 85 grams of total fat (1 gram per kilogram).

Mark increased his intake of fish, fruits, vegetables, nuts, and seeds in order to address some specific nutritional concerns. He was low in a number of nutrients, including vitamin C, vitamin K, vitamin E, chromium, molybdenum, potassium, zinc, and biotin. In addition, he learned to time and combine protein, fat, and carbohydrate in order to control his appetite and keep his metabolic rate as high as possible. He bumped up his fluid intake as well. I advised him to eat an egg yolk a day and five fish meals a week. I added flaxseed meal to his diet in order to increase his intake of linolenic acid and fiber. Mark had not been fueling his body well before exercising, so we emphasized better recovery nutrition.

His initial diet contained 7 bread or starch servings, 5 fruits, 3 servings of low-fat milk, 5 vegetables, 12 servings of very lean protein, 6 servings of lean protein, 1 medium-fat protein, 9 fat servings, and 11 teaspoons (46 grams) of added sugar at certain times of the day as part of his exercise recovery period. From April 2005 to January 2006, Mark made some rather dramatic improvements in his weight, body composition, and overall mood as we gradually increased his calories and his nutrition over time. Table 5.1 illustrates his progress and shows what can be accomplished by integrating the Power Eating principles into your lifestyle.

Mark ultimately dropped from 34.5 pounds (15.6 kilograms) of fat and 147.1 pounds (66.7 kilograms) of muscle to 22.2 pounds (10.1 kilograms) of fat and 155.8 pounds (70.7 kilograms) of muscle (a 6.5 percent change in the ratio of muscle to fat)—exactly the direction you want to head with your body composition. Obviously, he did well with a program of increasing calories, making incremental changes in nutrition, and personalizing his program. His case study is a practical picture of the positive changes that can happen with this approach.

Table 5.1   Mark's Power Eating Progress

Weigh-in dates	Weight	Body composition (% body fat)	Calories per day before weigh-in	Daily nutrients before weigh-in
Initial weigh-in: April 28, 2005	187 lb (85 kg)	19	2,900	159 g protein; 286 g carbohydrate; 115 g total fat; 15 g alcohol
June 14, 2005	178 lb (81 kg)	13.6	2,600	185 g protein; 204 g carbohydrate; 85 g total fat
August 22, 2005	172 lb (78 kg)	12.5	2,814 (added 2 bread servings and 1 fat serving every day)	185 g protein; 316 g carbohydrate; 90 g fat
January 4, 2006	178 lb (81 kg)	12.5	3,002 (added 2 fruits and 1 tbsp added sugar) to eventually 3,400 calories	At 3,002 calories: 185 g protein; 363 g carbohydrate; 90 g fat
Currently maintaining				At 3,400 calories: 185 g protein; 463 g carbohydrate; 90 g fat

Sport Nutrition Fact Versus Fiction:
Are Diet Pills a Shortcut to Cutting Up?

In recent years, a flood of different diet pills has hit the market. They are available in two major forms, including prescription drugs and over-the-counter pills (which include certain dietary supplements). Here's a general look at both categories.

Prescription Drugs

Depending on the drug, these agents work as appetite suppressors or fat blockers. Drugs such as sibutramine (Meridia), diethylpropion (Tenuate), and phentermine (Adipex-P, Fastin, Anoxine-AM, and so forth) affect chemicals in the brain that short-circuit the desire to eat. Sibutramine also helps stimulate the metabolism. These drugs are prescribed primarily for people who are considered obese, defined as being at least 20 percent over ideal weight. No ethical physician should recommend or prescribe them for anyone fewer than 10 pounds over a healthy weight.

The chief prescription fat blocker on the market is orlistat (Xenical), which works in the intestines to partially block fat from being absorbed. A side effect of orlistat is that it may interfere with the absorption of fat-soluble vitamins, namely vitamins A, D, E, and K. In January 2006, an FDA advisory panel of outside experts approved a recommendation to sell a lower dose of Xenical without a prescription.

Although drugs like Meridia and Xenical have been shown in clinical trials to help dieters shed weight, prescription drugs do have side effects and may interfere with existing medical conditions. Make sure you're well informed about these side effects.

Over-the-Counter Diet Pills and Supplements

Products such as Xenadrine and Dexatrim were once formulated with a combination of ephedra (an herb) and caffeine to potentially increase metabolism. It was a fairly successful combination, but in 2003, the FDA banned the use of ephedra due to evidence that it increased the risk of heart attack. Today, despite ephedra's removal from the FDA banned supplement list, the formulations have replaced ephedra with mixtures of various nutrients. Some contain an ephedra-like substance called synephrine that is found in certain citrus fruits. Caffeine is still used in many formulations, as it is believed to increase metabolism and activate the breakdown of fatty acids in the body.

More than 50 individual dietary supplements and 125 proprietary products are now sold for weight loss. Ingredients like caffeine, guarana (an herb that contains caffeine), and synephrine (bitter orange) are designed to rev up your metabolism. Certain fibers such as guar gum, glucomannan, and psyllium reportedly suppress your appetite by making you feel full. Other supplements claim to slow down fat production in the body, including hydroxycitric acid, green tea, and conjugated linoleic acid (CLA). Chitosan, a natural fat blocker made from shellfish, supposedly prevents fat from being absorbed.

The claims for these products sound too good to be true, and most of the time, they are. The research supporting their claims is scant, so there's no guarantee that they will even work. I advise against diet pills. As an exerciser and strength trainer, you have the best weapons available to fight body fat: high-energy eating habits and exercise that builds calorie-burning muscle and stokes your metabolic fires.

6

Hydrating for Heavy-Duty Workouts

Quick: What's the most critical nutrient for growth, development, and health?

If you guessed water, congratulations! People frequently overlook the importance of water in their diet, and most don't even consider water an essential nutrient. Without enough water and other fluids, though, you'll die within a week.

Although water does not provide energy in the same way carbohydrate and fat do, it plays an essential role in energy formation. As the most abundant nutrient in your body, water is the medium in which all energy reactions take place. Thus, you need ample fluids for fuel and stamina. You get those fluids from a variety of sources—the foods you eat; the beverages you consume; and the plain, pure water you drink. Here's a closer look at the importance of water and other fluids in the diet.

Water: An Essential Nutrient

The fluids in your body form a heavily trafficked river through your arteries, veins, and capillaries that carries nutrients to your cells and waste products out of the body. Fluids fill virtually every space in your cells and between each cell. Water molecules not only fill space, but they also help form the structures of macromolecules such as proteins and glycogen. The chemical reactions that keep you alive occur in water, and water is an active participant in those reactions.

It's hard to say enough good things about water. It makes up about 60 percent of the body's weight in adults. As the primary fluid in your body, water serves as a solvent for minerals, vitamins, amino acids, glucose, and many other nutrients. Without water, you can't even digest these essential nutrients, let alone absorb, transport, and use them.

In addition to carrying nutrients throughout the body, water transports waste products out of the body. It is a part of the lubricant in your joints that keeps them moving. And when your body's temperature begins to rise, water acts as the coolant in your radiator. Enough said! You can see why water is so vital to health.

Temperature Regulation

Your body produces energy for exercise, but only 25 percent of that energy is actually used for mechanical work. The other 75 percent is released as heat. The extra warmth produced during exercise causes your body to heat up, raising your core temperature. To get rid of that extra heat, you sweat. As sweat evaporates, your blood and body cool. If you couldn't cool off, you would quickly succumb to heat stress caused by the increase in your body's core temperature.

Fat Burning

Drinking more water can actually help you stay lean. Your kidneys depend on water to do their job of filtering waste products from the body. In a water shortage, the kidneys need backup, so they turn to the liver for help. One of the liver's many functions is mobilizing stored fat for energy. By taking on extra assignments from the kidneys, the liver can't do its fat-burning job as well. Fat loss is compromised as a result.

In addition, water can help take the edge off hunger so that you eat less, and it has no calories. If you are on a high-protein diet, water is required to detoxify ammonia, a by-product of protein energy metabolism. And, as you burn off stored fatty acids as energy, you release any fat-soluble toxins that have been benignly stored in your fat cells. The more fluid you drink, the more you dilute the toxins in your bloodstream, and the more rapidly they exit from the body.

Muscle Strength and Control

Ever wonder why some days you're so pooped you can't pump iron? One reason may be dehydration. To move your muscles, you need water. Of all the places in the body, water is found in highest concentrations in metabolically active tissues such as muscle and is found in lowest concentrations in relatively inactive tissues such as fat, skin, and some parts of bone. Muscles are controlled by nerves. The electrical stimulation of nerves and contraction of muscles occur as a result of the exchange of electrolyte minerals dissolved in water (sodium, potassium, calcium, chloride, and magnesium) across the nerve and muscle cell membranes.

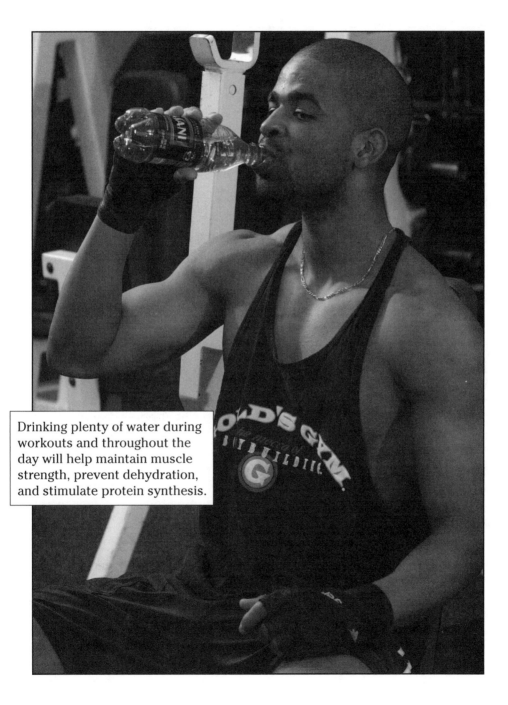

Drinking plenty of water during workouts and throughout the day will help maintain muscle strength, prevent dehydration, and stimulate protein synthesis.

If you're low on water or electrolytes, muscle strength and control are weakened. A water deficit of just 2 to 4 percent of your body weight can cut your strength-training workout by as much as 21 percent—and your aerobic power by a whopping 48 percent. Your body's thirst mechanism kicks in when you've lost 2 percent of your body weight in water. But by that time, you're already dehydrated. To prevent dehydration, you must get yourself on a scheduled plan to drink often throughout the day. (See the drinking schedule on page 104.)

If gaining muscle is your goal, you should care about cell volumization, or the hydration state of your muscle cells. In a well-hydrated muscle cell, protein synthesis is stimulated and protein breakdown is decreased. On the other hand, dehydration of muscle cells promotes protein breakdown and inhibits protein synthesis. Cell volume has also been shown to influence genetic expression, enzyme and hormone activity, and metabolism.

Joint Lubrication

Water forms the makeup of synovial fluid, the lubricating fluid between your joints, and cerebrospinal fluid, the shock-absorbing fluid between vertebrae and around the brain. Both fluids are essential for healthy joint and spine maintenance. If your diet is water deficient, even for a brief period, less fluid is available to protect these areas. Strength training places tremendous demands on the joints and spine, and the presence of adequate protective fluid is essential for optimum performance and long-term health.

Mental Performance

When it comes to peak mental capacity, whether at the office or in competition, your hydration state will affect your performance. Dehydration, in particular, decreases mental energy; causes fatigue, lethargy, light-headedness, and headaches; and can certainly make you feel down. In a study of subjects' abilities to perform mental exercises after dehydration induced by heat stress, a fluid loss of only 2 percent of body weight caused reductions of up to 20 percent in arithmetic ability, short-term memory, and the ability to visually track an object. With that powerful proof, you should be motivated to stay well hydrated to keep your mental energy high and your focus sharp.

Disease and Illness Prevention

Probably the most surprising fact about water is the effect that chronic, mild dehydration has on health and disease. It was a practice of Hippocrates to recommend large intakes of water to increase urine production and decrease the recurrence of urinary tract stones. Today, approximately 12 to 15 percent of the general population will form a kidney stone at some time in life. Many factors can modify the risk factors for developing stones. Of these, diet—especially fluid intake—is the only one that can be easily changed and that has a marked effect on all aspects of urinary health.

A little-known fact is that low water intake is a risk factor for certain types of cancers. One study found that patients with urinary tract cancer (bladder, prostate, kidney, and testicle) drank significantly smaller quantities of fluid compared with healthy controls.

In another study, researchers discovered that women who drank more than five glasses of water a day had a 45 percent lower risk of colon cancer compared with those who consumed two or fewer glasses a day. For men, the risk was cut by 32 percent when they drank more than four glasses a day versus one or fewer glasses a day.

Why does adequate water intake appear to have an anticancer effect? One theory holds that the more fluid you drink, the faster you flush the toxins and carcinogenic substances out of the body, and the less chance there is for them to be resorbed into the body or to be concentrated long enough to cause tissue change.

Even more fascinating, a pilot study reported that the odds of developing breast cancer were reduced by 79 percent, on average, among water drinkers. In this case, maintaining a dilute solution within the cells possibly reduces the potency of estrogen and its ability to cause hormone-related cancers, according to the theory proposed by the authors of this research.

Mild dehydration can also be a factor in the occurrence of mitral valve prolapse, a defect of one of the heart valves that controls the flow of blood between chambers of the heart. Mitral valve prolapse is a relatively harmless condition, but in a small percentage of cases, it may cause rapid heartbeat, chest pain, and other cardiac symptoms. In a study of 14 healthy women with normal heart function, mitral valve prolapse was induced by mild dehydration and resolved with rehydration.

How Much Water Do You Need?

Nearly all the foods you eat contain water, which is absorbed during digestion. Most fruits and vegetables are 75 to 90 percent water. Meats contain roughly 50 to 70 percent water. And beverages such as juice, milk, and glucose–electrolyte solutions are more than 85 percent water. On average, you may consume about 4 cups (1 liter) of water daily from food alone, but this is true only if you're eating an abundance of fruits and vegetables, which are the major food sources of water.

Most people are walking around in a moderately dehydrated state. You need 8 to 12 cups (2-3 liters) of fluids daily—even more to replace the fluid you lose during exercise. Of these 8 to 12 cups, make sure at least 5 of them are pure water.

You lose about a quart (4 cups, or 1 liter) of water per hour of exercise, depending on your size and perspiration rate. When you're working out moderately in a mild climate, you are probably losing 1 to 2 quarts (1-2 liters), or 2 to 4 pounds (1-2 kilograms), of fluid per hour through perspiration. That means that a 150-pound (68-kilogram) person can easily lose 2 percent of the body's weight in fluid (3 pounds, or 1 kilogram) within an hour. If exercise is more intense or the environment is more extreme, fluid losses will be greater. Thus, you can see how easily you become dehydrated.

If you don't replenish fluid losses during exercise, you will fatigue early and your performance will be diminished. If you don't replenish fluid after exercise, your performance on successive days will decay, and your long-term health may be at risk.

Moreover, according to the National Athletic Trainers' Association (NATA), dehydration:

- impairs your physical performance in less than an hour of exercise—or sooner if you start working out in a dehydrated state;
- cuts your performance by as much as 48 percent; and
- increases your risk of developing symptoms of heat illness, such as heat cramps, heat exhaustion, and heatstroke.

In addition to exercise, many other factors increase water requirements, including high heat, low humidity, high altitude, high-fiber foods, illness, travel, and pregnancy.

What about you? Are you dehydrated? Table 6.1 lists the early and severe warning signs of dehydration and heat stress.

Table 6.1 Symptoms of Dehydration and Heat Stress

Early signs	Severe signs
Fatigue	Difficulty swallowing
Loss of appetite	Stumbling
Flushed skin	Clumsiness
Heat intolerance	Shriveled skin
Light-headedness	Sunken eyes and dim vision
Dark urine with strong odor	Painful urination
Dry cough	Numb skin
Burning in stomach	Muscle spasm
Headache	Delirium
Dry mouth	

It's easy to monitor yourself for early signs of dehydration:

- Check your urine. It should be relatively odorless and no darker in color than straw. If it's a golden or deep color with a strong odor, you're dehydrated and need to consume more water.
- Weigh yourself without clothing before and after exercise. For every pound (.5 kilogram) lost during exercise, you've lost 2 to 3 cups (473-710 milliliters) of fluid. Any weight lost during exercise is fluid loss and should be replaced by fluids as soon after exercise as possible.
- A sore throat, dry cough, and hoarse voice are all signs of dehydration.
- A burning sensation in your stomach can signal dehydration.
- Be aware of muscle cramps. No one knows for sure what causes muscle cramps, but a shortfall of water may be an important factor. Muscle cramps are more apt to occur if you're doing hard, physical work in the heat and don't drink enough fluids. You can usually alleviate the cramps by moving to a cool place, drinking fluids, and replacing electrolytes with a glucose–electrolyte solution.

Drinking Schedule for Strength Trainers

You usually can't rely on thirst to tell you when to drink fluids. By the time your thirst mechanism kicks in during exercise, you've already lost 1 to 2 percent of your body weight as sweat. You need to drink water at regular intervals whether you're thirsty or not, and you need to do so every day. Remember, if you fail to drink enough fluids one day, your body can't automatically rehydrate itself the next. You'll be doubly dehydrated and possibly begin to show some signs of dehydration.

For workouts, here's a schedule that will keep you well hydrated. If you are an athlete, you can also refer to the recommendations from the NATA in table 6.2.

- **Before exercise.** Drink at least 16 ounces (2 cups, or 473 milliliters) of fluid two to three hours before exercise. Then, drink 8 ounces (1 cup, or 237 milliliters) of fluid immediately before exercise to make sure the body is well hydrated. In very hot or cold weather, you need even more water: 12 to 20 ounces (1.5-2.5 cups, or 296-708 milliliters) of fluid 10 to 20 minutes before exercise. Exercising during cold weather elevates your body temperature, and you still lose water through perspiration and respiration.
- **During exercise.** Drink 7 to 10 ounces (207-296 milliliters) every 10 to 20 minutes during exercise, and more in extreme temperatures. Although this might seem tough at first, once you schedule it into your regular training rou-

tine, you'll quickly adapt to the feeling of fluid in your stomach. In addition, the fuller your stomach is, the faster it will empty. Dehydration slows the rate at which your stomach will empty. Make regular water breaks part of your training.

- **After exercise.** This is the time to replace any fluid you've lost. Weigh yourself before and after exercise; then drink 2 to 3 cups (473-710 milliliters) of fluid within two hours after exercise for every pound (.5 kilogram) of body weight you've lost. Continue to drink an additional 25 to 50 percent more fluid for the next four hours.

Table 6.2   Fluid Replacement for Athletes: Practical Applications
Fluid guidelines
Before exercise
2-3 h before, drink 17-20 oz (503-708 ml) of water or sport drink.
10-20 min before, drink 7-10 oz (207-296 ml) of water or sport drink.
During exercise
Athletes benefit from drinking fluid with carbohydrate in many situations.
If exercise lasts more than 45 min or is intense, fluid with carbohydrate (sport drink) should be provided during the session.
A 6%-8% carbohydrate solution maintains optimal carbohydrate metabolism.
During events when a high rate of fluid intake is necessary to sustain hydration, carbohydrate composition should be kept low (less than 7%) to optimize fluid delivery.
Fluids with salt (sodium chloride) are beneficial for increasing thirst and voluntary intake as well as offsetting losses.
Cool beverages at temperatures of 10-15 degrees C (50-59 degrees F) are recommended.
Every 10-20 min, drink 7-10 oz (207-296 ml) of water or a sport drink. Athletes should be encouraged to drink beyond their thirst.
After exercise
Within 2 h, drink enough to replace any weight loss from exercise; drink approximately 20 oz (708 ml) of water or sport drink per pound (.5 kg) or weight loss.
Within 6 h, drink an additional 25%-50% more than weight loss from exercise.

Best Sources of Water

The easiest way to get water is right from your faucet. But reports of contaminated tap water are of concern to many people—and with good reason. The water supply in some areas contains contaminants such as lead, pesticides, and chlorine by-products that exceed recommended limits. A good move is to buy a water purifier, which filters lead and other contaminants from tap water. Some filters attach right to the tap; others can be installed as part of the entire water system. One of the most convenient and economic filtering methods is the pour-through filter you can place in a special pitcher and put right in your refrigerator. If you use a filtration product that removes fluoride from your water, discuss this concern with your dentist, because fluoride can support good dental health.

Another option is to purchase bottled water. There are hundreds of brands, the most popular of which offer spring water and mineral water. Spring water is taken from underground freshwater springs that form pools on the surface of the earth. Mineral water comes from reservoirs located under rock formations. It contains a higher concentration of minerals than most sources. Well water is another type of bottled water, which is tapped from an aquifer. Well, mineral, and spring waters still may contain some contaminants. For this reason, federal regulations are tightening on the bottled-water industry.

Distilled water, also labeled as purified water, is another type of bottled water. It has been purified through vaporization and is then condensed. A drawback of distilled water is that it does not contain any minerals. In addition, fluoride is missing from many bottled waters. However, several brands now add back a mineral package, making it more nutritious and usually better tasting.

Some people like seltzer water. This is a sparkling water that is bubbly because of the addition of pressurized carbon dioxide. Many of these products are flavored and contain sucrose or fructose. While carbonated waters are fine to drink throughout the day, they are not desirable during exercise. The gas from the bubbles takes up space in your stomach and makes you feel fuller, decreasing the amount of total fluid you will drink during and after exercise.

Regardless of what type of water you drink, be sure to drink the 8 to 12 cups (2 to 3 liters) or more of fluids you need daily to stay well hydrated, and make at least 5 of these cups (1 liter) pure water.

Designer Waters

Water now comes in more varieties than ever before. Today, there's fortified water, fitness water, herbal water, oxygen-enriched water, electrolyzed water—the list goes on. Welcome to the world of designer waters. While they may taste great, watch out for unsubstantiated claims on the labels, and for what I call "clear soda pop" masquerading as water. Some sweetened waters have almost as much sugar as a can of soda. Read the ingredients and nutrition labels to make informed choices.

- **Fortified water.** Featuring a splash of flavor and sweetness, these waters are fortified with predissolved vitamins and minerals. Some are formulated for people who want to drink their supplements, others for active people who drink water during workouts and want a little more flavor than plain water provides.

Fortified waters are not to be confused with sport drinks or glucose–electrolyte solutions, which are packed with more carbohydrate energy and higher amounts of electrolytes than specialty waters contain.

- **Fitness water.** These designer waters contain some vitamins, but with only 10 calories per serving. They are meant to be used when you want some flavor in your water but don't need a glucose–electrolyte solution or extra calories.

- **Herbal water.** Fairly new on the water front are herb-enhanced waters. You can now swill water containing such popular herbs as echinacea, ginkgo biloba, Siberian ginseng, ginger, or Saint-John's-wort. These beverages are a good option if you want the benefits of medicinal herbs without popping pills. Generally, herb-enhanced waters have a hint of flavor without sugar, calories, or carbonation.

Be aware of how many servings you consume of herbal or fortified waters, along with other sources of the same herbs, vitamins, and minerals. You might easily take in too much of these substances. And because the herbal part of the food industry is yet to be regulated, there's no guarantee that you're getting the ingredients listed on the label.

- **Oxygen-enriched water.** These beverages are said to be enhanced with up to 40 times the normal oxygen concentration found naturally in water. Available flavored or unflavored, they claim to boost energy by increasing oxygen saturation in the red blood cells. To date, though, there's no published medical evidence to validate such claims. There appears to be no value in them other than as another good source of water.

- **Electrolyzed water.** This category describes water that has been separated into alkaline and acid fractions. The alkaline fraction is bottled for drinking with a pH of about 9.5, compared with other bottled waters in which pH ranges from 6 to 8. The process removes contaminants and most of the total dissolved solids but leaves in electrolytes such as calcium, magnesium, potassium, sodium, and bicarbonates. Claims for electrolyzed water include smoother taste, healthier water, improved hydration ability, electrolyte availability, and antioxidant properties. Aside from smoother-tasting water, the scientific research into most of these claims is in its infancy. Keep an eye on this research.

Are Sport Drinks Superior to Water?

In some cases, yes. For general types of exercise lasting less than one hour, water is still the best sport drink around. The nutrient you most need to replace during and after these types of workouts is water.

Glucose–electrolyte solution drinks (also known as sport drinks) do have their place, mostly during high-intensity intermittent exercise and exercise lasting more than 45 minutes, and they are especially useful for endurance and ultraendurance athletes. These products are a mixture of water, carbohydrate, and electrolytes. Electrolytes are dissolved minerals that form a salty soup in and around cells. They conduct electrical charges that let them react with other minerals to relay nerve impulses, make muscles contract or relax, and regulate the fluid balance inside and outside cells. In hard workouts or athletic competitions lasting 45 minutes or longer, electrolytes can be lost through sweat. For a comparison of the various ingredients in these sport drinks, see table 6.3.

Where glucose–electrolyte solutions may have an edge over water is in their flavor. A lot of people don't drink much water because it doesn't taste good to them. Soldiers participating in a study at the U.S. Army Research Institute of Environmental Medicine were given the choice of drinking plain chlorinated water, flavored water, or lemon-lime glucose–electrolyte solution drinks. Most soldiers chose the glucose–electrolyte solutions or flavored water over plain water. If you don't need the extra carbohydrate and electrolytes, one way to sneak more water in and still get the flavor is to dilute your glucose–electrolyte solution or use one of the new flavored fitness waters. But remember, you will not get the performance-enhancement effect for exercise over one hour if you do this.

If you're an avid water drinker and really like water, you'll benefit just as much from water as you will from using a glucose–electrolyte solution, unless you're exercising an hour or more. But if you don't like water or tend to avoid it during exercise, try a filtered water or bottled water, which both have a different taste. Or try a glucose–electrolyte solution that contains less than 8 percent carbohydrate and some sodium. Another idea is to put some powdered sport drink mix into your water, although the powdered mixes sometimes don't taste as good as their premixed counterparts. At the very least, if a glucose–electrolyte solution encourages you to drink more, it has done its job.

Table 6.3 Replacement Beverage Comparison*

Beverage	Carbohy-drate (%)	Sodium (mg)	Other ingredients	Calories
1st Ade	7	55	Phosphorus	60
10K	6.3	55	Chloride, phosphorus, vitamin C	60
Accelerade	7	128	Protein	80
Allsport	8	55	Chloride, phosphorus, calcium	70
Cytomax	4-6	53	L-glutamic acid, inosine, L-glutamine (chloride, magnesium)	66
Endura	6.2	46	Chloride, calcium, magnesium, chromium	60
Enervitene	3-9	2.5-7.5	guar seed	30-90
Exceed	7.2	50	Chloride, magnesium, calcium	70
Extran Thirst-quencher	5	260	Sodium chloride, tripotassium citrate	45
Gatorade	6	110	Chloride, phosphorus	50
GU20	5	120	Sodium citrate, potassium citrate	50
Hydra Fuel	7	25	Chloride, phosphorus, magnesium, vitamin C, chromium	66
Performance	7	490	Sodium citrate, beet juice color, citric acid, sodium chloride, magnesium citrate, potassium citrate	66
Powerade	8	55	Chloride	70
Quickick	7	100	Chloride, phosphorus, calcium	67
RevengePro	4	85	Protein, ribose, ginseng, glucosamine, willow bark, feverfew, periwinkle, quercetin, creatine alpha-ketoglutarate, phosphatidylcholine, guarana, fish oil, coenzyme Q10, B-vitamin blend, chromium polynicotinate	100
Sustained Energy	10-12	37	Protein, L-carnosine, L-carnitine complex, choline	114
Ultima Replenisher	2	37.5	Coenzyme Q10, choline, inositol, pine bark, grape seed, bilberry, ginseng, green tea	12.5

*Per 8 oz or 237 ml serving.

Is Juice a Good Sport Drink?

Juices are a source of fluids. Orange juice, for example, is nearly 90 percent water and is full of vitamins and minerals. Although juices count as part of your fluid requirement, you'll feel at your best if you base your daily fluid plan on at least 5 cups (1 liter) of water and use juice to help you attain your minimum 8 to 12 cups (2 to 3 liters) of total fluids.

There are some cautions to consider regarding juice as a fluid in your training diet. In recent years, there has been a lot of hype surrounding the health benefits of fruit and vegetable juices. The makers of commercial juicing machines claim fresh juices are a panacea for all kinds of ills, from digestive upsets to cancer. But is it better to drink your five servings of fruits and veggies every day rather than eat them? No way!

In most juices, the pulp has been removed from the fruit or vegetables to make the juice. That means all-important fiber has also been subtracted, because the pulp is where you find the fiber. Granted, some juice machines boast that their process keeps the pulp in the juice to retain the important fiber and concentrate the nutrients. These products are excellent choices for a once-a-day juice. But they still do not replace whole fruit.

Freshly squeezed juice is often touted as a better source of nutrients than commercial juices. But commercially prepared juices that are frozen and refrigerated properly are only slightly lower in nutrients than fresh juice. If you don't buy fresh produce, don't store it properly at home, and don't drink your freshly squeezed juice immediately, your homemade juice may even be lower in nutrients than a well-made frozen or refrigerated brand.

Whether they are cooked, squeezed, dried, or raw, fruits and vegetables need to be a big part of your diet. If using a juice machine is one way of eating more fruits and vegetables and is enjoyable for you, go for it. But remember the drawbacks, and don't use juice as your only source of fruits and vegetables.

If you want to drink juice to rehydrate your body, dilute it with water by at least twofold. A cup (237 milliliters) of orange or apple juice plus 2 cups (356 milliliters) of water will provide a 6 to 8 percent carbohydrate solution, similar to a sport drink formulation. Don't use this combination during exercise, however, because of its fructose content. The body doesn't use fructose as well as the combination of sugars in a regular sport drink. In addition, some people are fructose sensitive and may experience intestinal cramping after drinking juice. As I noted earlier, juice may interfere with fluid absorption if consumed during exercise. Instead, drink your juice–water mix as part of your fluids an hour or more after exercise. The addition of water will speed the emptying of the fluid from your stomach and thus rehydrate your body more rapidly, and the carbohydrate will help replenish glycogen.

Hydration Danger Zones

It's hard to imagine that water could be bad for you, but just like everything else, too much water at the wrong place or the wrong time can actually be harmful. Moderation is the key, even when we're talking about water.

Overhydration

When considering your water intake, you must also consider overhydration. Hydration is a delicate balance between fluids and minerals. The concentration of sodium and other minerals (collectively known as electrolytes) in the bloodstream must fall within a very narrow range, or it can affect muscle contractions. That includes the most important muscle: your heart.

When you take in too much water relative to the amount of electrolytes in your body, the result will eventually be a condition called *hyperhydration* or *hyponatremia*. The problem is that the blood has become too dilute, which is just as dangerous as dehydration. During dehydration there are high levels of electrolytes without enough fluids. Surprisingly, the symptoms of dehydration and hyperhydration are basically the same.

Hyperhydration occurs more frequently than you might think, particularly in endurance events like marathons and triathlons. Not nearly as well documented is the possibility of bodybuilders hyperhydrating due to high intakes of purified water combined with very low food and sodium intakes during a cutting diet. While no occurrences of hyponatremia have been documented in strength trainers not participating in another sport, you should be aware that very high intakes of purified water over an extended period of time may put you at risk. Whether you're training for an endurance event or preparing for a strength-training competition, you can avoid hyponatremia with a few simple precautions.

If you're training for your first marathon or triathlon, don't cut all salt out of your diet (though, as a general rule, most of us could get away with a lot less than we currently take in). If the day is cooler or less humid than you expected, compensate by drinking less than you'd planned during the event.

Go for sport drinks over pure water. Don't think you have to match the more highly trained competitors drink for drink. Their sweat is different from yours, containing more water and fewer electrolytes. Your body is leaking sodium, while theirs are holding onto it. If you see pretzels being handed out along the course of a distance race, help yourself, assuming you're not sodium sensitive and you don't have high blood pressure. The extra sodium will prevent you from becoming hyperhydrated.

When you are dieting to make weight prior to a competition, don't overdo the water. Drink water with minerals in place of purified water, or don't remove all the sodium from your diet. As long as you are eating, your risk of hyponatremia is remarkably diminished.

What Not to Drink

Certain types of beverages should be shunned during exercise, according to the NATA in its position paper on fluid replacement for athletes. These beverages include fruit juices, carbohydrate gels (always consume these with extra water), sodas, and glucose–electrolyte solutions with carbohydrate levels greater than 8 percent. Such beverages slow fluid absorption and may cause gastrointestinal problems. The NATA also discourages the consumption of beverages containing caffeine, alcohol, and carbonation, because they stimulate excess urine production and thus dehydrate your body.

Alcohol

It has been a long time since a client has asked me whether drinking beer is a good way to replenish fluids and carbohydrate. But clients frequently ask whether alcohol will hurt their exercise performance, and even more frequently, they want to know whether drinking a little bit of alcohol may actually be heart healthy. Thanks to an ever-growing body of scientific research and knowledge, here are some answers to those questions and more.

• **What's in alcohol?** Alcohol is a carbohydrate, but it's not converted to glucose as other kinds of carbohydrate are. Instead, it is converted into fatty acids and thus is more likely to be stored as body fat. So if you drink and train, alcohol puts fat burning on hold. It's not your friend if you're trying to stay lean.

Pure alcohol supplies 7 calories per gram and nothing else. In practical terms, a shot (1.5 ounces, or 44 milliliters) of 90-proof gin contains 110 calories, and 100-proof gin contains 124 calories. Beer has a little more to offer, but not much. On the average, a 12-ounce (355-milliliter) can of beer contains 146 calories, 13 grams of carbohydrate, traces of several B-complex vitamins, and, depending on the brand, varying amounts of minerals. Light beer and nonalcoholic beer are lower in calories and sometimes carbohydrate. All table wines have similar caloric content. A 3.5-ounce (104-milliliter) serving of table wine contains about 72 calories, 1 gram of carbohydrate, and very small amounts of several vitamins and minerals. Sweet or dessert wines are higher in calories, containing 90 calories per 2-ounce (59-milliliter) serving.

• **What are alcohol's side effects?** Today, alcohol is the most abused drug in the United States. Ten percent of users are addicted, and 10 to 20 percent are abusers or problem drinkers. Alcohol is a central nervous system depressant. Compared with other commonly used substances, alcohol has one of the lowest effective dose–lethal dose ratios. In other words, there's a small difference in the amount of alcohol that will get you drunk and the amount that will kill you. The reason that more people don't die from alcohol intoxication is that the stomach is alcohol sensitive and rejects it by vomiting.

Acute alcohol intoxication results in tremors, anxiety and irritability, nausea and vomiting, decreased mental function, vertigo, coma, and death. In large amounts, alcohol causes the loss of many nutrients from the body, including thiamin, vitamin B6, and calcium. Furthermore, chronic alcohol abuse has negative effects on every organ in the body, particularly the liver, heart, brain, and muscle, and can lead to cancer and diseases of the liver, pancreas, and nervous system.

Don't drink alcohol in any form if you're pregnant. It can cause birth defects. Drinking alcohol in large amounts can also lead to accidents, as well as social, psychological, and emotional problems.

• **How does alcohol affect exercise performance?** Because alcohol depresses the central nervous system, it impairs balance and coordination and decreases exercise performance. Strength and power, muscle endurance, and aerobic endurance are all zapped with alcohol use. Alcohol also dehydrates the body considerably.

• **Is alcohol really heart healthy?** Research has found that daily consumption of one drink per day can do your heart good by positively affecting the levels of good cholesterol (HDL) in your blood. The higher your HDL levels, the lower your risk of heart disease.

However, excessive alcohol intake increases your chance of developing heart disease. More than two drinks a day can raise your blood pressure and contribute to high triglycerides, a risk factor for heart disease. Drinking large amounts of alcohol on a habitual basis can also cause heart failure and lead to stroke.

Alcohol consumption contributes to obesity, another major risk factor in the development of heart disease. Extra pounds are hard on your heart, and the higher your weight climbs, the greater your risk. Being overweight also raises blood pressure and cholesterol, which are risk factors themselves.

• **Is a drink a day good prevention?** The risks of alcohol outweigh its positives. If you drink alcoholic beverages, do so in moderation, with meals, and when consumption does not put you or others in harm's way. Moderation is defined as no more than one drink per day for women and no more than two drinks per day for men. One drink is 12 ounces (355 milliliters) of regular beer, 5 ounces (296 milliliters) of wine, and 1.5 ounces (44 milliliters) of 80-proof distilled liquor. However, exercising, quitting smoking, and lowering your blood cholesterol through a healthy diet are better ways to prevent heart disease without any added risks.

Sport Nutrition Fact Versus Fiction:

Do Soft Drinks Rehydrate the Body?

If given the option, many people would choose a soft drink over water to rehydrate themselves following workouts. And who can blame them? Soft drinks taste good, seem to quench thirst, and are generally refreshing.

But soft drinks are among the worst choices for rehydration. Soft drinks are laced with huge amounts of sugar—roughly the equivalent of 10 teaspoons (46 grams) per can. Because of their sugar content, soft drinks are absorbed less rapidly than pure water. The sugar in them keeps the fluid in your stomach longer, so less water is available to your body. Rather than rehydrating your system, soft drinks can make you feel even thirstier. Also, the sugar can trigger a sharp spike in insulin, followed by a fast drop in blood sugar. This reaction can leave you feeling tired and weak. In addition, the sugar in soft drinks is high-fructose corn syrup, which does not replenish glycogen as rapidly as other forms of carbohydrate. Fructose also can cause cramps in people who are sensitive to it.

What about sugar-free soft drinks? These beverages contain artificial sweeteners, which remain controversial. Furthermore, all soft drinks are, of course, carbonated, and carbonation produces gas. Who wants a gassy stomach, especially during a workout?

Diluting a soft drink isn't a good option either. Even in a diluted concentration, soft drinks have nothing beneficial to offer. As far as rehydration is concerned, no fluids—including artificially sweetened soft drinks—have yet been proven to do a better job than plain old water or a good glucose–electrolyte solution.

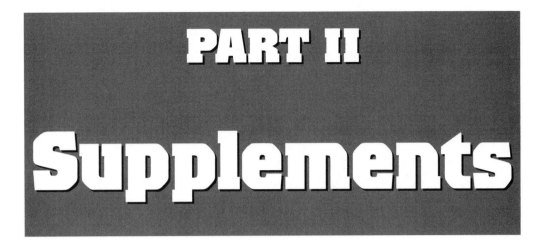

PART II
Supplements

Now that you've built your nutrition foundation and have your diet down to a science, it's time to consider supplements. Of course, supplements are just that—extras that you can add to your well-designed food plan. In addition, supplements play an important role as convenient tools in our busy lives:

- Perhaps there are critical foods that you can't eat or don't like. Supplements can fill in the nutritional gaps left by excluding such foods.
- Or, perhaps your schedule is so busy that you don't have time to prepare food immediately after exercise when your body really needs it for muscle growth—supplements to the rescue!
- And maybe you want to gain just a little competitive edge. There are a few supplements that work powerfully to give you that edge.

This section reviews the most popular supplements used by strength-training athletes. Using the most current scientific research, I evaluate the usefulness of these supplements as well as any potential for harm. Use my rating system to help decide for yourself which products meet their marketing claims, which ones have potential and which one don't, and which products are potentially harmful.

7

Vitamins and Minerals for Strength Trainers

Want to get ripped, shredded, striated, and vascular? Every supplement company says they've got the product for you. You have probably stood in the supplement aisle for hours, reading ingredients and wondering which ones really work. Ads for supplements certainly promise dramatic results. However, scientists have only begun to research the nutritional requirements of muscle building. The research is promising, but the whole story on what works and what doesn't is not in yet.

Among the many pills and potions on store shelves are vitamins and minerals. Quite possibly, you may need extra amounts of both. Research shows that most Americans fall short of the requirements for many key nutrients, including vitamins C, E, and B_{12}; folic acid; zinc; and magnesium, which is why a growing number of Americans are turning to supplements. A survey by the Centers for Disease Control and Prevention (CDC) shows that more than 60 percent of the general population takes supplements daily.

Furthermore, the American Medical Association (AMA) recommends that everyone take a multivitamin and mineral supplement daily; doing so has been shown to help prevent chronic illnesses such as cancer, heart disease, and osteoporosis. Even people who eat five daily servings of fruits and vegetables may not get enough of certain vitamins for optimum health. Most people, for instance, cannot get the healthiest levels of folate and vitamin D and E from their diets.

Hard workouts increase your nutritional needs, as does dieting. That's why you may want to add certain vitamins and minerals to your nutritional arsenal. From a sport science perspective, if you are deficient in vitamins and minerals, your performance can suffer. Research shows that if you've taken in less than one-third of the daily required amount of certain B vitamins (B_1, B_2, and B_6) and vitamin C, you can lose aerobic power and strength in a matter of weeks. Taking a multivitamin and mineral supplement isn't going to help you lift more, run faster, or build more muscle, but it will help prevent deficiencies that could impair your performance.

Keep in mind that vitamin and mineral supplements should not replace food. With the right planning, your body can get almost all the nutrients it needs from a balanced diet. What's more, your body absorbs nutrients best from food. However, if you would like the insurance, a good move is to take a daily antioxidant multivitamin containing 100 percent of the daily values for vitamins and minerals. These formulations help you cover your nutritional bases and contain nutrients that have special value to strength trainers.

A word of caution: Be sure to choose a product made by a reputable company such as a pharmaceutical company. Also, look for products that carry the USP (United States Pharmacopeia) certification on the label. The reason is that many products are adulterated with stimulants that are either intentionally or unintentionally laced with other ingredients that are not on the label of the product. The USP label ensures that only the items on the label are in the product. These ingredients might be stimulants (often intentionally put in products to make people feel good after they take the product) or even steroid-like compounds. Vitamin products produced in the same factory where drugs are made might unintentionally wind up containing traces of those drugs if both were manufactured in proximity to each other. It's rare, but it does happen.

Daily Reference Intake

A new way of rating the amounts of the nutrients we need for good health is the DRI. It expands on and includes the familiar RDA, but whereas the RDAs target nutrient deficiencies, the DRIs aim to prevent chronic diseases (see chapter 1).

Applied to vitamins, minerals, and protein taken by men and women in specific age groups, the DRIs contain three different rating sets appropriate for discussion here: the RDAs, a set of values that help us maintain our health; the tolerable upper intake levels (UL), which establish ceilings to help us avoid taking too much of a nutrient; and adequate intakes, or AIs, which are estimates of average intakes that seem healthy and won't harm health. For the purposes of this book, I will place all nutrient recommendations under the heading of DRIs.

Antioxidants

There has been a lot of excitement in strength sports about antioxidants—beta-carotene, vitamin C, and vitamin E and the minerals selenium, copper, zinc, and manganese. Antioxidants help fight free radicals, chemicals that are produced naturally by the body and that cause irreversible damage (oxidation) to cells. Free radical damage can leave your body vulnerable to advanced aging, cancer, cardiovascular disease, and degenerative diseases such as arthritis. The exercise-related functions of the key antioxidants are summarized in table 7.1.

Certain environmental factors such as cigarette smoke, exhaust fumes, radiation, excessive sunlight, certain drugs, and stress can increase free radicals. And, ironically, so can the healthy habit of exercise. During respiration, cells pick off electrons from sugars and add them to oxygen to generate energy. As these reactions take place, electrons sometimes get off course and collide with other molecules, creating free radicals. Exercise increases respiration, which produces more free radicals. Scientists are still studying why this happens and how to better defend against it; however, exercise also induces the production of enzymes that fight free radicals.

Body temperature, which tends to rise during exercise, may be another factor in generating free radicals. A third possibility is the increase in catecholamine production during exercise. Catecholamines are hormones released in response to muscular effort. They increase heart rate, let more blood get to muscles, and provide the muscles with fuel, among other functions.

Another source of free radical production is the damage done to the muscle cell membrane after intense exercise, especially eccentric exercise such as putting down a heavy weight or running downhill. In a domino-like series of chemical reactions, free radicals hook up with fatty acids in cell membranes to form substances called *peroxides*. Peroxides attack cell membranes, setting off a chain reaction that creates many more free radicals. This process is called *lipid peroxidation* and can lead to muscle soreness. The point is, several complex reactions occur with exercise, and each one may accelerate free radical production.

Beta-Carotene

Beta-carotene is a member of a group of substances known as carotenoids. There are hundreds of carotenoids in nature, found mostly in orange and yellow fruits and vegetables and dark green vegetables.

Once ingested, beta-carotene is converted to vitamin A in the body on an as-needed basis. As an antioxidant, beta-carotene can destroy free radicals after they're formed, and it has been shown to reduce muscle soreness by minimizing exercise-induced lipid peroxidation. With less soreness, you may be able to work out more times a week.

Table 7.1 Key Antioxidants

Vitamins

Beta-carotene

Exercise-related function	May reduce free radical production as a result of exercise and protect against exercise-induced tissue damage; complements antioxidant function of vitamin E.
Best food sources	Carrots, sweet potatoes, spinach, cantaloupe, broccoli, any dark green leafy vegetable, and orange vegetables and fruits.
Side effects and toxicity	None known because the body carefully controls its conversion to vitamin A. Daily intakes of 20,000 IUs from either food or supplements over several months may cause skin yellowing. This disappears when the dosage is reduced.
DRIs for adults	No established limits. 2,500 IUs daily from supplements is safe. You can get the same amount from a large carrot.

Vitamin C

Exercise-related function	Maintains normal connective tissue; enhances iron absorption; may reduce free radical damage as a result of exercise and protect against exercise-induced tissue damage.
Best food sources	Citrus fruits and juices, green peppers, raw cabbage, kiwi fruit, cantaloupe, and green leafy vegetables.
Side effects and toxicity	The body adapts to high dosages. Dosages higher than 250 mg daily may harm immunity. Dosages between 5,000 mg and 15,000 mg daily may cause burning urination or diarrhea.
DRIs for adults	Women, 75 mg; pregnant women, 85 mg; lactating women, 120 mg; men, 90 mg. Also, 110 milligrams for female smokers and 130 milligrams for male smokers.
*UL for adults	2,000 mg.

Vitamin E

Exercise-related function	Involved in cellular respiration; assists in the formation of red blood cells; scavenges free radicals; protects against exercise-induced tissue damage.
Best food sources	Nuts, seeds, raw wheat germ, polyunsaturated vegetable oils, and fish liver oils.
Side effects and toxicity	None known.
DRIs for adults	15 mg; lactating women, 19 mg.
UL for adults	1,000 mg.

Minerals

Selenium

Exercise-related function	Interacts with vitamin E in normal growth and metabolism; preserves the elasticity of the skin; produces glutathione peroxidase, an important protective enzyme.
Best food sources	Cereal bran, Brazil nuts, whole-grain cereals, egg yolk, milk, chicken, seafood, broccoli, garlic, and onions.
Side effects and toxicity	5 mg a day from food has resulted in hair loss and fingernail changes. Higher dosages are linked to intestinal problems, fatigue, and irritability.

Minerals	
Selenium, *continued*	
DRIs for adults	Women, 55 mcg; pregnant women, 60 mcg; lactating women, 70 mcg; men, 55 mcg.
UL for adults	400 mcg.
Copper	
Exercise-related function	Assists in the formation of hemoglobin and red blood cells by aiding in iron absorption; required for energy metabolism; involved with superoxide dismutase, a key protective antioxidant enzyme.
Best food sources	Whole grains, shellfish, eggs, almonds, green leafy vegetables, and beans.
Side effects and toxicity	Toxicity is rare.
DRIs for adults	Women and men, 900 mcg; pregnant women, 1,000 mcg; lactating women, 1,300 mcg.
UL for adults	10,000 mcg.
Zinc	
Exercise-related function	Involved in energy metabolism and immunity.
Best food sources	Animal protein, oysters, mushrooms, whole grains, and brewer's yeast.
Side effects and toxicity	Dosages higher than 20 mg a day may interfere with copper absorption, reduce HDL cholesterol, and impair the immune system.
DRIs for adults	Women, 8 mg; pregnant women, 11 mg; lactating women, 12 mg; men, 11 mg.
UL for adults	40 mg.
Manganese	
Exercise-related function	Involved in metabolism; involved with superoxide dismutase, a key protective antioxidant enzyme.
Best food sources	Whole grains, egg yolks, dried peas and beans, and green leafy vegetables.
Side effects and toxicity	Large dosages can cause vomiting and intestinal problems.
DRIs for adults	Women, 1.8 mg; pregnant women, 2.0 mg; lactating women, 2.6 mg; men, 2.3 mg.
UL for adults	11 mg.
Lipids	
Coenzyme Q10	
Exercise-related function	A coenzyme for mitochondrial enzymes of the oxidative phophorylation pathway essential for ATP production; a potent antioxidant that decreases oxidative damage to tissues.
Best food sources	Organ meats, beef, soy oil, sardines, mackerel, and peanuts.
Side effects and toxicity	None known.
DRIs for adults	No established limits. Doses of 30-300 mg per day have been used in clinical studies of heart failure patients.

*UL refers to tolerable upper intake levels, which have been established for vitamins and minerals. These levels represent the maximum intake of a nutrient that is likely to pose no health risks.

However, most clinicians now advise against supplementing with beta-carotene. Here is why: People who took supplemental beta-carotene while enrolled in a large cancer-prevention trial called the Carotene and Retinol Efficacy Trial, or CARET, continued to have increased rates of lung cancer six years after the trial was stopped early and the supplements discontinued, according to a long-term follow-up of trial participants. The results add to earlier evidence from this study and a second large prevention trial that, contrary to earlier expectations, not only do beta-carotene supplements not prevent lung cancer in people at high risk for the disease, they appear to increase rates of the disease, particularly among smokers. These findings hint that there is some adverse reaction going on in the body, and because of it, it is wise to get your beta-carotene from vegetables instead.

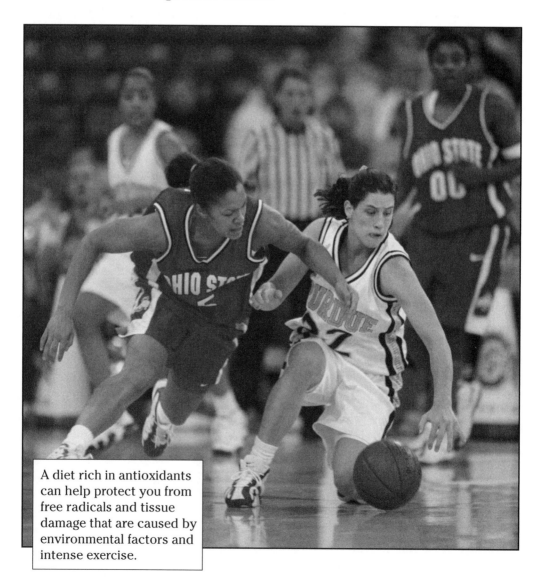

A diet rich in antioxidants can help protect you from free radicals and tissue damage that are caused by environmental factors and intense exercise.

Vitamin C

Vitamin C, or ascorbic acid, is a nutrient that can be synthesized by many animals, but not by humans. It's an essential component of our diets and functions primarily in the formation of connective tissues such as collagen. Vitamin C is also involved in immunity, wound healing, and allergic responses. As an antioxidant, vitamin C keeps free radicals from destroying the outermost layers of cells.

If you work out regularly or train for athletic competition, you know that a cold or respiratory infection can sideline you pretty fast. Fortunately, researchers have found that supplementing with 500 milligrams daily of vitamin C appears to cut the risk of upper respiratory tract infections. This benefit may be due to the antioxidant effect of vitamin C or to its overall immune-boosting capability.

Supplementing with vitamin C will improve your performance, but only if you are deficient in this nutrient. Supplementation does not enhance performance if you already eat a healthy, nourishing diet that is high in citrus fruits (which are high in vitamin C) and other fruits and vegetables.

Vitamin E

Many studies on antioxidants and exercise have focused on vitamin E, which resides in muscle cell membranes. Part of its job is to scavenge the free radicals produced by exercise, saving the tissues from damage. There is so much research in this area that I'd like to summarize some of the findings for you. A few studies on vitamin E have found benefits to supplementation:

- A daily 800-milligram vitamin E supplement protected against muscle damage and free radical production in subjects aged 55 and older who exercised by walking or running downhill.
- Supplementation appears to prevent the destruction of oxygen-carrying red blood cells. That means your muscles benefit from improved or sustained oxygen delivery during exercise.
- Supplementation may improve exercise performance at high altitudes; however, this benefit has not been observed at sea level.

Other studies on vitamin E have not shown benefits:

- Two months of vitamin E supplementation at 800 IUs a day actually increased oxidative stress and levels of homocysteine (a protein in the blood that can have heart-damaging effects) in triathletes.
- Supplementation with vitamin E (1,200 IUs daily) was not effective at preventing muscle damage or oxidative stress in untrained men who performed strength training for the first time. Several studies have found the same results.

- A review study of relevant research conducted on vitamin E since 1985 concluded that vitamin E supplementation does not appear to decrease exercise-induced lipid peroxidation.

Beyond sport performance, vitamin E has been widely studied as a nutrient that may help prevent chronic disease, which is why it has been recommended so widely and in such high doses. Recent findings, however, have reversed these recommendations. In one long-running study involving some 7,000 volunteers taking 400 IUs daily, vitamin E supplementation failed to reduce the risk of heart disease and cancer and actually may have increased the risk of heart disease in people with diabetes or preexisting heart problems. In a second study, the same dose of vitamin E nearly tripled the risk of new cancers among 540 patients undergoing cancer treatment.

Sounds pretty grim, but the better news is that taking 200 IUs of vitamin E appears safe. This is the dosage now being recommended. Some people can get the recommended daily intake of 30 IUs by eating foods rich in vitamin E, including nuts, sunflower seeds, and vegetable oils.

If you supplement your diet with vitamin E, choose a natural form of the nutrient over a synthetic version. Labeled as *d-alpha tocopherol,* natural vitamin E is isolated from soybean, sunflower, corn, peanut, grapeseed, and cottonseed oils. Synthetic vitamin E, labeled as *dl-alpha tocopherol,* is processed from substances found in petrochemicals. A recent review of 30 published studies on vitamin E concluded that the natural version is absorbed better by the body than the synthetic version.

Avoid taking supplemental vitamin E if you are taking anticlotting drugs such as low-dose aspirin or Coumadin, since vitamin E can further thin your blood.

Coenzyme Q10

Coenzyme Q10 (CoQ10) is actually a lipid that acts like a vitamin and is an essential component in the body's production of energy. But it is also an antioxidant that has been widely studied. CoQ10 is present in every single cell in the body and is found in the greatest concentration in the heart muscle, where it probably improves oxygen uptake at the cellular level. CoQ10 supplementation has been effective in the treatment of heart failure. Because of its role in energy production and oxygen uptake, CoQ10 has been theorized to improve aerobic performance. However, studies have shown otherwise, and one study even found that supplementation actually impaired performance.

CoQ10 is naturally present in small amounts in a variety of foods but is particularly high in organ meats such as heart, liver, and kidney, as well as in beef, soy oil, sardines, mackerel, and peanuts. According to Dr. Peter H. Langsjoen from the University of Washington, "To put dietary CoQ10 intake into perspective, 1 pound [.5 kilogram] of sardines, 2 pounds [.9 kilogram] of beef, or 2 1/2 pounds [1.1 kilograms] of peanuts, provide 30 mg of CoQ10." It has no known toxicity or side effects.

The small CoQ10 doses of 30 to 45 milligrams per day in the initial studies were associated with measurable clinical responses in patients with heart failure. More recent studies have used higher doses with improved clinical response, again in patients with heart failure. The use of CoQ10 for prevention of illness and possibly enhancement of performance is an extremely important question which, to date, does not have an answer.

Antioxidant Supplements and Exercise

An antioxidant cocktail may help prevent oxidative stress, a condition in which free radicals outnumber antioxidants and which may result in damage to muscle tissues, according to a study from the Washington University School of Medicine in St. Louis. For one month, unexercised medical students took high doses of antioxidants daily: 1,000 IUs of vitamin E, 1,250 milligrams of vitamin C, and 37.5 milligrams of beta-carotene. The doses were divided into five capsules a day. Some of the subjects took placebos.

Before supplementation, the students ran at a moderate pace on a treadmill for about 40 minutes, followed by 5 minutes of high-intensity running to exhaustion. The same exercise bout was repeated after supplementation.

The researchers discovered that oxidative stress caused by exercise was high before supplementation. In other words, there was a lot of tissue damage going on. With antioxidants, there was still some oxidative stress caused by exercise, but it wasn't as great. The researchers concluded that taking antioxidants offered protection against tissue damage. When you can reduce this damage, you might be able to optimize competitive sport performance. But like much research with supplements, other studies have come up with different results: that antioxidant supplementation does not appear to prevent exercise-induced muscle tissue damage.

Much of the research in antioxidant supplementation has been done with endurance athletes. But what about strength trainers? If you work out consistently, you are tearing down a lot of tissue, and muscles generate free radicals during and after exercise. For these reasons, there may be some benefit for strength trainers to take antioxidant supplements in order to help protect against the potential onslaught of free radicals.

Most of the people I have worked with eat diets that are deficient in vitamin E and other antioxidants. One of the reasons is that active, health-conscious people typically go on diets that are low in fat, but dietary fat from vegetable oils, nuts, and seeds is one of the best sources of vitamin E. What's more, some active people, particularly strength trainers, limit their intake of fruit. They incorrectly believe that the fructose in fruit will end up as body fat. But by cutting out fruits, they cut out foods that are loaded with beta-carotene and vitamin C.

Antioxidant Supplements and Performance

If you take antioxidants, will you be able to work out longer and harder? Whether antioxidant supplementation really improves performance hasn't been adequately nailed down by research. If you are undernourished—that is, you have a vitamin deficiency—you will definitely feel better and perform better by correcting that deficiency. But if your diet is already high in antioxidants, supplementing with extra antioxidants may not make much of a difference in your performance.

The amounts of vitamin C and beta-carotene that seem to be protective are easily obtained from food. To get enough of these two vitamins, follow my Power Eating recommendations in chapters 12 through 15 and throughout the book. Strive to eat three or more servings of vegetables and two or more servings of fruits every day.

As for vitamin E, a supplement of 100 to 200 IUs per day is safe and adequate. To boost your intake of the other antioxidants, be sure your daily vitamin and mineral supplement contains antioxidants.

B-Complex Vitamins

In this family of nutrients, there are eight major B-complex vitamins—thiamin, riboflavin, niacin, vitamin B_{12}, folic acid, pyridoxine, pantothenic acid, and biotin—that work in accord to ensure proper digestion, muscle contraction, and energy production. Although these nutrients do not enhance performance, training and diet do alter the body's requirement for some of them. If you are active and you restrict your calories, or if you make poor nutritional choices, then you put yourself at risk for deficiencies, particularly of thiamin, riboflavin, and pyroxidine. Table 7.2 summarizes the exercise-related functions of the B-complex vitamins.

Thiamin

Thiamin helps release energy from carbohydrate. Thiamin, along with pyridoxine and vitamin B_{12}, are believed to be involved in the formation of serotonin, a feel-good chemical made in the brain. Serotonin helps elevate mood and induce relaxation. Large doses of these vitamins (60 to 200 times the daily requirement) have been shown to help fine motor control and performance in pistol shooting. It remains to be seen whether supplementation with these vitamins would affect performance in precision sports that depend on fine motor control.

The amount of carbohydrate and calories in your diet determines your dietary requirement for thiamin. By eating a well-balanced, carbohydrate-dense diet, you generally get all the thiamin you need. The best food sources of thiamin are unrefined cereals, brewer's yeast, legumes, seeds, and nuts.

There is one possible exception, however. Are you taking a carbohydrate supplement to increase calories? If so, you may need extra thiamin, particularly if your carbohydrate formula contains no thiamin. For every 1,000 calories of carbohydrate you consume from a formula, you need to add .5 milligram of thiamin to your diet.

Dieting and erratic eating patterns can leave some nutritional gaps, too. To be on the safe side, be sure to take a daily multivitamin that contains 100 percent of the DRI for thiamin or up to 1.2 milligrams of the nutrient. It is not a good idea to exceed the upper limit (UL) recommendation for any B vitamins.

Riboflavin

Like thiamin, riboflavin helps release energy from foods. Also like thiamin, your dietary requirement of riboflavin is linked to your caloric and carbohydrate intake. As a strength trainer, you need to consume at least .6 milligram of riboflavin for every 1,000 calories of carbohydrate in your diet, and some athletes may need even more. Riboflavin is easily lost from the body, particularly in sweat. In a study of older women (aged 50 to 67), researchers at Cornell University discovered that exercise increases the body's requirement for riboflavin. An earlier study at Cornell found that very active women required about 1.2 milligrams of riboflavin a day. However, increasing riboflavin intake did not improve performance.

Foods rich in riboflavin include dairy products, poultry, fish, grains, and enriched and fortified cereals. A daily multivitamin containing 100 percent of the DRI or up to 1.3 milligrams of riboflavin will help prevent a shortfall.

Niacin

Like the previously mentioned B-complex vitamins, niacin is involved in releasing energy from foods. Supplementing with extra niacin is not a good idea and may be harmful, according to a great deal of research. For example, supplementation with extra niacin may block the release of fat from fat tissue, causing premature reliance on the use of stored carbohydrate and depletion of muscle glycogen. It may also impair aerobic performance. Excessive amounts of niacin could also possibly contribute to liver damage.

The amount of niacin you need each day is linked to your caloric intake. For every 1,000 calories you eat daily, you need 6.6 milligrams of niacin, or 13 milligrams for every 2,000 calories. If you are using a carbohydrate formula that contains no niacin, make sure you take 6.6 milligrams of niacin for every 1,000 calories that you supplement. The best food sources of niacin are lean meats, poultry, fish, and wheat germ. Taking a multivitamin every day will help you guard against deficiencies.

Table 7.2   Vitamin B Complex

Thiamin (B₁)

Exercise-related function	Carbohydrate metabolism; maintenance of nervous system; growth and muscle tone.
Best food sources	Brewer's yeast, wheat germ, bran, whole grains, and organ meats.
Side effects and toxicity	None known.
DRIs for adults	Women, 1.1 mg; pregnant women, 1.4 mg; lactating women, 1.4 mg; men, 1.2 mg.

Riboflavin (B₂)

Exercise-related function	Metabolism of carbohydrate, protein, and fat; cellular respiration.
Best food sources	Milk, eggs, lean meats, and broccoli.
Side effects and toxicity	None known.
DRIs for adults	Women, 1.1 mg; pregnant women, 1.4 mg; lactating women, 1.6 mg; men, 1.3 mg.

Niacin

Exercise-related function	Cellular energy production; metabolism of carbohydrate, protein, and fat.
Best food sources	Lean meats, liver, poultry, fish, peanuts, and wheat germ.
Side effects and toxicity	Liver damage, jaundice, skin flushing and itching, nausea.
DRIs for adults	Women, 14 mg; pregnant women, 18 mg; lactating women, 17 mg; men, 16 mg.
UL for adults	35 mg.

Vitamin B₁₂

Exercise-related function	Metabolism of carbohydrate, protein; and fat; formation of red blood cells.
Best food sources	Meats, dairy products, eggs, liver, and fish.
Side effects and toxicity	Liver damage, allergic reactions.
DRIs for adults	Women, 2.4 mg; pregnant women, 2.6 mg; lactating women, 2.8 mg; men, 2.4 mg.

Folic acid

Exercise-related function	Regulation of growth; breakdown of protein, formation of red blood cells.
Best food sources	Green leafy vegetables and liver.
Side effects and toxicity	Gastric problems; can mask certain anemias.
DRIs for adults	Women, 400 mcg; pregnant women, 600 mcg; lactating women, 500 mcg; men, 400 mcg.
UL for adults	1,000 mcg.

Pyridoxine (B_6)	
Exercise-related function	Protein metabolism; formation of oxygen-carrying red blood cells.
Best food sources	Whole grains and meats.
Side effects and toxicity	Liver and nerve damage.
DRIs for adults	Women aged 19-30, 1.3 mg; women aged 31-70, 1.5 mg; pregnant women, 1.9 mg; lactating women, 2 mg; men aged 19-30, 1.3 mg; men aged 31-70, 1.7 mg.
UL for adults	100 mg.
Pantothenic acid	
Exercise-related function	Cellular energy production; fatty acid oxidation.
Best food sources	Found widely in foods.
Side effects and toxicity	None known.
DRIs for adults	Women, 5 mg; pregnant women, 6 mg; lactating women, 7 mg; men, 5 mg.
Biotin	
Exercise-related function	Breakdown of fat.
Best food sources	Egg yolks and liver.
Side effects and toxicity	None known.
DRIs for adults	Women, 30 mcg; pregnant women, 30 mcg; lactating women, 35 mcg; men, 30 mcg.
Choline	
Exercise-related function	May improve fatigue and performance in aerobic sports.
Best food sources	Egg yolks, nuts, soybeans, wheat germ, cauliflower, and spinach.
Side effects and toxicity	None known.
DRIs for adults	Women, 425 mg; pregnant women, 450 mg; lactating women, 550 mg; men, 550 mg.
UL for adults	3,500 mg.

Vitamin B_{12}

Vital to healthy blood and a normal nervous system, vitamin B_{12} is the only vitamin found primarily in animal products. It works in partnership with folic acid to form red blood cells in the bone marrow.

If you are a vegetarian who eats no animal foods, you must be sure to get enough vitamin B_{12}. Fermented and cultured foods such as tempeh and miso contain some B_{12}, as do vegetarian foods fortified with the nutrient. The safest approach is to supplement with a multivitamin containing 3 to 10 micrograms of vitamin B_{12}.

If you are over 50 years old, your ability to absorb vitamin B_{12} from food may be limited. The Institute of Medicine recommends that you consume foods fortified with B_{12} or take a vitamin B_{12} supplement.

Folic Acid

Folic acid is the vitamin that, with B_{12}, helps produce red blood cells in the bone marrow. Found in green leafy vegetables, legumes, and whole grains, it also helps reproducing cells to synthesize proteins and nucleic acids.

Folic acid first attracted attention for its role in pregnancy. During pregnancy, folic acid helps create red blood cells for the increased blood volume required by the mother, fetus, and placenta. Because of folic acid's role in the production of genetic material and red blood cells, a deficiency can have far-reaching consequences for fetal development. If the fetus is deprived of folic acid, birth defects can result. Folic acid intake is so important to women in their childbearing years that foods are now being fortified with it. The most recent finding is that for pregnant women, it is also important to take a multivitamin supplement in order to get enough folic acid.

There is renewed excitement over folic acid because of its protective role against heart disease and cancer. It reduces homocysteine, a proteinlike substance, in the tissues and blood. High homocysteine levels have been linked to heart disease. Scientists predict that as many as 50,000 premature deaths a year from heart disease can be prevented if we eat more folic acid.

Recent scientific experiments have revealed that folic acid deficiencies cause DNA damage resembling the DNA damage in cancer cells. This finding has led scientists to suggest that cancer could be initiated by DNA damage caused by a deficiency in this B-complex vitamin. Other studies show that folic acid suppresses cell growth in colorectal cancer. It also prevents the formation of precancerous lesions that could lead to cervical cancer, a discovery that may explain why women who don't eat many vegetables and fruits (good sources of folic acid) have high rates of this form of cancer.

Stress, disease, and alcohol consumption all increase your need for folic acid. You should make sure that you're getting 400 micrograms a day of this vitamin, a level that is found in most multivitamins.

Pyridoxine

Pyridoxine, also known as vitamin B_6, is required for the metabolism of protein. It's also vital in the formation of red blood cells and the healthy functioning of the brain. The best food sources of pyridoxine are protein foods such as chicken, fish, and eggs. Other good sources are brown rice, soybeans, oats, and whole wheat.

Researchers in Finland found that exercise alters pyridoxine requirements somewhat. They learned this by testing the blood levels of various nutrients in a group of young female university students who followed a 24-week exercise program.

Ever feel anxious before an athletic competition? If so, try supplementing with a cocktail of pyridoxine, thiamin, and vitamin B_{12}. By increasing levels of serotonin—a mood-elevating chemical in the brain—this trio has been found to reduce anxiety and thus improve competitive performance.

The DRI for pyridoxine in women aged 19 to 50 is 1.3 milligrams; for women aged 51 and older, 1.5 milligrams; for pregnant women, 1.9 milligrams; for lactating women, 2 milligrams; for men aged 19 to 50, 1.3 milligrams; and for men aged 51 and older, 1.7 milligrams. If you're wondering whether your own requirement for pyridoxine falls within safe bounds, rest assured that it probably does. A training diet that contains moderate amounts of protein will give you all the pyridoxine you need. In other words, there's no need to supplement. Besides, large doses (in excess of 50 milligrams a day) can cause nerve damage.

Pantothenic Acid

Pantothenic acid participates in the release of energy from carbohydrate, fat, and protein. Because this vitamin is so widely distributed in foods (particularly meats, whole grains, and legumes), it is rare to find a deficiency without a drop in other B-complex vitamins. They all work as a team.

The safe range of intake for pantothenic acid is 4 to 7 milligrams a day. Exercise does affect pantothenic acid metabolism, but only to a slight degree. By following my strength-training nutrition plan in chapters 12 to 15, you'll take in plenty of this vitamin to cover any extra needs you might have from exercise.

Biotin

Biotin is involved in fat and carbohydrate metabolism. Without it, the body can't burn fat. Biotin is also a component of various enzymes that carry out essential biochemical reactions in the body. Some good sources of biotin are egg yolks, soy flour, and cereals. Even if you don't get the 30 to 100 micrograms you need daily from food, your body can synthesize biotin from intestinal bacteria. So there's no reason to supplement with extra biotin.

Together with choline and inositol, two other B-complex members, biotin is often found in lipotropic (prevents or reduces fat accumulation in the liver) supplements promoted as fat burners. However, there is no credible evidence that biotin or any other supplemental nutrient burns fat.

Some research shows that biotin levels are low in active people. No one is sure why, but one explanation may have to do with exercise. Exercise causes lactic acid, a waste product, to build up in working muscles, and biotin is involved in the process that breaks down lactic acid. The more lactic acid that accumulates in muscles, the more biotin is needed to break it down. But don't rush out to buy a bottle of biotin. There is no need to supplement with this vitamin, because your body can make up for any marginal deficiencies on its own.

Some strength trainers are in the habit of concocting raw-egg milkshakes. Raw egg white contains avidin, a protein that binds with biotin in the intestine and prevents its absorption. Eating raw eggs on a consistent basis can thus lead to a biotin deficiency. But once eggs are cooked, the avidin is destroyed, and there is no danger of blocking biotin absorption.

Choline

Present in all living cells, choline is another B-complex vitamin. It is synthesized from two amino acids, methionine and serine, with help from vitamin B_{12} and folic acid. Choline works together with inositol, another lipotropic dietary factor, to prevent fat from building up in the liver and to shuttle fat into cells to be burned for energy.

Choline is involved in the formation of acetylcholine in the body. Acetylcholine is a neurotransmitter, a chemical that sends messages from nerves to nerves and nerves to muscles. If acetylcholine is reduced in the nervous system, then fatigue may set in.

Researchers at MIT studied runners before and after the Boston Marathon and found a 40 percent drop in their plasma choline concentrations. They don't know why this happened; however, they speculated that choline is used up during exercise to produce acetylcholine. Once choline is depleted, there's a corresponding drop in acetylcholine production, and when production falls off, the ability to do muscular work falls off. Or so the theory goes.

Some research suggests that choline supplementation (1.5 to 2 grams daily) may improve performance in athletes who do not get enough of this vitamin in their diet. One study showed that supplementation with choline and carnitine (a vitamin-like nutrient) reduced lipid peroxidation in women who followed a walking program for 21 days.

However, other research shows that choline supplementation has no measurable effect on performance. It has been tested in aerobic exercise and on marathon runners, but did not improve performance or cut running times.

Normally, your body can easily manufacture enough choline for good health as long as you eat a balanced, nutrient-rich diet. Choline is found in egg yolks, nuts, soybeans, wheat germ, cauliflower, and spinach. Lately, I've worked with a number of athletes who have a low intake of choline. Often just adding an egg yolk a day is a great strategy to bump up your choline intake.

Other Vitamins

The fat-soluble vitamins A, D, and K are rarely promoted as exercise aids, most likely because they're toxic in large doses. Vitamin A, or retinol, is found primarily in animal sources such as liver, fish, liver oils, margarine, milk, butter, and eggs. Vitamin A is involved in the growth and repair of tissues, maintenance of proper vision, and resistance against infection. It also helps maintain the health of the skin and mucous membranes. Massive doses in excess of the DRI can cause nausea, vomiting, diarrhea, skin problems, and bone fragility, among other serious problems.

Vitamin D is unique because it is also a hormone your body can manufacture on its own when your skin is exposed to sunlight; it is called the sunlight vitamin because of this reaction. Just 10 to 15 minutes a day in the sun without sunscreen a few days a week supplies sufficient amounts of vitamin D. If you can't get out in the sun, live in northern climates where there is not much sunlight, or frequently wear sunscreen, you may need to take supplements. Unfortunately, the body's ability to manufacture vitamin D appears to decrease with age, so older adults may need to get more vitamin D through diet (fortified milk and fatty fish have good amounts) or supplements, whether they're exposed to ample sunlight or not. Do not take high doses because they can be toxic; the DRI for your gender and age is the proper amount (see table 7.3).

The only vitamin your body makes naturally, vitamin D promotes the absorption and balance of calcium in the body, strengthens bones and teeth, boosts the immune system, fosters normal muscle construction, and may prevent some types of cancer.

There is also a connection between vitamin D and weight management. Vitamin D helps your body better absorb calcium, which has a fat-burning effect. So for calcium to assist in fat-burning, your body requires sufficient vitamin D. On the other hand, if the calcium levels in your body are low, a hormone called *parathyroid hormone (PTH)* and vitamin D increase in response to the shortage and trick your body into thinking it is starving. Consequently, you may pack away more calories in the form of fat and put on extra weight when this imbalance occurs.

As for vitamin K, its primary function is to assist in the process of normal blood clotting. It is also required for the formation of other kinds of body protein found in the blood, bone, and kidneys. However, research has revealed another side to vitamin K that most people have never seen: It is vital for building healthy bones, which is why a number of calcium supplements are now being formulated with vitamin K. With a shortfall of vitamin K, bone can become weakened because of insufficient levels of osteocalcin, a protein involved in bone hardening. In one study with female athletes, 10 milligrams daily of vitamin K decreased the process of bone breakdown and increased bone formation. These improvements were measured by looking at the amount of osteocalcin (an indicator of bone formation), as well as by-products of bone breakdown, in the bloodstream and urine.

A vitamin K deficiency is extremely rare, and there's usually no need for supplementation unless recommended by your physician. The best food sources are dairy products, meats, eggs, cereals, fruits, and vegetables. The functions of vitamins A, D, and K and their possible roles in exercise performance are summarized in table 7.3.

Table 7.3   Vitamins A, D, and K

Vitamin A

Exercise-related function	Growth and repair; building of body structures.
Best food sources	Liver, egg yolks, whole milk, and orange and yellow vegetables.
Side effects and toxicity	Digestive system upset, damage to bones and certain organs.
DRIs for adults	Women, 700 mcg; pregnant women, 770 mcg; lactating women, 1,300 mcg; men, 900 mcg.

Vitamin D

Exercise-related function	Normal bone growth and development.
Best food sources	Sunlight, fortified dairy products, and fish oils.
Side effects and toxicity	Nausea, vomiting, hardening of soft tissues, kidney damage.
DRIs for adults	Women aged 19-50, 5 mcg; women aged 51-70, 10 mcg; women aged 70+, 15 mcg; pregnant women, 5 mcg; lactating women, 5 mcg; men aged 19-50, 5 mcg; men aged 51-70, 10 mcg; men aged 70+, 15 mcg.
UL for adults	50 mcg.

Vitamin K

Exercise-related function	Involved in glycogen formation, blood clotting, and bone formation.
Best food sources	Vegetables, milk, and yogurt.
Side effects and toxicity	Allergic reactions, breakdown of red blood cells.
DRIs for adults	Women, 90 mcg; men, 120 mcg.

Minerals and Performance

Minerals found naturally in food are particularly important to exercisers and athletes because of their involvement in muscle contraction, normal heart rhythm, oxygen transport, transmission of nerve impulses, immune function, and bone health. If you are not adequately nourished with minerals, a deficiency could harm your health, and this in turn could adversely affect your performance. What follows is a look at various minerals that can have a bearing on your performance. The functions of these vital minerals and others are summarized in table 7.4.

Electrolytes

The tissues in your body contain fluids both inside cells (intracellular fluid) and in the spaces between cells (extracellular fluid). Dissolved in both fluids are electrolytes, which are electrically charged minerals or ions. The electrolytes work in concert, regulating water balance on either side of the cell membranes. Electrolytes also help make muscles contract by promoting the transmission of messages across nerve cell membranes. Electrolyte balance is critical to optimal performance and overall health. The two chief electrolytes are sodium and potassium. Sodium regulates fluid balance outside cells, whereas potassium regulates fluids inside cells.

Sodium is obtained mostly from salt and processed foods. On average, Americans eat 2 to 3 teaspoons (12 to 18 grams) of salt every day—far too much for good health. A healthier sodium target is 500 milligrams (the minimum requirement) to 2,400 milligrams per day, or no more than 1 1/4 teaspoons (1.6 grams) of table salt each day.

Although some sodium can be lost from sweat during exercise, you don't have to worry about replacing it with supplements. Your usual diet contains enough sodium to replace what was lost. What's more, the body does a good job of conserving sodium on its own.

Severe sodium depletion, however, can occur during ultraendurance events such as triathlons that last more than four hours. Consuming 1/2 to 3/4 of a cup (119-178 milliliters) of sport drink every 10 to 20 minutes, along with adding salty foods to the diet, is enough to replenish an endurance athlete's need for sodium. Thus, during an endurance event lasting longer than three hours, you want to have a sport drink containing 200 to 300 milligrams of sodium per 8 ounces (237 milliliters). To restore fluid balance during recovery after endurance exercise, you need sodium in your beverage since it lets water enter your cells.

Drinking too much plain water (overhydration), however, can cause sodium and other electrolytes to become overly diluted. This imbalance can negatively affect performance.

Potassium works inside cells to regulate fluid balance. Potassium is also involved in maintaining a regular heartbeat, helping muscles contract, regulating blood pressure, and transferring nutrients to cells.

In contrast to sodium, potassium is not as well conserved by the body, so you should be sure to eat plenty of potassium-rich foods such as bananas, oranges, and potatoes. You need between 1,600 and 2,000 milligrams of potassium a day, which can be easily obtained from a diet plentiful in fruits and vegetables.

To get cut, some competitive bodybuilders use diuretics, drugs that increase the formation and excretion of urine in the body. This is a dangerous practice because diuretics can flush potassium and other electrolytes from the body. Life-threatening mineral imbalances can occur, and some professional bodybuilders have died during competition as a result of diuretic abuse. I can see no rational reason for taking diuretics for competitive purposes. The potential damage just isn't worth it.

Table 7.4   Major Minerals and Trace Minerals

Major

Calcium

Exercise-related function	A constituent of body structures; plays a part in muscle growth, muscle contraction, and nerve transmission.
Best food sources	Dairy products and green leafy vegetables.
Side effects and toxicity	Excessive calcification of some tissues, constipation, mineral absorption problems.
DRIs for adults	Women aged 19-50, 1,000 mg; women aged 51-70+, 1,200 mg; pregnant women, 1,000 mg; lactating women, 1,000 mg; men aged 19-50, 1,000 mg; men aged 51-70+, 1,200 mg.
UL for adults	2,500 mg.

Phosphorus

Exercise-related function	Metabolism of carbohydrate, protein, and fat; growth, repair, and maintenance of cells; energy production; stimulation of muscular contractions.
Best food sources	Meats, fish, poultry, eggs, whole grains, seeds, and nuts.
Side effects and toxicity	None known.
DRIs for adults	All women, 700 mg; men, 700 mg.
UL for adults	Women and men aged 19-70, 4,000 mg; aged 70+, 3,000 mg.

Potassium

Exercise-related function	Maintenance of normal fluid balance on either side of cell walls; normal growth; stimulation of nerve impulses for muscular contractions; conversion of glucose to glycogen; synthesis of muscle protein from amino acids.
Best food sources	Potatoes, bananas, fruits, and vegetables.
Side effects and toxicity	Heart disturbances.
DRIs for adults	No DRI, but a minimum requirement of 1,600-2,000 mg for sedentary adults and 3,500 mg for active adults.

Sodium

Exercise-related function	Maintenance of normal fluid balance on either side of cell walls; muscular contraction and nerve transmission; keeps other blood minerals soluble.
Best food sources	Found in virtually all foods.
Side effects and toxicity	Water retention and high blood pressure.
DRIs for adults	No DRI; a recommended safe minimum intake is 2,400 mg daily.

Chloride

Exercise-related function	Helps regulate the pressure that causes fluids to flow in and out of cell membranes.
Best food sources	Table salt (sodium chloride), kelp, and rye flour.
Side effects and toxicity	None known.
DRIs for adults	No DRI; a recommended safe minimum intake is 500 mg daily.

Magnesium

Exercise-related function	Metabolism of carbohydrate and protein; assists in neuromuscular contractions.
Best food sources	Green vegetables, legumes, whole grains, and seafood.
Side effects and toxicity	Large amounts are toxic.
DRIs for adults	Women aged 19-30, 310 mg; women aged 31-70+, 320 mg; pregnant women aged 19-30, 350 mg; pregnant women aged 31+, 360 mg; lactating women aged 19-30, 310 mg; lactating women aged 31+, 320 mg; men aged 19-30, 400 mg; men aged 31+, 420 mg.
UL for adults	350 mg from supplements alone.

Trace

Iron

Exercise-related function	Oxygen transport to cells for energy; formation of oxygen-carrying red blood cells.
Best food sources	Liver, oysters, lean meats, and green leafy vegetables.
Side effects and toxicity	Large amounts are toxic.
DRIs for adults	Women aged 19-50, 18 mg; women aged 51-70+, 8 mg; pregnant women, 27 mg; lactating women, 9 mg; men, 8 mg.
UL for adults	45 mg.

Iodine

Exercise-related function	Energy production; growth and development; metabolism.
Best food sources	Iodized salt, seafood, and mushrooms.
Side effects and toxicity	Thyroid enlargement.
DRIs for adults	150 mcg.
UL for adults	1,000 mcg.

Chromium

Exercise-related function	Normal blood sugar; fat metabolism.
Best food sources	Corn oil, brewer's yeast, whole grains, and meats.
Side effects and toxicity	Liver and kidney damage.
DRIs for adults	Women aged 19-50, 25 mcg; women aged 51+, 20 mcg; pregnant women, 30 mcg; lactating women, 45 mcg; men aged 19-50, 35 mcg; men aged 51+, 30 mcg.

Fluoride

Exercise-related function	None known.
Best food sources	Fluoridated water supplies.
Side effects and toxicity	Large amounts are toxic and can cause mottling of teeth.
DRIs for adults	All women, 3 mg; men, 4 mg.
UL for adults	10 mg.

Molybdenum

Exercise-related function	Involved in the metabolism of fat.
Best food sources	Milk, beans, breads, and cereals.
Side effects and toxicity	Diarrhea, anemia, and depressed growth rate.
DRIs for adults	45 mcg.
UL for adults	2,000 mcg.

(continued)

Table 7.4   Major Minerals and Trace Minerals, *continued*

Boron	
Exercise-related function	No clear biological function in humans has been identified.
Food sources	Fruit-based beverages and products, potatoes, legumes, milk, avocado, peanut butter, and peanuts.
DRIs for adults	None established.
Vanadium	
Exercise-related function	No clear biological function in humans has been identified.
Food sources	Mushrooms, shellfish, black pepper, parsley, and dill seed.
Side effects and toxicity	Large doses are extremely toxic and may cause excessive fatigue.
DRIs for adults	None established.

Other important minerals that can affect your performance include zinc and selenium, which are included in table 7.1 on page 120.

Soda and Phosphate Loading

Sodium bicarbonate, better known as baking soda, is a type of sodium used by athletes to delay muscular fatigue. The practice is called *soda loading,* and it neutralizes levels of lactic acid in the blood. Lactic acid accumulation makes muscles burn and eventually brings them to a point of fatigue. The ability of soda loading to neutralize lactic acid reduces muscle pain and can potentially prolong your workouts. The recommended dose is 300 milligrams per kilogram of body weight, taken with several glasses of water, about one to two hours before exercise. Generally, soda loading is safe but may cause nausea, bloating, and stomach cramps.

For a long time, athletes have experimented with phosphate loading as a way to extend performance. Phosphate is a type of salt made from phosphorus, the second most abundant mineral in the body. The supplement is usually taken in large doses several times daily a few days before competition. By some indications, phosphate loading increases oxygen availability from the blood and makes more glucose available to the working muscles—two advantages if you're a competitive athlete. One study found that phosphate supplementation improved oxygen uptake and improved performance on a bicycle ergometer. In addition, phosphate loading improves certain respiratory and circulatory factors, making phosphate useful for endurance athletes. The recommended dosage is generally 4 grams a day. But be forewarned: Phosphate loading can cause vomiting, upset the body's electrolyte balance, and lead to other untoward reactions.

Phosphates are constituents of some natural weight-loss supplements, too, since they may prevent a drop in metabolism by preserving thyroid hormone levels during severe dieting. A Polish study found that phosphate supplementation may even increase RMR in women on a diet of 1,000 calories a day, suggesting a fat-burning effect. More research is needed in this area, however.

Other Vital Minerals

Several other minerals could be low in your diet, particularly if you're a competitor and you frequently follow restrictive cutting diets.

Calcium

Ninety-nine percent of the calcium in the body is stored in the skeleton and teeth. The other 1 percent is found in blood and soft tissues. Calcium is responsible for building healthy bones, conducting nerve impulses, helping muscles contract, and moving nutrients in and out of cells. Exercise helps your body better absorb calcium. At the same time, high-intensity endurance exercise may cause your body to excrete calcium.

The chief sources of calcium in the diet are milk and other dairy products. However, almost every strength trainer and bodybuilder I have ever counseled has avoided dairy products like the plague during precompetition dieting. They believe that these foods are high in sodium, but I say that's nonsense. One cup (237 milliliters) of nonfat milk contains 126 milligrams of sodium and 302 milligrams of calcium. Two egg whites, a popular food in the diet of strength trainers and bodybuilders, contain 212 milligrams of sodium and only 12 milligrams of calcium. Sodium hardly seems to be a problem here, and there is no better low-fat source of calcium than nonfat milk.

So are milk and dairy products really your enemy? Absolutely not. As I pointed out earlier, milk in particular contains two proteins (whey and casein) that are involved in muscle building, fat burning, and recovery. (See chapter 2 for more information on these important milk proteins and how to use them.)

There's more to this story, however, and it has to do with the calcium in milk and dairy products. A number of studies show that this mineral may help you manage your weight. How? Calcium may assist the body in the breakdown of body fat. It appears that the more calcium a fat cell contains, the more fat the cell will burn.

In one widely publicized study, 32 obese adults were randomly assigned to one of the following diets for 24 weeks: (1) a standard diet containing 400 to 500 milligrams per day of calcium plus a placebo supplement; (2) a standard diet supplemented with 800 milligrams per day of calcium; or (3) a diet containing three servings per day of dairy products, providing 1,200 to 1,300 milligrams per day of calcium, plus a placebo supplement. Each diet cut calories by 500 calories a day. By the end of the experimental period, the average weight loss was 14.5 pounds (6.5 kilograms) with the standard diet, 19 pounds (8.5 kilograms) with the calcium-supplemented diet, and about 24.5 pounds (11 kilograms) with the high-dairy diet. Fat loss from the trunk region represented 19 percent of the total fat loss on the standard diet, 50 percent of total fat loss on the calcium-supplemented diet, and 66.2 percent of total fat loss on the high-dairy diet.

In sum, dietary calcium intake clearly enhanced weight loss and fat loss in obese subjects who followed a reduced-calorie diet. Interestingly, higher calcium intake increased the percentage of fat lost from the trunk region. Finally, consuming calcium in the form of dairy products was significantly more effective than taking calcium supplements. I have to add here, however, that the last finding, though significant, should be interpreted cautiously, since the study was funded by the National Dairy Council.

No one knows yet whether calcium from other foods such as leafy greens has the same effect. Additional research needs to be conducted to ascertain similar benefits. The take-home message is that if you're trying to drop weight, don't drop dairy products, and be sure to select low-fat products.

Overall, the calcium in dairy foods is essential to maintaining good health. With plenty of high-calcium foods, your diet provides the calcium needed to maintain healthy blood calcium levels. If you don't have enough in your diet, your body will draw calcium from bones to maintain blood calcium levels. As more and more calcium is removed from bones, they become brittle and break. The most susceptible areas are the spine, hips, and wrists. An exit of calcium from the bones can lead to the bone-weakening disease of osteoporosis. In women who develop the female athlete triad (disordered eating, menstrual irregularities, and weakened bones), low calcium intakes are common.

Female athletes, particularly those in weight-control sports, are often at risk of losing bone calcium. In a study I conducted at the 1990 National Physique Committee (NPC) USA Championships in Raleigh, North Carolina, female bodybuilders recorded their diets; were weighed and had their fat measured; and answered questions about their training, nutrition, and health.

None of the women ate or drank any dairy products for at least three months before competition, and most of them never used dairy products at all. None of them took calcium supplements, either.

Of these women, 81 percent reported that they did not menstruate for at least two months before a contest. The physical stress of training, the psychological stress of competition, the low-calorie diet, and the loss of body fat can all lead to a decrease in the body's production of estrogen. As in menopause, without enough estrogen, a woman stops menstruating. What's worse, no calcium can be stored in the bone when estrogen levels are low. Of course, these women were very lean, too. On average, they had 9 percent body fat. Extremely low body fat is another risk factor for loss of calcium from bones.

If your dietary practices regarding calcium mirror any of these, you must get calcium back into your diet by eating calcium-rich foods, namely, nonfat milk and dairy products. If for some reason you cannot or will not drink milk, try nonfat yogurts. They are equally high in calcium, and they often do not cause the intestinal problems that some people experience from milk. You can also obtain calcium from alternative sources if you are on a milk-free diet. Table 7.5 lists those sources.

Some people are lactose intolerant and can't digest milk. They lack sufficient lactase, the enzyme required to digest lactose, a sugar in milk that helps you absorb calcium from the intestine. If you are lactose intolerant, try taking an enzyme-replacement product such as Lactaid. These products replace the lactase you are missing and will digest the lactose for you. Another option is Lactaid milk. Available at most supermarkets, Lactaid milk is pretreated with the lactase enzyme.

Table 7.5 Alternative Sources of Calcium for Milk-Free Diets

Food	Amount	Calcium (mg)	Calories
Collards, frozen, cooked*	1/2 c (95 g)	179	31
Soy milk (fortified)	1 c (237 ml)	150	79
Mackerel, canned	2 oz. (56 g)	137	88
Dandelion greens, raw, cooked*	1/2 c (53 g)	74	17
Turnip greens, frozen, cooked*	1/2 c (72 g)	125	25
Mustard greens, frozen, cooked*	1/2 c (75 g)	76	14
Kale, frozen, cooked*	1/2 c (65 g)	90	20
Tortillas, corn	2	80	95
Molasses, blackstrap	1 tbsp (21 g)	176	48
Orange	1 large	74	87
Sockeye salmon, canned, with bone, drained	2 oz (56 g)	136	87
Sardines, canned, with bone, drained	2 medium	92	50
Boston baked beans (navy or pea bean), vegetarian, canned	1/2 c (127 g)	64	118
Pickled herring	2 oz (56 g)	44	149
Soybeans, cooked	1/2 c (90 g)	88	149
Broccoli, cooked	1/2 c (78 g)	36	22
Rutabaga (Swedish or yellow turnip), cooked, mashed	1/2 c (120 g)	58	47
Artichoke, cooked	1 medium	54	60
White beans, cooked	1/2 c (90 g)	81	124
Almonds, blanched, whole	1/4 c (36 g)	94	222
Tofu	2 oz (56 g)	60	44

*Frozen, cooked vegetable greens are higher in calcium than fresh, cooked greens. If you eat the fresh variety, you need to double your portion to get the same amount of calcium.

Table 7.6   A Day's Worth of Calcium

Food	Amount	Calcium (mg)	Calories
Orange juice, calcium fortified	1 c (237 ml)	300	112
Nonfat milk	1 c (237 ml)	301	86
Tofu	4 oz (113 g)	120	88
Low-fat yogurt, fruit	8 oz (226 g)	372	250
Mozzarella cheese, part-skim	1 oz (28 g)	229	73
Turnip greens cooked, chopped	1 c (72 g)	250	60
Total		**1,572**	**669**

Calcium supplements may be in order, too, particularly because three of every four Americans are believed to be deficient in calcium. The most bioavailable source of calcium as a supplement is calcium citrate. Calcium supplements are best taken with all of the other bone-building minerals such as magnesium, boron, and vitamin D.

The DRIs for calcium from food and supplements are as follows: women aged 19 to 50, 1,000 milligrams; women aged 51 to 70+, 1,200 milligrams; pregnant women, 1,000 milligrams; lactating women, 1,000 milligrams; men aged 19 to 50, 1,000 milligrams; and men aged 51 to 70+, 1,200 milligrams. The National Institutes of Health (NIH) recommends supplementation with calcium and vitamin D (which helps the body absorb calcium) by people not getting the DRIs, including women who develop the female athlete triad. If you have some calcium in your diet, don't take all 1,200 or 1,000 milligrams of calcium in a supplement. Too much calcium in the diet can cause kidney stones in some people.

For the prevention and treatment of osteoporosis in postmenopausal women, many physicians recommend 1,500 milligrams daily. Table 7.6 illustrates how to get a day's worth of calcium from food.

A word to women: If you have irregular menstruation, no menstrual cycle, or stop menstruating before a contest, you should see a good sports medicine physician or a gynecologist who is familiar with your sport. Loss of estrogen production at an early age can have a critical impact on your bone health. It's possible for osteoporosis to develop at a very early age.

Take care of your inside while you are taking care of your outside. Add some dairy to your diet, and you'll be standing straight and tall for many years to come.

Iron

The major role of iron is to combine with protein to make hemoglobin, a special protein that gives red blood cells their color. Hemoglobin carries oxygen in the blood from the lungs to the tissues. Iron is also necessary for the formation of myoglobin, found only in muscle tissue. Myoglobin transports oxygen to muscle cells to be used in the chemical reaction that makes muscles contract.

As a strength trainer or bodybuilder, you are constantly tearing down and rebuilding muscle tissue. This process can create an additional need for iron, a mineral that is enormously essential to human health. What's more, there seems to be a common increase in iron losses from aerobic exercises or sports that involve pounding of the feet, such as jogging, aerobic dancing, and step aerobics. Also at risk for low iron are women who exercise more than three hours a week, have been pregnant within the past two years, or eat fewer than 2,200 calories a day.

Low iron can impair muscular performance. A shortfall of iron can lead to iron-deficiency anemia, the final stage of iron loss, characterized by a hemoglobin concentration below the normal level. Athletic training does tend to deplete iron stores for a number of reasons, including physical stress and muscle damage. Another reason for low iron and iron-deficiency anemia is inadequate intake of iron. Studies on the diets of female athletes, who likely need to take in even more than the daily requirement (18 milligrams) to compensate for training-induced losses, indicate daily intakes of roughly 12 milligrams. Other possible reasons for low iron are losses that occur in the gastrointestinal tract, in sweat, and through menstruation.

Some people can have iron deficiency without anemia. This is characterized by normal hemoglobin but reduced levels of ferritin, a storage form of iron in the body. When iron is in short supply, your tissues become starved for oxygen. This can make you tire easily and recover more slowly. Several studies from Cornell University indicate that when untrained, iron-depleted women received an iron supplement during exercise training, they experienced greater increases in oxygen use and endurance performance. This goes to show how important iron is to performance. Taking iron supplements, however, will not enhance your performance if you have normal hemoglobin and iron status.

The best sources of dietary iron are liver and other organ meats, lean meat, and oysters. Iron is found in green leafy vegetables, too, although iron from plant sources is not as well absorbed as iron from animal protein.

Strength trainers and other active people tend to shy away from iron-rich meats because of their high fat content. But you can increase the iron in your diet without adding a lot of beef or animal fat. If you don't eat any meat at all, you must pay careful attention to make sure that you get the iron you need. Here are some suggestions:

• **Eat fruits, vegetables, and grains that are high in iron.** You won't get as much iron as from animal foods, but the plant foods are the lowest in fat. Green leafy vegetables such as kale and collards, dried fruits like raisins and apricots, and iron-enriched and fortified breads and cereals are all good plant sources of iron.

• **Enhance your body's absorption of iron** by combining high iron-containing foods with a rich source of vitamin C, which improves iron absorption. For example, drink some orange juice with your iron-fortified cereal with raisins for breakfast. Or sprinkle some lemon juice on your kale or collards.

- **Avoid eating very high-fiber foods at the same meal with foods high in iron.** The fiber inhibits the absorption of iron and many other minerals. Avoid drinking tea and taking antacids with high-iron foods; they also inhibit absorption of iron.

- **Try to keep or add some meat to your diet.** Lean red meat and the dark meat of chicken and turkey are highest in iron. Eating 3 to 4 ounces (85-113 grams) of meat three times a week will give your iron levels a real boost. And if you combine your meat with a vegetable source of iron, you will absorb more of the iron from the vegetables.

- **You might need an iron supplement.** Eight milligrams for men and 18 milligrams for women 19 to 50 years old, or 100 percent of the DRI for iron, may be a big help. Don't pop huge doses of iron, though. The more iron you take at one time, the less your body will absorb. Also, excess iron can lead to hemochromatosis, a disorder that causes iron buildup in major organs and eventual deterioration of liver function.

Because women are more prone to low iron, the United States Olympic Committee (USOC) recommends that female athletes undergo blood testing periodically to check hemoglobin status. If you think you might be deficient in iron, talk to your physician or a registered dietitian who specializes in sport nutrition. Self-medicating with large doses of iron can cause big trouble and is potentially dangerous.

Zinc

Zinc, one of the antioxidant minerals, is important for hundreds of body processes, including maintaining normal taste and smell, regulating growth, and promoting wound healing.

My research has found that female bodybuilders, in particular, don't get enough zinc in their diets. Zinc is an important mineral for people who work out. As you exercise, zinc helps clear lactic acid buildup in the blood. In addition, zinc supplementation (25 milligrams a day) has been shown to protect immunity during periods of intense training.

There is not much research on zinc supplementation and exercise performance. Interestingly, though, one study shows that if you're an endurance athlete who eats a diet that is rich in carbohydrate but low in protein and fat, you could be setting yourself up for a zinc deficiency, resulting in a loss of too much body weight, greater fatigue, and poor endurance.

Too much zinc might be a bad thing, however. It has been associated with lower levels of good cholesterol (HDL) and thus may increase your risk of cardiovascular disease. What's more, excess zinc over time may create mineral imbalances and produce undesirable changes in two substances involved in calcium metabolism: calcitonin, a hormone that boosts calcium in bones by drawing it from soft tissue, and osteocalcin, the key noncollagen protein needed to help harden bone.

By eating zinc-rich foods, you can get just the right amount, which is 8 milligrams a day for women and 11 milligrams a day for men. The best sources of zinc are meat, eggs, seafood (especially oysters), and whole grains. If you restrict your intake of meat, taking a multivitamin each day will help fill in the nutritional blanks.

Magnesium

Magnesium, a mineral that is in charge of more than 400 metabolic reactions in the body, has been touted as an exercise aid. One study hints at a link between magnesium and muscle strength. A test group of men were given 500 milligrams of magnesium a day, an increase over the DRI of 400 milligrams. A control group took 250 milligrams a day, significantly less than the DRI. After both groups weight trained for eight weeks, their leg strength was measured. The supplemented men got stronger, whereas the control group stayed the same. But many researchers are not yet convinced that magnesium is a strength builder. They caution that the magnesium status of the subjects before the study was unknown. That's an important point, because supplementing with any nutrient in which you are deficient is likely to produce some positive changes in performance and health. Basically, the current train of scientific thought on magnesium supplementation is that it does not affect aerobic power or muscle strength.

Magnesium promotes calcium absorption and helps in the function of nerves and muscles, including regulation of the heartbeat. The DRI for magnesium for men aged 19 to 30 is 400 milligrams, and for men 31 and older it is 420 milligrams per day. The DRI for women aged 19 to 30 is 310 milligrams, and for women 31 and older it is 320 milligrams.

Zinc–Magnesium Supplementation

Zinc–magnesium supplementation (ZMA) is widely marketed to strength athletes and bodybuilders as a muscle-building aid. While one small study investigated the effects of a supplement containing zinc, magnesium, and vitamin B_6 on the muscle strength and functional power of college football players and suggested positive results, more current research proves otherwise.

In a study conducted at Baylor University, 42 strength-training men supplemented with ZMA or a placebo before going to sleep at night over an eight-week period. Researchers tested the subjects' muscular endurance, strength, anabolic and catabolic hormone status, and body composition at intervals. The results indicated that the supplementation during training did not enhance any of these variables. It appears that ZMA is not an effective muscle-building product. For more on zinc and magnesium, see page 144.

The use of laxatives and diuretics can impair magnesium balance. If you use these products to make weight, beware that you can compromise your health and that you risk nervous system complications from fluid and electrolyte imbalances.

The best dietary sources of magnesium are nuts, legumes, whole grains, dark green vegetables, and seafood. These foods should be plentiful in your diet. You can also supplement these foods with a daily multivitamin formulated with 100 percent of the DRI for magnesium.

Boron

Boron is a trace mineral that has gained notoriety in recent years due to claims that it can build muscle mass by increasing testosterone in the body. The problem is that this theory is based on research with elderly women, not with athletes. I see no real point in supplementing with boron. You can get sufficient boron from fruits and vegetables.

Vanadium

Vanadyl sulfate is a commercial derivative of vanadium, a trace mineral found in vegetables and fish. The body needs very little vanadium, and more than 90 percent of it is excreted in the urine. At high doses, vanadium is extremely toxic and may cause excessive fatigue. To the knowledge of the medical community, no one has ever been diagnosed with a vanadium deficiency.

As a supplement, vanadyl sulfate is supposed to have a tissue-building effect by moving glucose and amino acids into the muscles faster and elevating insulin to promote growth, though the evidence for this has been found only in rats. Still, vanadyl sulfate is being aggressively marketed as a tissue-building supplement for strength trainers and athletes.

But does it work the magic it promotes? A group of researchers in New Zealand asked the same question. In a 12-week study, 40 strength trainers (30 men and 10 women) took either a placebo or a daily dose of vanadyl sulfate in amounts matched to their weight (.5 milligram per kilogram of body weight). So that strength could be assessed, the strength trainers performed bench presses and leg extensions in 1- and 10-repetition maximum bouts during the course of the experiment.

The findings of the study were that vanadyl sulfate did not increase lean body mass. There were some modest improvements in strength-training performance, but these improvements were short-lived, tapering off after the first month of the study. About 20 percent of the strength trainers experienced extreme fatigue during and after training.

Some research hints that vanadyl sulfate supplementation might help treat type 2 diabetes, but the results are conflicting. In my opinion, there's no reason to supplement with vanadyl sulfate. You can get the benefits it promises with the nutritional methods discussed elsewhere in this book.

Selenium

An antioxidant mineral, selenium works in partnership with vitamin E to fight damaging free radicals. Selenium is vital for a healthy immune system, boosting your defenses against bacteria and viruses, and it may reduce the risk of certain cancers, particularly in the prostate, colon, and lungs. As for performance, some studies have shown that selenium reduces lipid peroxidation after prolonged aerobic exercise, but this effect did not enhance athletic endurance in people who supplemented with selenium.

Selenium is found naturally in fish, meat, wheat germ, nuts (particularly Brazil nuts), eggs, oatmeal, whole-wheat bread, and brown rice. Most people have to make sure that they eat foods rich in selenium to get in enough. You can supplement, but carefully. There is a narrow margin between the DRI of 55 micrograms and the UL of 400 micrograms.

Quality Control

When you decide which vitamin and mineral supplements you need, stick to brands from well-known manufacturers. Avoid products from obscure, off-brand, or unknown international sources. There's so little regulation of the supplement industry that anything can be, or not be, in the products.

Products from unknown or nonestablished companies may have poor quality control and may not contain what is stated on the label. Lack of regulatory inspection can also lead to product contamination. These problems are less likely in products manufactured by recognized and well-established food supplement and pharmaceutical companies. Other important tips are to identify companies that do research on their own products and to ask your pharmacist for recommendations on quality supplements.

Food First

Always count on food first. Food is your body's best source of vitamins and minerals. Take the time to plan a healthy, well-balanced diet full of fruits, vegetables, grains, beans, lean meats, and nonfat dairy foods, and use the diet-planning guidelines in chapter 10. Along with dedicated training, a good diet with the correct balance of protein, the right kinds of carbohydrate, and the right kinds of fat is your best ticket to building a better body.

Aspartates: A Special Type of Mineral Supplement

If you perform a lot of aerobic exercise in addition to strength training, you may be interested in the use of aspartic acid salts for increasing endurance. The potassium and magnesium salts of aspartic acid, an amino acid composed of various substances, are called *aspartates*. Aspartate supplements are usually available in health food stores and fitness centers.

The feeling of fatigue you get during intense exercise is caused by a combination of factors, one of which may be the increased rate of ammonia production by the body. Aspartates turn excess ammonia, a by-product of exercise, into urea, which is consequently eliminated from the body.

Studies have shown that potassium and magnesium aspartates increase the endurance of swimming rats. Scientists speculate that the aspartates counteract energy-sapping increases in ammonia concentration.

But what about human exercisers? One study tested seven healthy men, all competitors in various sports, on a bicycle ergometer. At intervals during a 24-hour period before the test, four of the men took 5 grams of potassium aspartate and 5 grams of magnesium aspartate. The others took a placebo. During the test, the men pedaled at a moderately high intensity. The researchers took blood samples before, during, and after the test. A week later, the men participated in the same experiment but the conditions were reversed.

In the aspartate-supplemented group, blood ammonia concentrations were significantly lower than in the placebo group. Plus, endurance was boosted by about 14 percent in the aspartate group. On average, the aspartate group cycled a total of 88 minutes before reaching exhaustion, whereas the other group cycled about 75 minutes until exhaustion. The researchers noted, "The results of this study would suggest that potassium and magnesium aspartate are useful in increasing endurance performance."

Of course, this is only one study, and aspartates have not been widely researched in exercise science. Supplementing may or may not be useful. If you want to try supplementation, proceed with caution. Excess potassium or magnesium in the system may lead to water retention and mineral imbalances.

Sport Nutrition Fact Versus Fiction:
Chromium and Muscle Building

Chromium is a mineral that has been hyped as a safe alternative to anabolic steroids and as a muscle-building agent. Is there some hard fact behind the hype? Let's take a look.

Chromium is an essential trace mineral that helps insulin do one of its main jobs—transport glucose into cells. Chromium is also involved in the cellular uptake of amino acids. Its advocates say that increased doses of chromium can thus stimulate a higher uptake of amino acids, increasing the synthesis of more muscle mass. But that's quite a leap of faith. The exact way chromium works in the body is not entirely known.

What we do know about chromium is that you can lose it in urine as a result of exercise. A diet overloaded with simple sugars can force chromium from the body, too. However, the very small quantities of chromium we need for good health can be easily obtained from a good diet. Dietary sources include brewer's yeast, whole-grain cereals, meats, raw oysters, mushrooms, apples with skins, wine, and beer.

As for whether chromium supplementation (namely chromium picolinate) builds muscle mass, the evidence is conflicting. Some studies suggest that it increases lean body mass and even decreases body fat, others show it doesn't, and still others show no change. Most of the studies to date have been very poorly designed and flawed. They used inaccurate methods of measuring body composition, and they failed to assess chromium status before the research.

More recent research has not shown any benefits to taking chromium picolinate. One of the best and most well-controlled studies was conducted at the University of Massachusetts. Thirty-six football players were given either a placebo or 200 micrograms of chromium picolinate daily for nine weeks during spring training. During that period, they worked out with weights and ran for aerobic conditioning. Before, during, and after supplementation, the researchers assessed the players' diet, urinary chromium losses, girths of various body parts, percentages of body fat and muscle, and strength. Percentages of body fat and muscle were measured by underwater weighing, one of the most precise ways to measure body composition. The results? Chromium picolinate supplementation did not help build muscle, enhance strength, or burn fat. Incidentally, other forms of supplemental chromium, such as chromium chloride, have no effect on body composition or performance, either, according to the latest research.

A word of warning about chromium picolinate: A study released in 1995 suggested that supplementation with chromium picolinate may damage chromosomes, the bodies inside the cell nucleus that carry our genes. In the laboratory, researchers injected hefty amounts of chromium picolinate into hamster cells in dishes—about 3,000 times the normal safe amount you'd see in people supplementing with 200 micrograms a day. The chromosomes broke, and such breakage can lead to cancer. Other forms of chromium, namely chromium nicotinate and chromium chloride, did not cause this damage. Defenders of chromium picolinate responded by pointing out that the study was meaningless because such huge doses of chromium were used.

Chromium also causes the body to excrete other trace minerals and interferes with the metabolism of iron. Given these drawbacks and the fact that chromium picolinate doesn't live up to its claims, supplementation is walking a nutritional tightrope at best.

8

Muscle-Building Products

You train hard. You're building body-hard muscle. Still, you want to know: Isn't there something else—besides intense workouts and healthy food—that can help you gain a little faster, something that will give you a muscle-building edge with less effort?

Definitely. You can do several things to pack on lean muscle. Unfortunately, not all of them are safe—or legal. Anabolic steroids, though approved for medical use and available by prescription only, are among the most abused drugs among athletes. *Anabolic* means "to build," and anabolic steroids tend to make the body grow in certain ways. They do have muscle-building effects, but they're also dangerous. Once practiced mainly by elite athletes, abuse of anabolic steroids has spread to recreational and teen athletes and is now a national health concern. Research from the National Institute on Drug Abuse shows that in 2005, 1.2 percent of all eighth grade boys, 1.8 percent of all tenth grade boys, and 2.6 percent of all twelfth grade boys have used anabolic steroids in the past year. Table 8.1 lists some of the dangers associated with these drugs.

A trend related to anabolic steroid abuse is the use of androstenedione, a precursor or building block to testosterone, and others of its kind. Testosterone is the male hormone responsible for building muscle and revving up the sex drive. Although legal, androstenedione is not without side effects, including acne, hair loss in genetically susceptible people, abnormal growth of breast tissue (gynecomastia), negative blood cholesterol profiles that can lead to the increased risk of heart disease, and potentially reduced testosterone output. Use of this family of compounds may also result in a positive drug test.

Table 8.1 Health Dangers of Anabolic Steroids	
Liver disease	Masculinization in women
High blood pressure	Muscle spasms
Increased LDL cholesterol	Headache
Decreased HDL cholesterol	Nervous tension
Fluid and water retention	Nausea
Suppressed immunity	Rash
Decreased testosterone	Irritability
Testicular atrophy	Mood swings
Acne	Heightened or suppressed sex drive
Gynecomastia	Aggressiveness
Lowered sperm count	Drug dependence

In addition to using steroids and androstenedione, athletes use other types of drugs, including stimulants, pain killers, diuretics, and drugs that mask the presence of certain drugs in the urine. Some athletes also use synthetic growth hormone (GH) because they believe it will increase strength and muscle mass. However, GH has many horrific side effects, including progressive overgrowth of body tissues, coronary heart disease, diabetes, and arthritis. GH is one of more than 100 drugs that have been banned by the International Olympic Committee (IOC). The full list of banned substances appears in table 8.2. Notice that not one of these substances is nutritional; they are drugs, not foods.

My advice is to forget health-destroying drugs. There are some natural aids you can use to enhance muscle building, give you an extra edge in training, and keep your body in healthy balance.

Sport Supplements: Sorting Through the Confusion

On average, exercisers and athletes spend $45 million on sport supplements—a sum that's growing every year. With so many supplements on the market, how do you know which ones will help you, hurt you, or just waste your money?

With many products, the real hazards and nutritional implications are not based on what the supplement does, but what it doesn't do, and what other avenues of support it may impede. I call this the *laetrile effect.*

Laetrile, or amygdalin, is derived primarily from apricot pits and almonds. In the 1920s, a theory was formulated that laetrile could kill cancer cells. In the 1960s and 1970s, it became a popular cancer treatment promoted by nonmedical practitioners. Because it was not an approved medical treatment, patients seeking the cure had to travel to Mexico to acquire treatment. By 1982, medical science proved that laetrile was not effective against cancer.

Table 8.2 Drugs Banned by the IOC

Stimulants

Ameneptine, amfepramone, amiphenazole, amphetamine, bambuterol, bromontan, carphedon, cathine, cocaine, cropropamide, crotethamide, ephedrine, ethamivan, etilamphetamine, etilefrine, fencamfamin, fenethylline, fenfluramine, formoterol, heptaminol, mefenorex, mephentermine, mesocarb, methamphetamine, methoxyphenamine, methylenedioxyamphetamine, methylephedrine, methylphenidate, nikethamide, norfenfluramine, parahydroxyamphetamine, pemoline, pentetrazol, phendimetrazine, phentermine, phenylephrine, phenylpropanolamine, pholedrine, pipradrol, prolintane, propylhexedrine, pseudoephedrine, reproterol, salbutamol, salmeterol, selegiline, strychnine, terbutaline

Narcotics

Buprenorphine, dextromoramide, diamorphine (heroin), hydrocodone, methadone, morphine, pentazocine, pethidine

Anabolic agents

Androstenediol, androstenedione, bambuterol, boldenone, clenbuterol, clostebol, danazol, dehydrochlormethyltestosterone, dehydroepiandrosterone (DHEA), dihydrotestosterone, drostanolone, fenoterol, fluoxymesterone, formebolone, formoterol, gestrinone, mesterolone, methandienone, methenolone, methandriol, methyltestosterone, mibolerone, nandrolone, 19-norandrostenediol, 19-norandrostenedione, norethandrolone, oxandrolone, oxymesterone, oxymetholone, reproterol, salbutamol, salmeterol, stanozolol, terbutaline, testosterone, trenbolone

Diuretics

Acetazolamide, bendroflumethiazide, bumetanide, canrenone, chlorthalidone, ethacrynic acid, furosemide, hydrochlorothiazide, indapamide, mannitol (by intravenous injection), mersalyl, spironolactone, triamterene

Masking agents

Bromontan, diuretics (see previous group), epitestosterone, probenecid

Peptide hormones, mimetics, and analogues

ACTH, erythropoietin (EPO), hCG,* nGH, insulin, IGF-1, LH,* clomiphene,* cyclofenil,* tamoxifen*

Beta-blockers

Acebutolol, alprenolol, atenolol, betaxolol, bisoprolol, bunolol, carteolol, celiprolol, esmolol, labetalol, levobunolol, metipranolol, metoprolol, nadolol, oxprenolol, pindolol, propranolol, sotalol, timolol

*Prohibited in males only.

But in most cases, people who sought (and still seek) laetrile treatment did so by delaying standard medical treatment and at large financial expense, with no beneficial results but usually without harm from the treatment. However, by delaying or forgoing more proven treatment, these patients lost time, and their disease advanced. In some cases, the laetrile treatment was harmful and even deadly.

And so it is with many sport supplements. Looking for a shortcut, athletes and exercisers spend time and money on supplements that don't work while delaying the use of proven methods—good nutrition and intense training—to support their goals. Even worse, some supplements can be harmful and even deadly.

To help you sort through the confusion regarding sport supplements, I have developed a rating system for strength-training supplements and herbal supplements based on the concept of the laetrile effect:

Meets marketing claims. This supplement lives up to its marketing claims.

Possibly meets marketing claims. There is not yet enough research backing this supplement, although available data look promising.

Does not meet marketing claims. An abundance of negative data exists on this supplement.

Potentially harmful. This supplement does not meet marketing claims and is potentially harmful.

Now, here's a roundup of various sport supplements on the market, categorized according to this rating system. You can use table 8.3 at the end of the chapter to quickly refer to the ratings for all the supplements discussed in this chapter.

Meets Marketing Claims

The products in this category have numerous research studies that back up the marketing claims. In the right setting, these products work. When I say that the supplements meet their marketing claims, it doesn't mean that I recommend that you use them. It just tells you that what is claimed on the label is substantiated by research. You should choose to use or not use supplements based on your exercise goals, lifestyle, and attention to all the factors that support the enhancement of strength and power. Supplements will not help you if you don't have your diet, training, and rest dialed in.

Caffeine

Caffeine, a drug found in coffee, tea, soda, or over-the-counter pharmaceutical preparations, can have a wide range of effects depending on your sensitivity to it. You might feel alert and wide awake, or you might get the jitters. Your heart might race, or you might race to the bathroom (caffeine is a diuretic).

Caffeine lingers in the body, so even small amounts can accumulate over time. It has a half-life of four to six hours, meaning that it takes that long for the body to metabolize half the amount consumed. Because of its half-life, caffeine can become counterproductive. If you drink small amounts during the day, they add up, and you eventually reach a point at which your body has more caffeine than it can handle. By increasing anxiety or restlessness, caffeine reduces the body's ability to function. Other unwanted side effects include upset stomach, irritability, and diarrhea.

Caffeine also inhibits the absorption of thiamin (a vitamin important for carbohydrate metabolism) and several minerals, including calcium and iron. Women who consume caffeine regularly (4 or more cups [1 or more liters] of coffee a day or 330 milligrams of caffeine) and have a low intake of calcium in their diet (fewer than 700 milligrams a day) may run a greater risk of developing osteoporosis or brittle bone disease.

How It Works

Most research on caffeine has focused on endurance sports. The main finding is that for many endurance athletes, caffeine may extend performance. There are three theories that offer possible explanations. The first was originally thought to be the most plausible theory and has to do with caffeine's ability to enhance fat use for energy. Caffeine stimulates the production of adrenaline, a hormone that accelerates the release of fatty acids into the bloodstream. At the beginning of exercise, the muscles start using these available fatty acids for energy while sparing some of your muscle glycogen. Some research has supported this theory.

The second theory goes like this: Caffeine may directly affect skeletal muscle by altering key enzymes or systems that regulate carbohydrate breakdown within the cells. But the research on this theory has been conflicting and inconclusive.

The third theory may actually be at the root of why caffeine makes you perceive that you are doing less work than you really are during exercise. It states that caffeine, because of its direct effect on the central nervous system, might have the psychological effect of making athletes feel they are not working as hard, or it may somehow maximize the force of muscular contractions. We now know that caffeine can cross the blood–brain barrier and antagonize the effects of adenosine, the neurotransmitter that causes drowsiness by slowing down nerve cell activity. In the brain, caffeine looks like adenosine and can bind to adenosine receptors on brain cells. But caffeine doesn't have the same action as adenosine, so it doesn't slow down nerve cell activity. Instead, it stimulates brain chemicals to secrete epinephrine, the flight-or-fight hormone that makes you feel better while working out. Currently this is the prevailing theory most supported by the research.

Caffeine Use in Power Sports

Until recently, it was believed that caffeine doesn't help much if your sport skills relate mainly to strength and power. But Dr. Larry Spriet and his colleagues at the University of Guelph in Ontario might disagree. They have looked into the effect of caffeine on power sports. In one study, 14 exercisers did three bouts of exercise as hard as they could. Each bout was separated by six minutes of rest. The first two exercise bouts lasted two minutes each, and the third bout was performed to exhaustion. The exercisers were tested twice, once with caffeine and once with a placebo. In the third bout, they were able to exercise longer with caffeine (4.93 minutes with caffeine versus 4.12 minutes with the placebo). Caffeine clearly boosted performance in short-term, intense exercise.

The mechanism behind this effect isn't exactly clear, but the researchers were able to rule out one possibility. By taking blood samples and muscle biopsy specimens, they found that in this instance caffeine did not spare muscle glycogen, as was previously thought.

Ground-breaking new research shows that caffeine can increase strength by triggering the release of epinephrine from the adrenal glands, resulting in improved muscle contraction. When this happens, perceived exertion is reduced, letting you push more weight without making a conscious decision to work harder. Basically, it seems that caffeine can improve strength over time, which of course leads to greater muscle mass. Caffeine is a bona fide ergogenic aid: A large collection of studies shows that it can improve exercise performance by 22 percent. More good news: The amount of coffee it takes to enhance performance—about 16 ounces (473 milliliters), or 2 cups—does not have a dehydrating effect on the body.

Well-Trained Athletes Do Best

Studies also show that caffeine works best as a power booster if you're well conditioned. Proof of this comes from experiments with swimmers, whose sport is anaerobic as well as aerobic. Highly trained swimmers improved their swimming velocity significantly after consuming 250 milligrams of caffeine and then swimming at maximal speed. Untrained, occasional swimmers didn't fare as well. The same group of researchers had previously conducted experiments with untrained subjects who cycled against resistance after supplementing with caffeine. Again, caffeine didn't provide much of a performance boost in untrained individuals.

The Final Word on Caffeine

Caffeine may give you a kick for exercise (especially if you're in super shape), although no one has pinpointed exactly why and how. If you want to judge caffeine's effect on your own performance, start off with a little bit—maybe a cup or half a cup of coffee—before your workout. An 8-ounce (237-milliliter) cup of coffee contains between 100 and 150 milligrams of caffeine. See what happens, and compare it with the workouts when you don't consume caffeine beforehand. Overall, laboratory studies suggest that supplementing with doses of 3 to 6 milligrams per kilogram of body weight 30 to 60 minutes before exercise can enhance both power and endurance exercise in well-trained subjects. However, study results in the laboratory might not be the same as results in the real world of the gym.

Keep in mind, too, that caffeine may aggravate certain health problems, such as ulcers, heart disease, high blood pressure, and anemia, to name just a few. Stick to your doctor's advice. Above all, don't substitute caffeine for sound, commonsense nutritional practices for extending energy.

Carbohydrate–Protein Sport Drinks

Unimaginable as it may seem, it is within your control to retool your body for more lean muscle and less fat—and do it naturally—all with a simple formulation. Here's how: Immediately after your workout, drink a liquid carbohydrate supplement that contains protein, and you'll jump-start the muscle-building process, plus boost your energy levels.

This simple formula is 12 ounces (355 milliliters) of carbohydrate and protein in liquid form taken immediately after your strength-training routine. This is the time your body is best able to use these nutrients for muscle firming and fat burning. The supplement I use with my clients is my Kleiner's Muscle-Building formulas, featured in chapter 16. For a long time, I've used these formulas with many of my bodybuilding clients, and soon after they begin drinking the formulas, we observe a major shift in their body composition from less fat to more muscle.

How It Works

How does this formula help muscles get stronger and firmer? Exercise, of course, is the initial stimulus. You challenge your muscles by working out, and they respond with growth. But for muscle building to take place, muscles need protein and carbohydrate in combination to create the right hormonal climate for muscle growth.

What happens is this: Protein and carbohydrate trigger the release of insulin and GH in your body. Insulin is a powerful factor in building muscle. It helps ferry glucose and amino acids into cells, reassembles those amino acids into body tissue, and prevents muscle wasting and tissue loss. GH increases the rate of protein production by the body, spurring muscle-building activity, and it also promotes fat burning. Both hormones are directly involved in muscle growth. Your body is primed for growth thanks to this simple muscle-gain formula.

Scientific Proof

Research into the effect of carbohydrate–protein supplements on athletes and exercisers supports what I've observed for years. Here are some examples:

- In one scientific study, 14 normal-weight men and women ate test meals containing various amounts of protein (in grams): none (a protein-free meal), 15.8, 21.5, 33.6, and 49.9, along with 58 grams of carbohydrate. Blood samples were taken at intervals after the meal. The protein-containing meals produced the greatest rise in insulin compared with the protein-free meal. This study points out that protein has an insulin-boosting effect.

- In another study, nine experienced male strength trainers were given water (which served as the control), a carbohydrate supplement, a protein supplement, or a carbohydrate–protein supplement. They took their designated supplement immediately after working out and again two hours later. Right after exercise and throughout the next eight hours, the researchers drew blood samples to determine the levels of various hormones in the blood, including insulin, testosterone, and GH.

  The most significant finding was that the carbohydrate–protein supplement triggered the greatest elevations in insulin and GH. The protein works hand in hand with postexercise carbohydrate to create a hormonal climate that's highly conducive to muscle growth.

- If you've started strength training later in life, consuming protein after your workout is very important. Researchers in Denmark instructed a group of men (aged 74 and older) to have a protein drink consisting of 10 grams of protein, 7 grams of carbohydrate, and 3 grams of fat either immediately after or two hours after each training session. The study lasted 12 weeks. By the end of the study, the best gains in muscular growth occurred when the subjects consumed liquid protein immediately after their workouts. The point here seems to be that the sooner you replenish with protein, the better results you can obtain.

More Energy

If you supplement with a carbohydrate–protein beverage after your workout, you'll notice something else: higher energy levels. Not only does this nutrient combination stimulate hormone activity, it also starts replenishing muscle glycogen, which means more muscle energy. The harder you can work out, the greater your muscular gains.

When protein is added to the supplement mix, your body's glycogen-making process accelerates faster than if you just consumed carbohydrate alone.

Some intriguing research proves this point. In one study, nine men cycled for two full hours during three different sessions to deplete their muscle glycogen stores. Immediately after each exercise bout and again two hours later, the men drank a straight carbohydrate supplement, a straight protein supplement, or a carbohydrate–protein supplement. By looking at actual biopsy specimens of

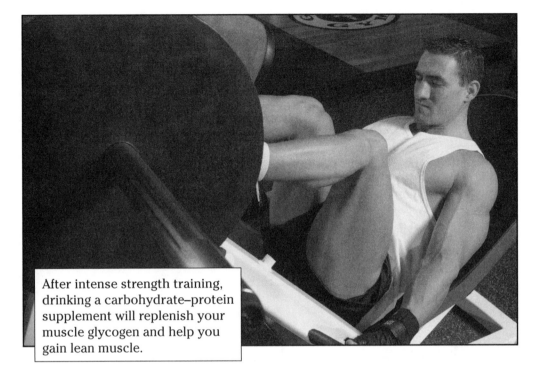

After intense strength training, drinking a carbohydrate–protein supplement will replenish your muscle glycogen and help you gain lean muscle.

the muscles, the researchers observed that the rate of muscle glycogen storage was significantly faster when the carbohydrate–protein mixture was consumed.

Why such speed? It's well known that eating carbohydrate after prolonged endurance exercise helps restore muscle glycogen. When protein is consumed along with carbohydrate, there's a surge in insulin. Biochemically, insulin is like an acceleration pedal. It races the body's glycogen-making motor in two ways. First, it speeds up the movement of glucose and amino acids into cells, and second, it activates a special enzyme crucial to glycogen synthesis.

In another study, a group of athletes performed enough exercise to deplete their glycogen reserves. Afterward, part of the group consumed a carbohydrate–protein supplement; the other consumed a 6 percent glucose–electrolyte solution. Both groups exercised again. Endurance-wise, the carbohydrate–protein group outlasted the other group by 66 percent.

In a similar study, eight endurance-trained cyclists performed two two-hour exercise bouts designed to deplete their glycogen stores. After exercise and again two hours later, they consumed either a carbohydrate–protein supplement or a carbohydrate-only formula. The carbohydrate-protein formula contained 53 grams of carbohydrate and 14 grams of protein, while the carbohydrate formula contained 20 grams of carbohydrate. The effects of the carbohydrate–protein supplement were quite remarkable: Glucose levels rose by 17 percent, and insulin levels increased by 92 percent. Furthermore, there was 128 percent greater storage of muscle glycogen when athletes took the carbohydrate–protein supplement compared with when they took the carbohydrate-only formula.

Scientific research indicates that for hard trainers, the optimal combination of protein and carbohydrate after exercise is one part protein to three parts carbohydrate, or approximately 45 to 50 grams of carbohydrate and 15 grams of protein. A question often arises as to whether you should eat your postexercise meal or drink it in the form of a carbohydrate–protein supplement. Let's turn to some scientific data for the answer. Researchers at Ithaca College in Ithaca, New York, tested whether a whole-foods meal, a supplemental drink of protein and carbohydrate, a carbohydrate-only beverage, or a placebo would have any effect on insulin, testosterone, or cortisol levels following resistance training. The bottom line of the study was that the supplemental drink of protein and carbohydrate had the most effect, but mostly in terms of increasing insulin levels. As I noted before, insulin is essential for driving the manufacture of glycogen, so it looks like your best meal after a workout is one that is in liquid form. That's why my clients love my smoothies! You can find a variety of smoothie recipes in chapter 16.

Creatine

Creatine is one of the most important natural fuel-enhancing supplements discovered thus far for strength trainers. Unlike a lot of supplements, creatine has been extensively researched, with more than 500 studies conducted to date. Of these studies, 300 have focused on the performance-enhancing value of creatine, and about 70 percent of these studies report positive effects. These exciting experiments show that creatine produces significant improvement in sports that require high levels of strength and power, including strength training, rowing, and cycling sprints. Another big plus for creatine: Several studies have shown gains in body mass averaging 2 to 4 pounds (.5-1 kilogram), as well as decreases in body fat. It was once thought that this increase was mostly water weight, but now we're seeing that a significant amount of the gain is pure muscle and only a small portion is water.

Creatine received the following endorsement from a 1995 review article in the *International Journal of Sport Nutrition,* a respected publication in sport nutrition: "Creatine should not be viewed as another gimmick supplement; its ingestion is a means of providing immediate, significant performance improvements to athletes involved in explosive sports."

Sound good? You bet. Who wouldn't prefer a bona fide natural supplement like creatine over synthetic, dangerous compounds like steroids? Creatine is the ticket to greater strength and improved muscularity.

How It Works

Creatine is a substance produced in the liver and kidneys at a rate of about 2 grams a day from arginine, glycine, and methionine, three nonessential amino acids. About 95 percent of the body's creatine travels by the blood to be stored in the muscles, heart, and other body cells. Inside muscle cells, it's turned into creatine phosphate (CP), a compound that serves as a tiny energy supply, enough for several seconds of action. CP thus works best over the short haul in activities such as strength training that require short, fast bursts of activity. CP also replenishes your cellular reserves of ATP, the molecular fuel that provides the power for muscular contractions. With more ATP around, your muscles can do more work.

As a strength trainer, you load creatine into your muscles just as endurance athletes do with carbohydrate. Consequently, you can push harder and longer in your workouts because creatine boosts the pace of energy production in your muscle cells. Creatine supplementation doesn't build muscle directly. But it does have an indirect effect: You can work out more intensely, and this translates into muscle gains. Once in the muscles, creatine appears to induce swelling, which in turn may influence carbohydrate and protein metabolism.

The Latest Word on Creatine

There are more than 500 articles investigating the influence of creatine supplementation on strength, power, and athletic performance. A new area of creatine research, how creatine may influence medical conditions involving the nervous system, has greatly increased the number of publications addressing the possible benefits of creatine supplements. Here's the rundown of what the most current scientific literature says regarding creatine supplementation:

• By supplementing with creatine, lacto-ovo vegetarians (who typically have lower stores of creatine in their bodies) can increase their muscular stores of creatine to levels similar to those of people who eat meat and experience better synthesis of ATP.

• Supplementing with creatine has been shown to increase bone mineral content and bone density in older men who engage in strength training. This benefit may be related to enhanced muscle mass and strength due to taking the creatine. Men tend to lose both muscle mass and bone mass as they age, so this finding is quite promising in terms of quality of life as men age.

• Amateur swimmers who supplemented with creatine (5 milligrams) twice a day for seven days were able to sprint faster in the last 50 meters of a 400-meter swimming competition. This finding hints that creatine might give you a final surge of energy in the last leg of a race.

• During sleep deprivation, creatine levels decrease in the brain. Creatine supplementation, however, had a positive effect on sleep and mood in an experiment involving subjects who took 5 grams of creatine four times a day for seven days immediately before the experiment.

• More and more, creatine is being tested in medical settings to see if it can enhance muscle recovery. Sometimes, the findings are promising; other times, they are not. In one study, researchers looked into the effect of strength training and creatine supplementation on patients with myasthenia gravis, a chronic autoimmune neuromuscular disease characterized by varying degrees of weakness of the skeletal (voluntary) muscles of the body. They found that both interventions promoted gains in strength and in muscle mass. In another study, creatine supplementation was not found to help muscle strength when given before knee arthroplasty, nor did it help with recovery afterward.

How Much?

Creatine supplements swell the ranks of creatine in your muscles, giving the working muscles another fuel source in addition to glycogen from carbohydrate. The question is, how much creatine do you need? You do get creatine from food—roughly 1 gram a day. But that's not enough to enhance strength-training performance.

Creatine usually comes in a powdered form as creatine monohydrate. Scientific research shows that taking four 5-gram doses a day (about a teaspoon) for five days will do the trick (or .3 gram per kilogram of body weight per day). This is typically called the *loading phase.* During your maintenance phase, 2 to 5 grams (or .03 gram per kilogram of body weight) a day—about half a teaspoon—will keep your muscles saturated with enough extra creatine. The logic that if a small dose is good, a large dose is better isn't a good idea. The body has a ceiling on the amount of creatine that it will store in the muscles. If you keep taking more, creatine will not continue to load in the muscles.

Since creatine levels will be maintained in your muscles for about 3 weeks, another strategy is to cycle on and off creatine rather than using the loading maintenance phases. Start with a dose of 5 grams per day for about 6 weeks. It will take a little longer to reach saturation levels compared to the loading dose, but the end results are virtually the same. Cycle off the creatine for about 3 weeks, and then go back on it again. Your muscle levels and training results will remain high during the off period. This strategy will lighten the strain on your wallet, while still giving you competitive results.

The question of when to supplement with creatine has been answered somewhat in research. A Canadian study conducted over a six-week period found that when you supplement with creatine after working out, it can increase muscle size. This particular study focused on arm muscle, and the effect was more pronounced in men than in women. On the other hand, taking creatine before intense aerobic exercise improved energy production during exercise. More testing in terms of creatine timing is needed, but this study opens some intriguing possibilities for when to take creatine.

Creatine is nontoxic, and studies have been unable to find any negative side effects to its use when dosage recommendations are followed. It does not interfere with normal body fluid shifts that occur when exercising or competing in the heat—good news to endurance athletes who often train or compete in hot weather. But if you take too much at once, you can experience an upset stomach.

The only known side effect associated with creatine intakes of 1 to 10 grams per day is water weight gain. In addition, one report suggests that some people may experience muscle cramping and possibly muscle tearing when supplementing with creatine. However, these claims are unsubstantiated.

While loading with creatine, make sure to drink extra water. This may control any cramping that may occur. And you're asking for trouble if you belt down daily dosages of 40 grams or more. Such high doses may cause possible liver and kidney damage, according to some reports. Thus, creatine is ill advised if you have preexisting kidney disease (for example, renal dialysis or previous kidney transplant). In healthy people, however, creatine does not seem to adversely affect kidney function.

My stand has always been that you must have your nutrition, your training, and your rest dialed in before you add creatine to your program. Of course, always check with your physician before supplementing with creatine.

Supercharge With Creatine and Carbohydrate

Here's an important fact about creatine supplementation: Creatine works best in combination with carbohydrate. This combination boosts the amount of creatine accumulated in muscles by as much as 60 percent!

That's the key finding of a recent study. Investigators divided 24 men (average age was 24) into experimental and control groups. The control group took 5 grams of creatine in sugar-free orange juice four times a day for five days. The experimental group took the same dose of creatine followed 30 minutes later by 17 ounces (503 milliliters) of a solution containing carbohydrate. Muscle biopsies after the five-day test period showed that both groups had elevated creatine levels, but with one dramatic difference—creatine levels in the experimental group were 60 percent higher than in the control group. There were also higher concentrations of insulin in the muscles of the experimental group.

The implications of this study to strength trainers, athletes, and exercisers are enormous. Just think: By supplementing with creatine and carbohydrate at the same time, you're supercharging your body. With more creatine in your muscles, you have more power to strength train. The fact that the creatine–carbohydrate combination increases insulin is equally important. Insulin increases the uptake of glucose, which is ultimately stored as glycogen in the liver and muscles for fuel. The more glycogen you can stockpile, the more energy you'll have for exercise, including aerobics. The creatine–carbohydrate combination is a true energy booster for all types of exercise activity. Other studies have shown a similar benefit to combining creatine with protein and carbohydrate.

Glucose–Electrolyte Solutions

Glucose–electrolyte solutions are beneficial for athletes competing in high-intensity sports lasting less than one hour or events that last an hour or longer. These solutions do two things: Replace water and electrolytes lost through

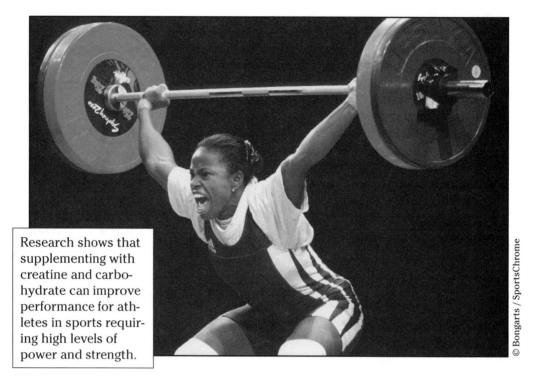

Research shows that supplementing with creatine and carbohydrate can improve performance for athletes in sports requiring high levels of power and strength.

© Bongarts / SportsChrome

sweat and supply a small amount of carbohydrate to the working muscles, decreasing the use of muscle and liver glycogen stores. During competition, athletes can thus run, bike, or swim longer because the supplemental carbohydrate has spared stored glycogen. Most drinks are about 6 to 8 percent carbohydrate. The carbohydrate may be glucose, a simple sugar; fructose, a fruit sugar; sucrose, ordinary table sugar (a blend of glucose and fructose); maltodextrin, a complex carbohydrate derived from corn; or a combination of these.

There's no evidence that electrolytes improve exercise performance for general workouts. For events lasting less than three hours, they're not required unless you have a mineral deficiency diagnosed by your physician or your daily sweat losses total more than 3 percent of your body weight, or 4.5 pounds (2 kilograms) in a 150-pound (68-kilogram) athlete. Endurance and ultraendurance athletes exercising more than three hours are among those who do need to replace electrolytes. But that is probably not you. If you are eating a diet rich in whole foods, you are getting enough of these minerals.

In addition to their ability to replenish fluids, electrolytes, and carbohydrate, glucose–electrolyte solutions may strengthen your immune system. This amazing news comes from Appalachian State University, where researchers put two groups of marathoners on some high-intensity treadmill exercise for two and a half hours. One group drank 25 ounces (739 milliliters) of a glucose–electrolyte solution (Gatorade) 30 minutes before exercise, 8 ounces (237 milliliters) every 15 minutes during exercise, and a final 25 ounces over a six-hour recovery period. The other group replenished fluids on the same schedule but with a noncarbohydrate placebo solution.

The researchers took blood samples from the marathoners and found that the Gatorade drinkers had lower levels of cortisol in their blood than the other exercisers did. Cortisol is a hormone that suppresses immune response. The head of the research team, Dr. David Nieman, was quoted in *Runner's World* as saying, "It seems that when blood glucose level stays up, cortisol level stays down, thus immune function remains relatively strong." Because this is just one study, obviously it offers no final and complete answers on the glucose–immunity connection. This research is intriguing, nonetheless.

In addition, other research has found that consuming a sport drink during aerobic exercise can enhance feelings of pleasure, meaning that you may not notice feelings of discomfort while working out. For people who don't like to exercise, sipping a sport drink may spark motivation simply because it makes them feel better.

Glucose–electrolyte solutions are designed primarily for endurance athletes. But they also have application for strength trainers in two important ways. First, if you train aerobically—particularly in the heat—these supplements prevent electrolyte and fluid depletion. Second, if you're training intensely for 45 minutes or more, extra fluid and fuel mean more energy.

A study conducted by Dr. Greg Haff at Appalachian State University examined the muscle glycogen levels and performance effect of supplementing with a glucose beverage or placebo just before and during resistance exercise. There was significantly less muscle glycogen degradation in the supplemented group versus the placebo group (15 percent versus 19 percent) after resistance exercise. Although this group of researchers has previously reported improvements in successive bouts of resistance exercise when subjects were supplemented with a glucose beverage, in this study no improvements in the single bout of resistance exercise were observed.

What About Carbohydrate Gels?

Carbohydrate gels are highly concentrated carbohydrate with a pudding-like consistency that is usually packaged in single-serve pouches. Designed for athletes and exercisers participating in endurance activity, these products are usually a mixture of simple carbohydrate with flavoring, and some are formulated with protein as well. These gels are quickly absorbed into the bloodstream and thus are a good source of immediate food energy, particularly during extended exercise. Carbohydrate gels that contain protein have been found in research to extend performance longer than plain carbohydrate gels and may be a better choice. When using these gels, make sure you take in sufficient water to process the carbohydrate and protein and to prevent dehydration.

There has also been speculation on whether these drinks have any influence on oxidative damage in the aftermath of exercise. In strength trainers who were given a sport drink or a placebo, researchers could find no difference in oxidative stress. Sport drinks apparently don't help heal muscle damage following exercise. Adding protein to a sport drink in the form of amino acids has been shown to help with muscle recovery and muscle protein synthesis, however, particularly in novice strength trainers who drank a sport drink spiked with 6 additional grams of amino acids. The mixture significantly elevated insulin concentrations for an anabolic effect and decreased levels of the stress hormone cortisol, decreasing the stress effects of exercise on the body. Adding protein to these drinks has been shown to reduce the mental fatigue involved in exercise as well.

The best time to swill one of these drinks is during an aerobic workout or during any period of exertion, especially if you're exercising or working in hot weather. That's when fluid loss is greater than any other time of the year. You can lose more electrolytes, too, although the concentration of these minerals in sweat gets weaker the fitter you are. You also burn more glycogen working out in the heat—another good reason to quench your thirst with a glucose–electrolyte solution.

Weight-Gain Powders

You've seen them: huge cans brightly labeled with alluring product descriptions such as "weight gainer," "solid mass," "lean mass enhancer," or "muscle provider." These products belong to a group of supplements known as weight-gain powders. Most contain various combinations of carbohydrate, protein, amino acids, vitamins, minerals, and other ingredients thought to enhance performance. The manufacturers of these products claim that their specific formulations will help you pack on muscle.

But do they? Actually, no one knows for sure. However, in 1996 a group of researchers at the University of Memphis put two weight-gain powders to the test. One was Gainers Fuel 1000, a high-calorie supplement that adds about 1,400 calories a day to the diet (290 grams of carbohydrate, 60 grams of protein, and 1 gram of fat). Although the supplement contains many other ingredients, it's formulated with two minerals that have been hyped as muscle builders: chromium picolinate and boron.

Chromium picolinate is linked to muscle growth because it increases the action of insulin. But that's where the association ends. There's no valid scientific evidence that chromium directly promotes muscle building. (For more on chromium picolinate, see chapter 7.)

Boron has been touted as a supplement that promotes muscle growth by increasing the amount of testosterone circulating in the blood. But experiments have failed to verify this claim. In one recent study, 10 male bodybuilders took 2.5 milligrams of boron daily while 9 male bodybuilders took a placebo. Both groups performed their regular bodybuilding routines for seven weeks. Lean mass, strength, and testosterone levels increased in all 19 men to the same relative degree. Boron supplementation didn't make a bit of difference. It was the training, pure and simple, that did the trick.

Back to the 1996 study on weight-gain powder: The second supplement investigated was Phosphagain. It adds about 570 calories a day to the diet (64 grams of carbohydrate, 67 grams of protein, and 5 grams of fat). As with most weight-gain powders, Phosphagain contains lots of other ingredients that are rumored to build muscle. Among the most notable are creatine (see the previous section), taurine, nucleotides, and l-glutamine. An amino acid found in muscles, taurine has been found in animal studies to enhance the effectiveness of insulin. Nucleotides are the building blocks of RNA and DNA; in Phosphagain, they are derived from the RNA in yeast. Nucleotides are fundamental to metabolism and integral to the cell division and replication involved in growth and development. As for l-glutamine, an amino acid, it theoretically regulates the water volume in cells and the protein-making process in muscles.

To check the effects of Gainers Fuel 1000 and Phosphagain on muscle growth, the University of Memphis researchers selected 28 strength-trained men around the age of 26. None was currently taking anabolic steroids, and none had a history of steroid use. The subjects had been training for an average of six years.

The researchers assigned them to one of three groups: a third of the men took a maltodextrin supplement three times a day (maltodextrin is a carbohydrate derived from corn); a third took two servings a day of Gainers Fuel 1000 according to the manufacturer's directions; and the remaining third took three servings a day of Phosphagain according to the manufacturer's directions. None knew which supplement they were taking. They all continued their normal workouts and diets during the course of the study. In addition, they were told to not take any other supplements two weeks before the study and until the study was over.

Here's a summary of what the researchers discovered:

- Both the maltodextrin supplement and Gainers Fuel 1000 promoted modest gains in muscle mass in combination with a strength-training program.

- In the group that supplemented with Gainers Fuel 1000, fat weight and percent body fat increased significantly.

- Phosphagain supplementation was more effective in promoting muscle gains than either maltodextrin or Gainers Fuel 1000 during strength training. In fact, muscle gains were significantly greater with Phosphagain, according to lead researcher Dr. Richard Kreider. The men who supplemented with Phosphagain did not gain any additional fat.

Before you draw your own conclusions, let me emphasize: It's still up in the air as to exactly which ingredients in Phosphagain were responsible for these results. More tests are needed on weight-gain powders in general as well as on the individual ingredients they contain in order to confirm these findings. But, carbohydrate with some protein (weight-gain powders contain both) taken at the proper times is an important supplement to a muscle-building diet. Also, the creatine in Phosphagain could have been a factor in the results.

Weight-gain powders are helpful for increasing calories when you can't increase your calories from food alone. But keep in mind that these products are often quite high in calories (500 to 1,000 calories). Sure, those calories can help you gain weight, but that weight might wind up as fat. It is far easier to control your body composition by controlling your protein, carbohydrate, and fat ratios yourself.

Possibly Meets Marketing Claims

These products have some early research that looks promising, but there is not yet enough data for a definitive answer. In the end, they may or may not work. I suggest that you keep your eye on the magazines and research publications, because these are the supplements that will be in the news.

Arginine

Arginine is an amino acid taken by athletes for a number of reasons. Supposedly, arginine activates the secretion of GH, which drives muscle growth, but no studies have demonstrated this benefit. Arginine is involved in the synthesis of creatine. However, that is not a good reason to supplement with arginine; just take creatine.

Arginine is also the chief ingredient in most nitric oxide (NO) products. NO works as a hemodilator that relaxes smooth muscle in the arteries. This helps reduce blood pressure and increase blood flow to the muscles, possibly delivering more nutrients and oxygen for enhanced muscle growth. So far, though, there is little evidence to support a muscle-building effect of arginine. Additional research is needed to better evaluate the role of arginine for strength trainers.

Be careful with arginine supplementation—too much may damage the pancreas. At least one case study in the scientific literature indicates that arginine supplementation has been associated with pancreatitis, or inflammation of the pancreas.

Beta-Alanine

Billed as the next creatine, beta-alanine is a naturally occurring nonessential amino acid. It is a component of carnosine, anserine, and pantothenic acid (a

B-complex vitamin). Carnosine and anserine are protein-like compounds that seem to be concentrated in actively contracting muscles.

Beta-alanine appears to be a buffering agent, meaning that it prevents certain enzymatic reactions that increase lactic acid in working muscles and therefore dampens the burn in your muscles when you work out. This means that you might be able to perform extra reps or sprint longer before muscle burn forces you to quit. The more beta-alanine in your muscles, the better you should be able to perform. Supplementing with beta-alanine, therefore, can perhaps enhance performance in high-intensity workouts.

Beta-alanine also increases carnosine in the muscle. Research shows that muscles with higher carnosine levels may produce greater force and contract harder for longer periods, which ultimately leads to better muscular development and endurance. Carnosine, which is also available from eating meat, appears to work by preventing the buildup of chemical by-products during strenuous exercise.

Expect to see beta-alanine in a number of different supplement formulas, even mixed with creatine. Already, one study has shown that beta-alanine combined with creatine delayed the onset of muscular fatigue better than beta-alanine or creatine alone.

Beta-Hydroxy-Beta-Methylbutyrate

Found in grapefruit, catfish, and other foods, beta-hydroxy-beta-methylbutyrate (HMB) is a breakdown product of leucine, a BCAA. The body produces it naturally from proteins containing leucine.

Studies show that HMB may be anticatabolic; that is, it inhibits the degradation of muscle and protein in the body, so you can possibly train harder on successive days. Preliminary research on HMB indicates that 1.5 to 3 grams a day of HMB can assist with increasing muscle mass, decreasing body fat, and boosting strength levels if you are just beginning a strength-training program. But there are few benefits for well-trained athletes, according to research.

Branched-Chain Amino Acids

The BCAAs are leucine, isoleucine, and valine. During endurance exercise, levels of these amino acids fall, which may contribute to fatigue during competition. Emerging but limited research suggests that supplementation with BCAAs may enhance performance, particularly if you compete in endurance events. One study found that marathoners who consumed a sport drink containing BCAAs increased their performance by as much as 4 percent. Not all studies have shown a positive effect, however.

Here are some guidelines based on what is currently known about BCAA supplementation: Dosages of 4 to 21 grams daily during training and 2 to 4 grams per hour with a 6 to 8 percent glucose–electrolyte solution before and during prolonged exercise have been shown to improve physiological and psychological responses to training. In other words, athletes felt better mentally and physically during exercise. Theoretically, BCAA supplementation during hard training may help reduce fatigue, too, as well as prevent protein degradation in your muscles. You can buy BCAAs in a bottle, but you can also find them in dairy products and in whey protein powder. Refer to chapter 2 for more information on BCAAs in food.

According to Richard B. Kreider, PhD, in *Overtraining in Sport* (Human Kinetics, 1998), "In our view, the greatest potential application of BCAA supplementation is to help athletes tolerate training to a greater degree rather than a performance enhancement supplement."

Carnitine

Found in red meat and other animal products, carnitine is a proteinlike substance once thought to be an important vitamin. Now scientists know carnitine is not an essential nutrient because the liver and kidneys can synthesize it without any help from food. Most people consume between 50 and 300 milligrams of this nutrient each day from food. Even if you don't eat that much carnitine, your body can produce its own from the amino acids lysine and methionine. About 98 percent of the body's carnitine is stored in the muscles.

The main job of carnitine in the body is to transport fatty acids into cells to be burned as energy. Because of this role, many theories have been floated regarding carnitine's potential benefits to exercisers. One theory is that carnitine boosts exercise performance by making more fat available to working muscles, thus sparing glycogen. Another theory has it that carnitine, because of its role in cellular energy processes, reduces the buildup of waste products such as lactic acid in the muscles, thereby extending performance. Theories aside, what does scientific research show?

Numerous studies have evaluated the benefits of carnitine supplementation in both patient and athletic populations. With varying results, some studies indicate that carnitine (.5 to 2 grams a day) may increase fat oxidation and improve cardiovascular efficiency during exercise. New research suggests that supplemental carnitine can help you burn more of the fat found in muscle. It has also been shown to enhance carbohydrate metabolism. The ability to use more fat and stored carbohydrate from the muscle would certainly give you a tremendous competitive advantage for endurance activity. More research is needed, however, to see if carnitine really has these effects.

Research also shows that carnitine taken in partnership with choline reduces lipid peroxidation and conserves vitamin E and vitamin A in the body. Similarly, carnitine alone has been found to enhance the antioxidant capacity in rats during prolonged exercise, so there may be a protective effect of carnitine on the immune system.

There is a lot to watch in carnitine research. One study looked at infusing carnitine into the muscle cells along with insulin. The theory is that if you can get carnitine directly into muscle cells, then it will burn fat. It's possible that at some future date, researchers will discover that taking carnitine with a carbohydrate (like we do with creatine) will somehow allow you to direct it to muscle cells.

One thing we know for sure is that supplementation definitely improves performance in carnitine-deficient people and may be helpful for vegan athletes prone to low muscle levels of carnitine. However, there is little support for the belief that well-nourished, healthy athletes benefit from carnitine supplementation in energy metabolism, exercise capacity, or body composition.

I see no real danger in trying carnitine, and we shouldn't count it out just yet. According to research, there are no ill effects with doses ranging from 500 milligrams a day to 6 grams a day for up to a month. But there is no research to suggest that taking more than 2 grams a day makes any difference. Large doses of 4 grams per day can cause diarrhea.

A word of caution: Some supplement preparations contain a mixture of L-carnitine and D-carnitine. The L-carnitine form appears to be safe; D-carnitine, on the other hand, can cause muscular weakness and excretion of myoglobin, the oxygen-transporting protein in the blood. If you supplement with carnitine, use products that contain L-carnitine only.

Carnosine

In 1984, sports scientists noted that elite sprint athletes had unusual abilities to perform anaerobic activities for significantly longer than one would predict based on general principles of muscle physiology. The buildup of the by-products of anaerobic exercise create an acidic environment in the muscle, which leads to fatigue. Scientists postulated that sprint athletes had an enhanced buffering capability, giving them a competitive edge. Carnosine was identified as one of the intracellular buffers possibly contributing to enhanced performance.

Today, carnosine is being added to supplements for exactly this purpose—preventing the buildup of chemical by-products during strenuous exercise that lower the pH environment of the muscle cell and lead to fatigue. Theoretically, by maintaining a higher pH, exercise time and performance can be enhanced. While the theory is sound, studies to date have not found improvements in exercise performance in human subjects supplementing with carnosine. The animal research is promising, and carnosine deserves your attention as a newcomer on the supplement scene.

Coenzyme Q10 (Ubiquinone)

Found in the mitochondria (energy factories) of cells, coenzyme Q10 (CoQ10), or ubiquinone, plays a central role in a series of chemical reactions that transport oxygen and produce energy. It also works as an antioxidant and thus may help destroy free radicals, particularly during aerobic exercise.

In addition, supplemental CoQ10 has been used successfully in patients with heart disease. As for its benefits for athletes and exercisers, the verdict is still out, though I've placed it in the "possibly useful" category due to its effectiveness in treating heart disease. For more information on CoQ10, refer to chapter 7.

A few studies have shown that CoQ10 may enhance aerobic performance in people who don't exercise. But in one study, trained triathletes took 100 milligrams of CoQ10, 500 milligrams of vitamin C, 100 milligrams of inosine, and 200 IUs of vitamin E for four weeks, and no change in their endurance capacity was found.

It is important to add that CoQ10 in high doses may be harmful. In one study, supplementation with 120 milligrams daily for 20 days resulted in muscle tissue damage, possibly because of increased oxidation.

Conjugated Linoleic Acid

Derived from safflower oil, this supplement is promoted as a fat-burning, muscle-toning, energy-boosting agent. There has been a groundswell of research on this supplement. For example, in observing the action of CLA on isolated fat cells, researchers found that it encourages the breakdown of fat and stifles lipoprotein lipase, a fat-storage enzyme. In addition, CLA ferries dietary fat into cells where it is burned for energy or used to build muscle. Another observation: CLA investigators say that the supplement does not shrink fat cells (like dieting does), but rather, it keeps them from enlarging. Enlarged fat cells are the main reason we get pudgy.

Ever since CLA was shown to reduce body fat in animals, researchers have attempted to verify whether it does the same in humans. In one study, published in the *Journal of Nutrition,* CLA clearly banished pounds in a group of 60 overweight volunteers. They took either a placebo or CLA for 12 weeks; the CLA dosage ranged from 1.7 grams to 6.8 grams daily. By the end of the experimental period, those who supplemented with 3.4 grams of CLA daily had dissolved their body fat by 6 pounds (2.5 kilograms) on average. The researchers concluded that supplementing with 3.4 grams a day may be enough to pare down fat and manage your weight effectively.

One of the most intriguing areas of CLA research focuses on its apparent ability to trim abdominal fat, which is good news if you are trying to lose your belly bulge. To date, evidence for this waist-trimming effect has been observed only in men, but that doesn't necessarily rule out the same benefit for women. Let's look at the research.

In a Swedish study published in 2001 in the *International Journal of Obesity and Related Metabolic Disorders,* 25 men with abdominal obesity (aged 39 to 64) took either 4.2 grams of CLA or a placebo every day. At the end of the four-week experiment, those who took CLA had reduced their waists by 1.4 centimeters, a reduction considered clinically significant by the researchers. The placebo group, by contrast, had insignificant reductions. The results of the study suggest that the effect of this safe and potentially helpful supplement on the reduction of abdominal fat is an avenue of research clearly worth further pursuit, particularly in women.

However, there is quite a bit of conflicting data on CLA. One reason is that there are different versions, or isomers, of CLA, and they all have different effects on the body. I believe we need to wait for more research on this supplement before running out to buy it by the box load.

Glucosamine Sulfate and Chondroitin Sulfate

The combination supplement of glucosamine sulfate and chondroitin sulfate is being sold as an arthritis cure. Although research into this combination is ongoing, there is good initial evidence that this supplement does help relieve the pain and ease the movement of arthritis sufferers—perhaps as effectively as nonsteroidal anti-inflammatory drugs (NSAIDS), without the long-term negative side effects.

One study of athletes with cartilage damage in their knees showed that 76 percent had complete resolution of symptoms and resumed full athletic training after 140 days of supplementation. However, there is no evidence demonstrating that glucosamine can repair damaged ligaments or tendons from sport-related injuries. More research is needed in this area, but supplementation with these compounds looks promising.

Glutamine

Glutamine is the most abundant amino acid in your body. Most of it is stored in your muscles, although significant amounts are found in your brain, lungs, blood, and liver. It serves as a building block for proteins, nucleotides (structural units of RNA and DNA), and other amino acids, and it is the principal fuel source for cells that make up the immune system.

Emerging evidence shows that glutamine may optimize recovery in at least four ways. Glutamine spares protein, stimulates the formation of glycogen, protects immunity, and enhances protein synthesis.

During intense exercise, the muscles release glutamine into the bloodstream. This can deplete muscle glutamine reserves by as much as 34 percent. Such a shortfall can be problematic, because a deficiency of glutamine promotes the breakdown and wasting of muscle tissue. But if sufficient glutamine is available, muscle loss can be prevented.

Glutamine also stimulates the synthesis of muscle glycogen. In a study involving subjects who cycled for 90 minutes, intravenous glutamine administered during a two-hour period after exercise doubled the concentration of glycogen in the muscles. It's not clear exactly how glutamine works in this regard, though. Scientists speculate either that glutamine itself can be converted into muscle glycogen or that it may inhibit the breakdown of glycogen.

In addition, glutamine is the chief fuel source for cells that make up the immune system. As noted, strenuous exercise depletes glutamine, and researchers believe that this shortage may be one of the reasons for the weakened immunity seen in hard-training athletes. Supplementing with glutamine may fend off infections that can sideline training.

Finally, glutamine assists with controlling hydration levels of cells, or cell volumization. By helping maintain cell volume, protein synthesis is stimulated and protein breakdown is decreased.

Glutamine thus may have benefits for anyone who wants to maximize performance, muscle repair, and immunity. The recommended dosage is between 5 and 15 grams a day.

Glycerol

Glycerol is a syrupy substance that causes the body to store water and curtail urine output. It is an ingredient in some sport drinks and is available as a supplement you can add to water. A few studies indicate that glycerol supplementation can superhydrate your body. Research on whether glycerol supplementation actually enhances performance is equivocal, but one recent study in Australia showed enhanced fluid retention (600 milliliters) and improved endurance performance (5 percent) by cyclists in a hot environment when supplemented with glycerol.

The recommended dosage is 1 gram of glycerol per kilogram of body weight, with each gram diluted in 20 to 25 milliliters of fluid.

Medium-Chain Triglyceride Oil

Processed mainly from coconut oil, medium-chain triglyceride oil (MCT oil) is a type of synthetic derived dietary fat that was first formulated in the 1950s by the pharmaceutical industry for patients who had trouble digesting regular fat. Still used in medical settings today, MCT oil is also a popular fitness supplement, marketed as a fat burner, muscle builder, and energy source.

At the molecular level, MCT oil is structured quite differently from conventional types of fat such as butter, margarine, and vegetable oil. Conventional fats are made up of long carbon chains, with 16 or more carbon atoms strung together, and are thus known as long-chain triglycerides (LCTs). Body fat is also an LCT. MCT oil, on the other hand, has a much shorter carbon chain of only 6 to 12 carbon atoms, which is why it is described as a medium-chain triglyceride.

As a result of this molecular difference, MCTs are digested, transported, and metabolized much more quickly than fatty acids from regular oil or fat and thus have some interesting properties. To begin with, MCTs are burned in the body like carbohydrate. Unlike conventional fat, MCTs are not stored as body fat but are shuttled directly into the cells to be burned for energy.

MCT oil is burned so quickly that its calories are turned into body heat during thermogenesis, which boosts the metabolic rate. The higher your metabolism, the more calories your body burns.

Does that mean if you take MCT oil you can rev up your metabolism and therefore burn more fat? Researchers at the University of Rochester looked into this possibility. In an experiment involving seven healthy men, they tested whether a single meal of MCTs would increase the metabolic rate more than an LCT meal would. The men ate test meals containing 48 grams of MCT oil or 45 grams of corn oil given in random order on separate days. In the study, metabolic rate increased 12 percent over six hours after the men ate the MCT meals but increased only 4 percent after the LCT meals were consumed. What's more, concentrations of triglycerides in plasma (the liquid portion of blood) were elevated 68 percent after the LCT meal but did not change after the MCT meal. These findings led the researchers to speculate that replacing LCTs with MCTs over a long period of time might be beneficial in weight loss.

Other researchers aren't so sure. In a study at Calgary University in Alberta, Canada, healthy adults were placed on a low-carbohydrate diet supplemented with MCT oil. The researchers found that the diet had no real effect on elevating the metabolism. The calories burned over a 24-hour period were less than 1 percent of total caloric intake. However, there was a decrease in muscle protein burned for energy. Although MCT might not be a fat burner per se, it may help preserve lean mass by inhibiting its breakdown.

In most studies on MCT oil and fat burning, volunteers ingest huge amounts of the fat—usually 30 grams or more—to bring on metabolic-boosting results. Such amounts are not tolerable for most people, because too much MCT oil produces intestinal discomfort and diarrhea. In my opinion, taking such huge doses of MCT oil to spur fat burning just isn't practical.

There's another problem with using MCT oil to try to burn fat. The recommended way to take MCT oil is with carbohydrate, a practice that prevents ketosis. In ketosis, by-products of fat metabolism called *ketones* build up if carbohydrate isn't available to assist in the final stages of fat breakdown. But when MCTs are taken with carbohydrate, there is no effect on fat burning whatsoever. Here's why: Carbohydrate triggers the release of insulin, which inhibits the mobilization of fat for energy. Thus, there's simply no benefit to the use of MCT oil as a fat burner. You have to do it the old-fashioned way, by exercising and watching your diet.

Since MCT oil is processed in the body much like carbohydrate, it may help boost endurance. Case in point: At the University of Capetown Medical School in South Africa, researchers mixed 86 grams of MCT oil (nearly 3 tablespoons) with 2 liters of 10 percent glucose drink to see what effect it would have on the performance of six endurance-trained cyclists. The cyclists were fed a drink consisting of glucose alone, glucose plus MCT oil, or MCT oil alone. In the laboratory, they pedaled at moderate intensity for about two hours and then completed a higher intensity time trial. They performed this cycling bout on three separate occasions so that each cyclist used each type of drink once. The cyclists sipped the drink every 10 minutes. Performance improved the most when the cyclists supplemented with the MCT–glucose mixture. The researchers did some further biochemical tests on the cyclists and confirmed that the combination spared glycogen while making fat more accessible for fuel. Thus, when combined with carbohydrate, MCT oil may improve aerobic endurance performance by sparing muscle glycogen.

Another claim attached to MCT oil is that it helps you put on muscle; however, there are no controlled studies to prove this. Using some MCT oil to sneak in extra calories for harder workouts makes some sense, though. Go easy at first by taking 1/2 tablespoon to 1 tablespoon (7 to 15 milliliters) a day. Its fast absorption can cause cramping and diarrhea if you take too much. Before experimenting with MCT oil, get your doctor's okay.

N-Acetyl-Cysteine

NAC is an altered form of cysteine, an amino acid that helps the body synthesize glutathione (an antioxidant involved in boosting immunity). This supplement is used in the treatment of respiratory disorders, including acute and chronic bronchitis. What's more, it may help treat cardiovascular disease and might be useful in treating diabetes and some cancers.

In the exercise arena, NAC has been tested mostly in endurance sports. In one study, eight men took either NAC or a placebo while cycling for 45 minutes at a very high intensity meant to simulate a race. NAC improved performance by 26 percent, probably due to its ability to enhance oxygen-carrying molecules and to decrease oxidation in the muscle. It's too early to tell whether NAC will be a true performance-enhancing supplement, but it is worth watching.

Phosphatidylserine

Phosphatidylserine (PS) is a fat-soluble nutrient that is most concentrated in the brain, where it supports many crucial nerve cell functions, including mood and brain health. It is available as a supplement (extracted from soybeans), and it has been well studied. Here's what some of the research shows:

- Taking 300 milligrams daily of PS for a month helped young adults better cope with stress (from taking a mental arithmetic test).

- Male soccer players who supplemented with 850 milligrams of PS for 10 days increased their running time to exhaustion. This benefit probably has to do more with the ability of PS to reduce anxiety and improve mood than anything else, because the nutrient had no real effect on preventing muscle damage, oxidative stress, or lipid peroxidation. A study with cyclists looked at similar parameters and also found that PS has a positive effect on performance. Again, this may have occurred because of the ability of PS to improve mood. If your mood is good, you're naturally going to feel like exercising because you have better mental energy.

If you wish to supplement with PS, I suggest 750 milligrams daily. I believe that supplementation with PS may have some benefit in any brain health program.

Protein Supplements

Protein supplements are a convenient way to consume high-quality, fat-free, lactose-free protein after workouts or between meals. A variety of these supplements are on the market. Each has unique benefits to exercisers, strength trainers, and other athletes. Here's a rundown:

• **Bovine colostrum.** A clear premilk fluid and life's first food for every newborn mammal, colostrum is loaded with growth factors, amino acids, and bioactive protein that help the newborn develop in its first week of life.

Several brands are on the market, including one called Intact. Studies have been conducted on this low-heat processed colostrum for its role on athletic performance, showing promising results for strength and power improvements in repetitive bouts of exercise.

Colostrum is similar to whey protein in both protein efficiency ratio (PER) (3.0) and protein digestibility score (PDCAAS) (1.0). What's more, it is low in fat and free of lactose. Due to its naturally high content of insulin-like growth factors, colostrum is banned by the National Collegiate Athletic Association (NCAA) and the USOC. If you are not affected by these organizations, you might try colostrum for its easy digestibility if you are looking for any possible strength-building edge.

• **Egg protein.** The protein obtained from egg whites (ovalbumin) is considered the reference standard with which to compare types of protein. Egg protein was traditionally the protein of choice for supplements but is rather expensive. The PER of egg protein is 2.8; the PDCAAS is 1.0. If you like variety in your protein supplements, this one has value.

• **Soy protein.** Despite being low in the amino acid methionine, soy is an excellent source of quality protein. Soy protein concentrate (70 percent protein) and isolate (90 percent protein) are particularly good protein sources for vegetarians. Soy protein isolate also contains isoflavone glucosides, which have a number of potential health benefits. The PER of soy protein is 1.8 to 2.3; the PDCAAS is 1.0. The downside of soy protein is that it is not as effective at muscle building as whey protein. On the other hand, if you are a vegetarian or you don't consume milk proteins, soy protein is an excellent alternative for boosting protein intake, especially immediately after exercise.

• **Whey protein.** Whey is a component of milk that is separated from milk to make cheese and other dairy products. It is high in B-complex vitamins, selenium, and calcium. In addition, whey appears to boost levels of the antioxidant glutathione in the body.

Could whey protein possibly ward off oxidative stress? Yes—says at least one study. Twenty athletes (10 men and 10 women) took a whey protein supplement (20 grams a day) for three months. A control group supplemented with a placebo. Researchers assessed the athletes' power and work capacity during bouts of cycling. Both aspects of physical performance increased significantly in the whey-supplemented group, whereas there was no change in the placebo group. The researchers concluded that prolonged supplementation with a product designed to shore up antioxidant defenses resulted in improved performance.

Along with colostrum, whey protein represents the highest quality protein available in supplements. It is digested rapidly, allowing for fast uptake of amino acids. Also available are whey protein hydrolysate, ion exchange whey protein isolate, and cross-flow microfiltration whey protein isolate. Among these, there are subtle differences in the amino acid profiles, fat content, lactose content, and ability to preserve glutamine. It is unclear whether these small differences would have any impact on exercise performance. Using the isolated form of whey is a good idea if you want to reduce the amount of carbohydrate you consume. However, you will get less calcium and other minerals from this form of whey.

Ribose

Found in every cell of your body, ribose is a simple sugar that forms the carbohydrate backbone of DNA and RNA, the genetic materials that control cellular growth and reproduction, thus governing all life. Ribose is also involved in the production of ATP, the main energy-producing molecule of all living cells, and is one of its structural components. Cells need ATP to function properly.

Normally, your body can produce and recycle all the ATP it needs, especially when there is an abundant supply of oxygen. But under certain circumstances—namely ischemia (lack of blood flow to tissues) and strenuous exercise—ATP cannot be regenerated fast enough, and energy-producing compounds called *adenine nucleotides* may be lost from cells. This can impair muscle function and tax strength, because cells need adenine nucleotides to produce sufficient amounts of ATP.

In animal research, ribose supplementation increased the rate of nucleotide synthesis in resting and exercising muscles of rats by three to four times. Other animal studies have found that ribose can restore nucleotides to near normal levels within 12 to 24 hours of intense exercise.

Some medical studies indicate that ribose supplementation (10 to 60 grams a day) can increase ATP availability in certain patients and protect against ischemia in others. But what about athletes and exercisers? Does ribose, now marketed as a sport supplement, have any benefit? Two abstracts of research presented at the 2000 ACSM meeting have convinced me to move ribose to the "possibly meets marketing claims" category. Both studies indicate that ribose taken before, during, and after hard exercise quite possibly helps energize muscles and enhance power.

In one small study, six subjects consumed 2 to 10 grams of ribose. As a result, their blood glucose levels were maintained over 120 minutes, whereas subjects who took a placebo experienced no such benefit. This study hints that ribose may make more energy (blood glucose) available to working muscles.

The results of the second study were a little more convincing since it was an actual performance test. This study investigated whether short-term ribose supplementation improved anaerobic performance in eight young men compared with a taste-matched placebo. Subjects performed a series of six 10-second cycle sprints separated by 60-second rest periods.

There were two familiarization rides before the series of six and then four depletion rides and two posttest rides. Four 8-gram doses were given over a period of 36 hours, with a final dose given 120 minutes before posttesting. In four of six sprints, values for peak power were improved by 2.2 to 7 percent, and overall power improved by 2 to 10 percent. The researchers are now hoping to confirm these results in a larger study.

Supplemental ribose is available in sport drinks, energy bars, tablets, or powders. The usual recommended dosage is 3 to 5 grams daily as maintenance dose and 5 to 10 grams daily for hard-training athletes.

As a way to restore muscular energy, ribose looks promising. So stay tuned: There is much more to learn about this intriguing new supplement and what it holds for athletes and exercisers.

Taurine

One of the most abundant amino acids in the body, taurine is found in the central nervous system and skeletal muscle and is very concentrated in the brain and heart. It is manufactured from the amino acids methionine and cysteine, with help from vitamin B_6. Animal protein is a good source, but taurine is not found in vegetable protein.

Taurine appears to act on neurotransmitters in the brain. There have been reports on the benefits of taurine supplementation in treating epilepsy to control motor tics such as uncontrollable facial twitches. The effectiveness of taurine in treating epilepsy is limited, however, because it does not easily cross the blood–brain barrier.

Taurine is also an effective cellular protector against exercise-induced DNA damage. It appears to reduce muscle damage caused by exercise, therefore accelerating recovery between workouts. Other research indicates that supplemental taurine may improve exercise performance by increasing the muscles' force of contraction (strength). In addition, taurine may exert an insulin-like effect. Research hints that it might improve insulin resistance and help the body better use glucose. It also appears to reduce triglycerides and blood levels of harmful cholesterol.

With high-intensity exercise, blood levels of taurine increase, possibly due to its release from muscle fibers. Because of its association with neurotransmitters in the brain, taurine has recently been advocated as a supplement to enhance attention, cognitive performance, and feelings of well-being. One study investigated these possibilities with a supplement containing caffeine, taurine, and glucuronolactone (a natural detoxifier derived from carbohydrate metabolism), and found that these ingredients had positive effects on human mental performance and mood. But because a combination of ingredients was tested, there's no way of knowing how much of the effect was contributed by taurine alone.

Research into taurine is very limited, and many more studies need to be done to verify its benefits. However, due to the possible effectiveness of supplemented taurine in other populations, it is a supplement to watch.

Does Not Meet Marketing Claims

These products either have no scientific data or they have negative data, poor studies, or only animal studies to support their claims. You might still keep your eye on any research publications, but I wouldn't waste my money or my time on them.

- **Inosine** is a natural chemical that improves oxygen use, possibly by forcing additional production of ATP. However, research does not support claims that supplemental inosine increases physical power. If it really creates more ATP, it would give you more energy. But again, there is no research support for that claim.

- **Pyruvate**, or more specifically pyruvic acid, is made naturally in the body during carbohydrate metabolism and is involved in energy-producing reactions that occur at the cellular level. Pyruvate is also found in many foods in tiny amounts. The dietary supplements sold as pyruvate are derived from pyruvic acid, which is bonded to a mineral salt, usually calcium, sodium, or potassium. Little data support the claims that the dosages currently marketed to promote fat loss (.5-2 grams a day) affect fat loss or improve exercise performance. Nor is there enough research to support the effectiveness of newer supplements that pair pyruvate with creatine.

- **Tryptophan** is an amino acid supplement used by athletes to increase strength and muscle mass, although it does neither. Other people have used tryptophan to relieve insomnia, depression, anxiety, and premenstrual tension. In 1989, thousands of Americans developed a crippling illness called eosinophilia-myalgia syndrome after taking tainted tryptophan made by a Japanese chemical company. As a result, tryptophan was yanked from the market. There are some new tryptophan products on the market, but I feel that there is no reason to use them. If you'd like to give your brain a serotonin boost by consuming more tryptophan, try turkey and milk instead.

• **Zinc** and **magnesium** are mineral elements required in adequate amounts to maintain health and physiologic function, and they promote increased energy expenditure and work performance. Zinc and magnesium are being formulated together as a supplement and marketed as a strength-building formula. But to date no formally published studies have proved that this combination even works.

Potentially Harmful

These products have been shown to cause harm and are not worth the risk. All medications come with a ratio of risks versus benefits. Just because these products are potentially harmful doesn't necessarily mean that they don't work. What it does mean is that the risks outweigh any potential benefits.

• **Amino acid** supplements are heavily marketed to bodybuilders and other strength-training athletes with claims that they build muscle as a safe alternative to steroid drugs. But these supplements are bought not only by bodybuilders but also by average exercisers lured by promises that amino acids, the building blocks of protein, build lean mass and burn fat. While there is data to support the claims that essential amino acids taken after exercise will lead to increased muscle growth and strength, it requires 6 grams of essential amino acids. This is a very costly endeavor and is not without risks. The Federation of American Societies for Experimental Biology (FASEB) recently conducted an exhaustive search of available data on amino acids and concluded that insufficient information exists to establish a safe intake level for any amino acids in dietary supplements, and that their safety should not be assumed. Eighteen to 20 grams of whey protein will safely give you approximately 6 grams of essential amino acids.

• **Androstenedione** is a hormone that occurs naturally in the body and is a direct precursor to testosterone. Androstenedione is found in some plants, notably pollen, and in the gonads of mammals. Athletes take it to increase blood levels of testosterone for a strength- and muscle-building effect. Supposedly, it is safer than taking anabolic steroids. However, there has not been much reliable research to prove the marketing claims made by supplement companies that androstenedione really works.

• **Bee pollen** supplements sold are actually a loose powder of bee saliva, plant nectar, and pollen compressed into tablets of 400 to 500 milligrams or poured into capsules. Bee pollen also comes in pellets to be sprinkled on foods. It is rich in amino acids, with a protein content that averages 20 percent but ranges from 10 to 36 percent. Ten to 15 percent is simple sugars. There are traces of fats and minerals in bee pollen. Bee pollen has been marketed as an athletic supplement for improving physical performance. Some European studies have found benefits, but American studies have not.

Can bee pollen hurt you? Possibly. It does contain pollen so you could suffer an allergic reaction if you're prone to allergies, or worse, death from anaphylactic shock.

• **Dehydroepiandrosterone** (DHEA) is a steroid that's naturally secreted by the adrenal glands. Promoted as an antiaging product, DHEA is probably the most talked about, most hyped supplement on the shelves. Near-magical properties have been attached to DHEA, ranging from increased sex drive to enhanced immunity to weight loss to higher energy levels. Bodybuilders, strength trainers, and other athletes take it with the hope that it will build muscle and burn fat. But there's no real evidence to support this effect; in fact, research shows that supplementation with DHEA does not increase strength. As with all anabolic steroids, DHEA has side effects, including excessive hair growth and other virilizing effects in women and breast enlargement in men. A major concern with DHEA is that there have been no long-term human experiments with it.

• **Dimethylglycine** (vitamin B_{15}) is a dietary supplement rather than a vitamin. Dimethylglycine (DMG), often seen as vitamin B_{15}, supposedly increases aerobic power and endurance. However, there are no studies to substantiate these claims, and what most people don't realize is that supplements containing DMG may cause chromosome damage in cells.

• **Gamma butyrolactone** (GBL) is commercially available as an industrial solvent and is used as an ingredient in cleaners, solvents, paint removers, and engine degreasers. It is also sold as a natural supplement over the Internet and in some health food stores and gymnasiums, and it is marketed as a natural, nontoxic dietary supplement. Manufacturers of GBL claim that it builds muscle, improves physical performance, and acts as an aphrodisiac.

Although labeled as a dietary supplement, GBL and products containing it are illegal drugs marketed under various trade names, including Renewtrient, Revivarant, Blue Nitro, GH Revitalizer, Gamma G, and Remforce. The FDA has issued a recall on products containing GBL because of at least 55 adverse events, including one death. Read ingredient labels on supplements to make sure you avoid this substance.

• **Plant sterols** are naturally occurring steroids extracted from plants that are promoted to exercisers, strength trainers, and athletes. They include gamma oryzanol, found in rice bran oil; Smilax, an herbal extract that is advertised as a natural form of testosterone; beta-sitosterol, a lipid extract; and ferulic acid, another type of lipid extract. The research that has been done so far with these supplements indicates that they have no effect on body composition in people who exercise. Some people may be sensitive to these substances, which can cause allergies and possibly anaphylactic shock.

Table 8.3   Rating the Supplements

Supplement	Meets marketing claims	Possibly meets marketing claims	Does not meet marketing claims	Potentially harmful
Caffeine	•			
Carbohydrate–protein sport drinks	•			
Creatine	•			
Glucose–electrolyte solutions	•			
Weight-gain powders	•			
Arginine		•		
Beta-alanine		•		
Beta-hydroxy-beta-methylbutyrate (HMB)		•		
Branched-chain amino acids (BCAAs)		•		
Carnitine		•		
Carnosine		•		
Coenzyme Q10 (CoQ10)		•		
Conjugated linoleic acid (CLA)		•		
Glucosamine/chondroitin sulfate		•		
Glutamine		•		
Glycerol		•		
MCT oil		•		
N-acetyl cysteine (NAC)		•		
Phosphatidylserine (PS)		•		
Protein supplements		•		
Ribose		•		
Taurine		•		
Inosine			•	
Pyruvate			•	
Tryptophan			•	
Zinc–magnesium			•	
Amino acids				•
Androstenedione				•
Bee pollen				•
Dehydroepiandrosterone (DHEA)				•
Dimethylglycine (DMG; vitamin B_{15})				•
Gamma butyrolactone (GBL)				•
Plant sterols				•

Diet Is Still Key

Building fit, firm muscle isn't as easy as just exercising and supplementing; there's a lot more to it than that. You can't neglect a good diet. Learn how to develop your Power Eating plan in chapters 10 and 11, and refer to the sample strength-training diets in chapters 12 through 15. Above all, eat enough quality calories each day to fuel your body for exercise and activity.

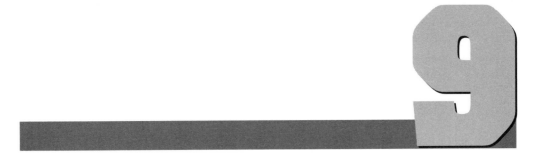

Performance Herbs

Herbs are the most popular self-prescribed medication. They now come in capsules, tablets, liquids, and powders. Of the $1.2 billion dietary supplement industry in the United States, $700 million is spent on herbal supplements alone. There is a lot of promotion of herbs as bodybuilding supplements. Yet there's little evidence that herbs can help you, and they may even do harm.

An herb is a plant or part of a plant valued for its medicinal qualities, its aroma, or its taste. Herbs and herbal remedies have been around for centuries. Even Neanderthal people used plants for healing purposes. About 30 percent of all modern drugs are derived from herbs. The information in this chapter can help guide you through the often-confusing maze of which herbs can be helpful and which may be harmful.

Natural, but Not Always Safe

It's a common but dangerous notion to think that because herbs are natural, they are safe. What separates plant-derived drugs from herbal supplements is careful scientific study. Makers of herbal supplements in the United States are not required to submit their products to the FDA, so there is no regulation of product quality or safety. Without the enforcement of standards, there is a meager chance that the contents and potency described on labels are accurate.

Some eye-opening proof of this was found in a study conducted at the UCLA Center for Human Nutrition. Researchers analyzed commercial formulations of saw palmetto, kava kava, echinacea, ginseng, and Saint-John's-wort. They purchased six bottles each of two lots of supplements from nine manufacturers and analyzed their contents. There were differences in what was actually in the product versus what was stated on the labels, particularly with echinacea and ginseng. Even the product labels varied in the information provided. Dosage recommendations and information about the herb often varied.

This study reflects an important problem with herbal products. When products are not standardized but are being tested in research for effectiveness, you can't really get conclusive evidence on what works and what doesn't, no matter how well a study is designed. What you may be taking may not be the same in any way as the extract that was tested.

Herbs are classified as food supplements by the FDA. Labeling them as medicines would require stringent testing to prove their safety and effectiveness. This costs millions of dollars per herb, an investment few manufacturers are willing to make.

Fortunately for consumers, supplements can no longer be labeled with unsubstantiated claims. The latest government regulations require that the supplement industry abide by the same food-labeling laws that govern packaged foods. This means that any supplement bearing a health claim must support the claim with scientific evidence that meets government approval. Any product marketed as a way to cure, modify, treat, or prevent disease is regulated as a drug by the FDA.

What you see on supplement labels now are structure and function claims. This means that manufacturers are allowed to make claims about the impact of dietary supplements on the structure or function of the body, but these claims must be truthful. An example of such a claim is, "Vitamin C is involved in immune function."

It's not uncommon to have an allergic reaction to drugs, even though these medicines have been tested and manufactured with strict safeguards. Therefore, it is even more likely that untested herbs, which are consumed in large amounts, may also produce allergic reactions. These reactions can sometimes be fatal. Herbs can interact with prescribed medications, too. If you're taking any medications, you should consult your physician, pharmacist, or dietitian before using any herbal supplement.

In addition, if you're scheduled for surgery and are taking herbal supplements, let your physician know well in advance of your operation. Certain herbs, particularly gingko biloba, garlic, ginger, and ginseng, interfere with normal blood clotting and can lead to excessive blood loss during surgery. Mood-boosting herbs such as Saint-John's-wort and kava kava dangerously heighten the sedative effects of anesthesia.

Pregnant and nursing mothers should avoid all herbal preparations. Ask your physician or dietitian about specific herbal teas, because even these can cause harmful reactions in a developing baby or nursing infant. Don't give herbal supplements or remedies to children, either. There is virtually no medical information about the safety of herbs for children. Your best intentions could be terribly harmful.

Because there's no universal quality-control regulation of the industry, the danger of chemical contamination of herbal supplements is real. Were the plants sprayed with any chemicals before harvesting or processing? Other toxic contaminants or banned or illegal substances may enter the product during processing as well. For instance, a study testing herbal products for prohibited anabolic androgen steroids and GH found that 15 percent contained prohormones (variants of hormones) that were not declared on the label. Most of these substances were manufactured in the United States but were sold in European countries. Products that are purchased by mail order from other countries are even more questionable than those purchased in the United States.

The following is a rundown of well-known herbs, either sold alone or as an ingredient in fitness supplements. I have classified these herbs in a manner similar to the classifications of sport supplements in chapter 8. According to current sport science research, some meet their marketing claims, and others are possibly useful. Table 9.1 on page 194 provides a quick reference for the effectiveness of the many performance herbs on the market.

Meets Marketing Claims

Much of this research has been conducted outside the United States, but experts agree that these products have been well-tested for their efficacy. Even so, herbs can act as powerful drugs. Approach them with the same respect as you would any prescription medication.

Buchu

Derived from a shrub native to South Africa, the leaves of this herb are usually made into a tea and other supplement forms. Buchu is a mild diuretic, and in that regard it may help rid your body of excess water weight. It is also an antiseptic that fights germs in the urinary tract.

Buchu is generally considered safe, although herbalists recommend taking no more than 2 grams two or three times a day.

Fo-Ti

Ancient Chinese herbalists swore that this member of the buckwheat family is one of the best longevity promoters ever grown. As herbalists see it, fo-ti exhibits different properties depending on the size and age of its root. A fist-sized 50-year-old plant, for example, keeps your hair from turning gray. A 100-year-old root the size of a bowl preserves your cheerfulness. At 150 years old and as large as a sink, fo-ti makes your teeth fall out so that new ones can grow in. And a 200-year-old plant restores youth and vitality. Or so the folk tales go.

Fo-ti has a reputation as a good cardiovascular herb. Supposedly, it lowers cholesterol, protects blood vessels, and increases blood flow to the heart. Fo-ti does act as a natural laxative, however, and in this regard it's probably a safe herb.

Guarana

Guarana is a red berry from a plant grown in the Amazon valley. It contains seven times the caffeine as coffee beans and is widely sold in health food stores as a supplement to increase energy. It is also found in energy drinks and energy waters. The supplement is made from the seeds of the berry.

Guarana is used in a number of natural weight-loss supplements. It is believed to increase thermogenesis (body heat) and thus stimulate the metabolism. Guarana may also cause the body to lose water because the caffeine it contains is a diuretic. As for a possible performance benefit, guarana has been shown to increase blood glucose in animals. Whether that holds true for humans, however, remains to be seen. A note of caution: If you're sensitive to caffeine, it's best to leave guarana alone.

Maté

Another caffeinated herb is maté. Touted as a natural upper, it has a caffeine content of 2 percent. Maté is found in some natural weight-loss supplements because it is believed to help control appetite. Like guarana, it is found in energy drinks and energy waters. It also has a mild diuretic effect and thus may produce temporary water weight loss. Medical experts say the herb is relatively safe when taken in small quantities for short periods of time.

Please keep in mind that both guarana and maté contain caffeine. I've had clients come to me, thrilled that they are off caffeine, only to find out that they've been drinking energy waters containing one of these herbs! They haven't quit caffeine at all; they went from caffeine in their coffee to caffeine in their herbal water. Read labels to watch out for these herbs.

Possibly Meets Marketing Claims

Research is still not clear on whether the claims made about these herbs are true—maybe they are, maybe they aren't. If you try these herbs, remember that you are being the guinea pig. It may be preferable to wait and see how the research pans out before trying them yourself.

Ciwujia

Ciwujia is the Chinese term for eleuthero, also known as Siberian ginseng. According to noted herbalist and author Christopher Hobbs, writing in his book *Ginseng: The Energy Herb* (Botanica Press, 1996), "With over 35 years of intense clinical and practical research behind it, eleuthero is taken by millions of Russians daily. It is used by the Russian Olympic team, especially weight lifters and runners. The extract was used by cosmonauts to adapt to radically different conditions in outer space. Among others, mountain climbers, sailors, and factory workers all use eleuthero regularly to increase adaptability, reduce sick days, and promote increased endurance."

Ciwujia is the herbal constituent of a number of performance-enhancing supplements. Despite its popularity, a recent study that reviewed the data on ciwujia concluded that supplementation up to 1,200 milligrams daily for one to six weeks does not enhance performance during exercise. A few studies have found that the herb may improve cardiovascular fitness and fat metabolism, but these studies are flawed and therefore not really valid. Ciwujia is questionable at best.

Echinacea

Echinacea is a member of the sunflower family. There are three species used medicinally—purpurea, angustifolia, and pallida. The German Commission E, Germany's equivalent to the U.S. FDA, has approved *Echinacea purpurea* as supportive therapy for colds and chronic infections of the respiratory tract. The Commission's monograph, a publication describing scores of herbs and their therapeutic applications, notes that echinacea preparations increase the number of white blood cells in the body. White blood cells destroy invading organisms, including cold viruses.

A stringent scientific review study of echinacea conducted in 2006 analyzed 16 trials of the herb. It concluded that some evidence has found that the aerial parts of *Echinacea purpurea* are effective for the early treatment of colds in adults, but that these results are not fully consistent.

Weakened immunity is often seen in athletes and highly active people—which is why many sport scientists recommend supplementing with echinacea. However, I am not one of them. One reason is that if you suffer from hay fever, taking echinacea puts you at risk for a severe reaction, even anaphylactic shock, a life-threatening allergic reaction. Allergies in general appear to be on the rise, so I believe that taking an herb like this is not worth the risk.

Don't supplement with echinacea if you have an autoimmune disease such as lupus or a progressive illness such as multiple sclerosis, because the herb may overstimulate your immune system and do further damage. Also, don't take echinacea orally for longer than eight weeks.

Green Tea

Derived from the leaves and leaf buds of an evergreen plant native to Asia, green tea is of interest to fitness-minded people because it may help encourage weight loss. Certain natural chemicals called *catechins* are abundant in green tea; animal and human studies show that these chemicals appear to increase fat burning and stimulate thermogenesis, the calorie-burning process that occurs as a result of digesting and metabolizing food.

Let's look at a few examples from the scientific literature. A study by Japanese researchers in 2001 reported that tea catechins (600 milligrams per day) taken with a standard diet for 12 weeks in men promoted weight loss, a decrease in BMI, and a decrease in waist circumference compared with subjects who consumed a placebo with a small amount of catechins.

To begin to understand the mechanisms of exactly what happens in the body and how the catechins work, these researchers conducted a more recent study of the effects of tea catechins on energy and fat metabolism in rats. The rats were fed an extract of catechins from green tea with a minimal amount of caffeine. The study results showed that the tea catechins helped suppress diet-induced obesity in rats that were fed a high-fat diet. Since minimal caffeine was available in the tea extract, the effect was attributed primarily to the tea catechins and not to caffeine. According to the researchers, the effects may be attributed in part to a stimulation of fat metabolism in the liver, and long-term tea consumption has the potential to influence the accumulation of body fat.

Most of the studies thus far have been conducted using green tea, and secondly oolong tea, so right now these would be your teas of choice. The amount that you need to consume isn't clear yet. A 1999 study in Maryland used 6 1/4 cups (1.5 liters) of tea per day for four days. The more recent Japanese study (just described) found successful results feeding 2 1/2 cups (591 milliliters) every day for 12 weeks. If you are sensitive to caffeine, you might want to start with the lower dose, and definitely don't drink the tea in the evening before bed.

Whether or not green tea pans out as an antiobesity agent, it's worth drinking for other reasons. Research has found that the natural chemicals in green tea may protect against periodontal disease, some cancers, and heart disease. Unless you're sensitive to caffeine, green tea or extracts containing it are very safe and probably beneficial to health.

Does Not Meet Marketing Claims

These products don't have enough research to back up the marketing claims. I wouldn't waste my money on them. At another time in history, this category would have been called "snake oil."

• **Burdock** is a relative of the dandelion and is often called a blood purifier, a diuretic, a treatment for skin diseases such as acne and psoriasis, and a diaphoretic (sweat producer). None of these claims has been verified scientifically, and no solid evidence exists that burdock has any useful therapeutic effects. In addition, there have been reports of poisonings caused by burdock tea contaminated with belladonna, a harmful herb.

• **Canaigre** is deceptively promoted as a less expensive American alternative to real ginseng (see page 193) but in no way is it related to ginseng, either botanically or chemically. Native to the southwestern United States and Mexico, canaigre has been recommended by herbal enthusiasts for a variety of problems ranging from lack of energy to leprosy. Trouble is, canaigre is potentially cancer causing because of its high content of tannin.

• **Citrus aurantium** (also known as bitter orange or synephrine) is the botanical name of the Chinese fruit zhishi. An alkaloid called *synephrine* is extracted from this fruit and used as an ingredient in numerous fitness supplements. Synephrine is a chemical cousin to ephedrine (an alkaloid found in the herb ephedra) but has few of ephedrine's adverse side effects. (See the section later on ephedra.) Synephrine is thought to suppress the appetite, increase the metabolic rate, and help burn fat by stimulating the action of fat-burning enzymes inside cells. To date, though, there are no published studies on synephrine as a fat burner.

• **Coleus forskohlii** is a member of the mint family and has been used extensively for many applications in Indian (ayurvedic) medicine. Its active ingredient, diterpene forskolin, activates adenylate cyclase, an enzyme that increases cyclic adenosine monophosphate (cAMP) in cells. The synthesis of cAMP influences many biological systems, including the breakdown of stored fat in animal and human fat cells. This enzyme also regulates the body's thermic response to food, increases the metabolic rate, and activates fat burning.

The theory behind using this herb is that if you can stimulate fatty acid metabolism, then you can lose body fat while saving lean muscle tissue. Even so, research on coleus forskohlii does not substantiate this effect, and the herb does not appear to promote weight loss.

• **Cordyceps** is a mushroom native to mountainous regions of China and Tibet, and it is unusual in that it grows on caterpillar larvae. Cordyceps is available as a performance supplement, believed to open breathing passages to let more oxygen circulate. With more oxygen available to cells, endurance increases. Research fails to substantiate this effect, however. Although cordyceps is described as safe and gentle, little information exists on its safety.

• **Damiana** comes from the leaves of a Mexican shrub. Around the turn of the century, it was touted as a powerful aphrodisiac. Closer scientific scrutiny of damiana revealed that it has no aphrodisiac properties or beneficial physiological action whatsoever.

- **Gotu kola**, a member of the parsley family, is a common weed, usually found growing in drainage ditches in Asia and orchards in Hawaii. A known effect of this herb is that it fights water retention by helping the body eliminate excess fluid. It is also a central nervous system stimulant and believed to be a lipotropic, or fat-burning, herb. Gotu kola is also a constituent of numerous cellulite-fighting supplements. However, the *Physician's Desk Reference (PDR) for Herbal Medicines* does not cite research supporting any of these claims for gotu kola.

Because of its stimulating effect, you should avoid gotu kola if you have any chronic medical conditions. Side effects may include insomnia and nervousness.

- **Hoodia** *(Hoodia gordonii)* is a spiny succulent that grows in the Kalahari Desert on the border of South Africa and Namibia. For thousands of years, it has been used by the Xhomani Bushmen, a people indigenous to the region, to stave off pain, hunger, and thirst during long-distance travel over the vast desert. In the 1960s, South African researches began studying the plant after the Xhomani revealed the plant's secrets to the South African army. Since then, hoodia has been studied for its various properties, including its ability to reduce weight by suppressing appetite. Only recently has it been introduced as a natural dietary supplement for weight control. But there haven't really been any human studies on hoodia, so we just don't know if the claims are valid.

- **Saw palmetto** is one of several plants approved in Germany to help men with benign prostatic hypertrophy (BPH), an enlargement of the prostate gland. Purportedly, saw palmetto increases urinary flow, cuts the frequency of urination, and makes it easier to pass urine. It is used by more than 2 million men in the United States to treat BPH. But does it work?

Well-designed research shows that the herb does not improve symptoms of BPH, nor does it help improve prostatitis, or chronic pelvic syndrome, which causes pain in the groin with or without urinary symptoms such as an urgency or frequency in the need to urinate.

- **Tribulus terrestris**, also known as puncture weed, is a popular strength-training herb. This herb is believed to be a natural steroid that increases testosterone, enhances muscle mass, and boosts strength. Unfortunately, it does none of these, according to recent research.

Potentially Harmful

These products have been shown to cause harm and are not worth the risk. While some of these products may offer a few benefits, the risks are not worth the benefits.

- **Ephedra** is the world's oldest known cultivated plant, also known as ma huang, Chinese ephedra, or Mormon tea, and is a short-acting stimulant and effective weight-loss aid, and may be found in some cold remedies. Ephedra in dietary supplements was banned by the FDA several years ago due to safety concerns, including its harmful effect on the cardiovascular system. In April 2005, however, a federal judge struck down the ban, saying that the FDA was regulating ephedra as a drug and not as a food. The ruling allows supplement companies to bring back ephedra, but most haven't because of the bad press. In fact, many supplement makers now proudly market their products as ephedra free.

Ephedra has a lot of side effects, including nervousness, agitation, and rapid heartbeat. It can make the heart race and blood pressure soar, and it can be lethal in people with heart conditions, high blood pressure, or diabetes.

- **Ginseng** has been used for thousands of years in the East as a tonic to strengthen and restore health. More recently, ginseng has been touted as a performance-boosting herb for exercisers and athletes. For background, ginseng comes from the root of a medicinal plant in the ginseng family (Araliaceae). There are various types of ginseng, including those in the Panax classification and a botanical cousin known as Siberian ginseng, or eleuthero, for short. *Panax ginseng* and eleuthero are approved medicines in Germany.

The main active constituents of the Panax species are plant steroids called *ginsenosides*. The active constituents of eleuthero are plant steroids known as eleutherosides, which differ in chemical structure from ginsenosides but have similar properties. The performance-enhancing effects of *Panax ginseng* in humans have been explored rather extensively, though studies have often yielded mixed results.

The most valid explanation for the conflicting research on ginseng is the wide variability found among commercial ginseng products.

It can be difficult to know what you're buying. In addition, taking ginseng is a questionable practice. There are known side effects of large doses and long-term use: high blood pressure, nervousness, insomnia, low blood pressure, sedation, painful breasts, breast nodules, and vaginal bleeding. In addition, ginseng reacts with many drugs.

- **Pau d'arco**, as an herbal agent, is found as a tea or in cosmetic preparations. The name *pau d'arco* refers to the bark of various species of trees. Pau d'arco is often billed as a cancer cure. Indeed, the bark contains a tiny amount of lapachol, an agent shown in research to have anticancer properties, but pau d'arco is potentially toxic and not to be fooled with.

- **Sassafras**, usually found as a tea, is a well-known herb that may sound like a cure-all. It has been promoted as a stimulant; a muscle relaxant; a sweat producer; a blood purifier; and a treatment for rheumatism, skin diseases, and typhus. However, none of these benefits has been supported or even documented by medical science. Furthermore, sassafras contains an oil called safrole, which is carcinogenic.

Table 9.1 Rating the Herbal Supplements				
Supplement	**Meets marketing claims**	**Possibly meets marketing claims**	**Does not meet marketing claims**	**Potentially harmful**
Buchu	•			
Fo-ti	•			
Guarana	•			
Mate	•			
Ciwujia		•		
Echinacea		•		
Green tea		•		
Burdock			•	
Canaigre			•	
Citrus aurantium			•	
Coleus forskohlii			•	
Cordyceps			•	
Damiana			•	
Gotu kola			•	
Hoodia			•	
Saw palmetto			•	
Tribulus terrestris			•	
Ephedra (ma huang)				•
Ginseng				•
Pau d'arco				•
Sassafras				•
White willow bark				•
Yohimbe				•

• **White willow bark**, derived from the willow trees native to central and southern Europe, contains an active ingredient called *salicin*. Salicin is a natural anti-inflammatory agent related to the compound used to make aspirin—which is why white willow bark has often been dubbed the "natural aspirin." If you are sensitive or allergic to aspirin, you should not be taking this herb. Both aspirin and white willow bark are a source of salicylates, which trigger allergic reactions in susceptible people.

• **Yohimbe** is an herb derived from the bark of an evergreen grown in West Africa. It is best known for its aphrodisiac properties, because it stimulates erection. An extract of the herb, yohimbine, is available as a prescription drug for treating erectile dysfunction.

Yohimbe stimulates the release of noradrenaline (norephedrine), a hormone that raises body temperature and helps liberate fatty acids from cells to be burned as fuel, and for this reason is included in some natural weight-loss supplements. However, very little research supports its use as a fat-burner. Yohimbe is considered a dangerous herb even by herbalists' standards. It can cause anxiety, elevated blood pressure, irregular heartbeats, headaches, painful erections, flushing, hallucinations, kidney failure, seizures, and death.

Precautions

If you're still curious and want to try an herbal supplement, do so with care by following these few precautions: Start with low doses. More is not necessarily better and could be dangerous. Take only one type of supplement at a time. Allow at least 24 hours in between supplements before changing the dosage or starting something new. Keep empty bottles on hand for a while so that if you have an adverse reaction, you can provide information about the supplement to your doctor.

Sport Nutrition Fact Versus Fiction:

Are Functional Foods the New Training Staple?

If you've ever bitten into a sport bar, swilled a glass of calcium-fortified orange juice, or slurped a soup beefed up with herbs such as Saint-John's-wort or echinacea, you've feasted on a functional food.

Technically, the term *functional food* refers to a food product that enhances performance or is beneficial to health. In its position paper on functional foods, the American Dietetic Association defines these products as "any modified food or food ingredient that may provide a health benefit beyond the traditional nutrients it contains."

Products that fit this definition include the following:

- Foods in which sugar, fat, sodium, or cholesterol have been reduced or eliminated. Fat-free cheese, reduced-sugar jam, or low-sodium soup are all examples. Functional foods like these are beneficial to people on restricted diets and may be helpful in preventing or controlling obesity, cardiovascular disease, diabetes, and high blood pressure.

- Foods in which naturally occurring ingredients have been increased. Breakfast cereal and pasta that have been enriched with additional fiber or vitamins are good examples. Foods modified in this way can play an important role in preventing disease.

- Foods enhanced with nutrients not normally present. Folic acid–enriched bread and soups or soft drinks spruced up with therapeutic herbs are good examples. Enriched foods help people take in higher levels of health-protective nutrients and can be important in maintaining general wellness.

- Probiotic yogurt and other dairy products to which special healthy bacteria have been added as a part of the fermentation process. These foods are believed to enhance healthy flora in the intestines, which improve digestion and prevent disease.

- Sport foods targeting the nutrient and energy needs of athletes and exercisers. These include sport drinks with added electrolytes; protein powders formulated with creatine, amino acids, and other nutrients; and sport bars packed with vitamins, minerals, or herbs. Functional foods like these are designed to provide energy, enhance muscle growth, and replenish nutrients lost during exercise.

Should you incorporate these foods into your diet if you're not already doing so?

The answer is yes, particularly if convenience is important and you're trying to enhance muscular health, strength, and growth. Sport foods, in particular, can help you achieve those goals. However, think of functional foods as supplements to your diet rather than substitutes for real food. Ultimately, the best way to fuel your body is always by eating a varied, nutrient-rich diet of lean protein and dairy products, fruits, whole grains, vegetables, and the right kinds of fat.

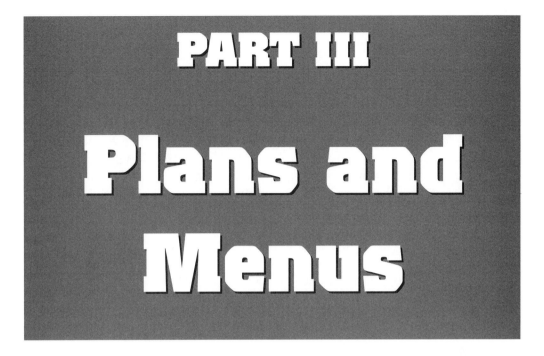

PART III

Plans and Menus

Here's where you put your knowledge to work. You have the foundation, the information, and hopefully, the inspiration. Now let's put it all into practice, designing your own personalized Power Eating plan. To begin, determine your goals: Do you want to maintain, build, lose fat, or cut? Are you in your off-season trying to gain, or approaching a championship and planning for a peak? Are you new to strength training or have you been training for years? Chapter 10 will walk you through the same steps that I take as I design a client's customized nutrition plan. With the information here, you can figure your calories and map out your protein, carbohydrate, and fat needs based on your personal goals, just as I would if you came to my office. Chapter 10 also provides you with the information you need to customize all of the menu plans presented later in this part. Chapter 11 gives you the ultimate competitive nutrition strategies on how to prepare your body to peak for competition. I've kept no top-level professional secrets from these pages—it's all here.

Each of the four diet strategies (maintenance, building, losing fat, cutting) in chapters 12 through 15 offers a menu plan designed especially for novice strength trainers or those who workout three to four times per week and for highly-muscled strength trainers who workout five or more times per week. The menu plans are also divided into plans geared for women and for men. The plans begin with the mathematical models that I designed to create the menus.

By plugging in your weight, you can create your own personalized diet plan. The menus in this section are provided as examples and are based on the needs of a 180-pound (82-kilogram) man and a 130-pound (59-kilogram) woman.

The menus are similar to each other in food choices so that you can easily move from one strategy to the next as your training goals change. Some menus place exercise in the morning and some in the late afternoon so that you can see how to customize your own menu to your training schedule. Always make sure to have a preworkout snack and a postworkout snack or meal. Menu planning takes some time and effort, but the results will be worth it!

Once you've designed your diet, have some fun with the recipes in chapter 16. This section includes my special power drinks, which I created for the clients and teams I've worked with over the years. These drinks can be used in place of liquid supplements. Add liquid or powdered supplements to them for an extra boost. My family and I particularly enjoy the smoothies, and we make them daily. They're a great way to sneak in extra protein and fruit servings. Don't miss the power breakfasts, either—they will give your day a tasty and energy-charged start.

Most of all, train hard and Power Eat!

10

Developing a Power Eating Plan

The Power Eating plan is based on several strategies. First, I determine the proper calorie level for the goal of the plan and then the right distribution of protein, fat, and carbohydrate to meet that goal. Menu development is based on a food group plan that I have tweaked just a bit based on state-of-the-art nutrition science. Food groups force you to have variety in your diet and at the same time allow you to personalize your program through food choices and exchanges between food groups. Use the sample diets as a starting point and then add or subtract servings to meet your protein, carbohydrate, and fat needs.

There are a lot of examples of fat servings, which is done purposely to give you the freedom to personalize your plan. Nonfat milk and very lean and lean protein sources are the primary choices included in the meal plans. This is to accommodate adding healthier fat from sources such as vegetable oils, nuts, and seeds in place of animal fat that is higher in saturated fat. You will also count any low-fat or fat-free protein supplements as very lean protein servings.

To use more medium-fat protein sources such as soy products, as well as the occasional high-fat protein source, just exchange one very lean protein serving plus one fat serving for one medium-fat protein serving. Exchange one lean protein serving plus one fat serving for one high-fat protein serving. Refer to the Nutrients per Food Group Serving chart to become proficient at food group exchanges. Remember that you can easily determine your fat grams once you have calculated your total calories, protein, and carbohydrate needs. All the leftover calories are fat calories. Divide fat calories by 9 to get your total fat grams per day.

You will also be able to add in teaspoons of sugar and sport drinks and learn how to use these to your advantage. These are high-glycemic foods that can assist you in muscle recovery.

A note on alcohol: Alcohol is metabolized more similarly to fat than any of the other macronutrients. Too much alcohol on a regular basis will slow your training, halt your fat loss, and even impair your health and safety. Thus, alcohol is not part of the Power Eating plan.

Creating Your Diet Plan

Once you have calculated your daily nutrient and calorie needs, use the table that follows to design your diet. This table shows the amount of nutrients in one serving from each food group. Make sure that you include choices from all of the food groups to ensure a well-balanced diet. Add liquid supplements to meet additional carbohydrate, protein, omega-3 fats, and calorie needs. Refer to the charts on serving size guidelines on pages 201 through 204 for a representation of foods and serving sizes for each food group.

Nutrients Per Food Group Serving				
Food groups	**Carbohydrate (g)**	**Protein (g)**	**Fat (g)**	**Calories**
Bread and starch	15	3	1 or less	72-81
Fruit	15	-	-	60
Milk				
Nonfat	12	8	0-1	80-89
Low fat	12	8	3	107
Added Sugar (1 tsp)	4	-	-	16
Vegetables	5	2	-	25
Meat and meat substitutes				
Very lean	-	7	0-1	35
Lean	-	7	3	55
Medium	-	7	5	75
Fat	-	-	5	45

Adapted from the American Diabetes Association and the American Dietetic Association, 1995, *Exchange Lists for Meal Planning.*

Knowing Your Portions

A portion is the amount of food used to determine the numbers of servings for each food group. It is not always the amount of food that you would think of as a serving, however. For example, one portion of cooked pasta is just 1/2 cup (70 grams). But if you have pasta for dinner, you would likely eat at least 1 cup (140 grams). One cup of pasta equals two servings from the bread and starch group.

Learning the portion sizes for servings is the foundation of success. It is the method by which calorie control is built into the Power Eating plan. If you are eating portions that are too large or too small, the plan will not work. Look at the following chart for a list of foods and serving sizes for each food group. In the beginning, you should refer to this chart frequently, as well as weigh and measure foods to get a handle on portion sizes. After a few weeks, you will be able to do it on your own.

Milk and Yogurt Group

A portion equals 90-110 calories.

Food	Size of one portion
Nonfat or low-fat milk	1 c (236 ml)
Evaporated nonfat milk	1 c (236 ml)
Nonfat dry milk powder	1/3 c (22g)
Plain nonfat yogurt	1 c (245 g)
Nonfat or low-fat soy or rice milk, fortified with calcium and vitamins A & D	1 c (236 ml)

Vegetable Group

Each portion contains 25 calories.

Food	Size of one portion
Most cooked vegetables	1/2 c (81 g)
Most raw vegetables	1 c (30-100 g)
Sprouts	1 c (30 g)
Vegetable juice	6 oz (177 ml)
Vegetable soup	1 c (236 ml)
Tomato sauce	1/2 c (118 ml)
Salsa (made without oil)	3 tbsp (45 g)

Fruit Group

A portion contains 60 calories.

Food	Size of one portion
Most fruits, whole	1 medium
Most fruits, chopped or canned in own juice	1/2 c (118 g)
Melon, diced	1 c (156 g)
Berries, cherries, grapes (whole)	3/4 c (80 g)
Fruit juice	1/2 c (118 ml)
Banana	1 small
Grapefruit, mango	1/2
Plums	2 each
Apricots	4 each
Strawberries (whole)	1-1/4 c (180 g)
Kiwi	1 each
Prunes, dried	3 each
Figs	2 each
Raisins	2 tbsp (28 g)
Juice—cranberry, grape, fruit blends (100% juice)	1/3 c (78 ml)
Cranberry juice cocktail (reduced calorie)	1 c (236 ml)

Bread and Starch Group

Each portion has 60 to 100 calories.

Food	Size of one portion
Bread	1 slice
Pita	1 small (1 oz)
Bagel, English muffin, bun	1/2 small (1 oz)
Roll	1 small
Cooked rice, cooked pasta	1/2 c (97 g)
Tortilla	6 in. round (15 cm)
Crackers, large	2, or 3-4 small
Croutons	1/3 c (13 g)
Pretzels, baked chips	1 oz (28 g)
Rice cakes	2 each
Cooked cereal	1/2 c (119 g)
Cold cereal, unsweetened	1/2-1 c (15-30 g)
Granola	1/2 c (30 g)
Corn, green peas, mashed potato	1/2 c (105 g)
Corn on the cob	1 medium
White or sweet potato baked with skin	1 small

Protein

Each protein portion contains about 35 to 75 calories. Very lean servings contain 35 calories and 0 to 1 grams of fat; lean, 55 calories and 3 grams of fat; and medium-fat, 75 calories and 5 grams of fat.

Food	Size of one portion
Very lean	
White meat skinless poultry	1 oz (28 g)
White fish	1 oz (28 g)
Fresh or canned tuna in water	1 oz (28 g)
All shellfish	1 oz (28 g)
Beans, peas, and lentils*	1/2 c (100 g)
Cheeses and processed sandwich meat with 1 gram of fat	1 oz (28 g)
Egg whites	2 each
Lean	
Select or choice grades of lean beef, pork, lamb, or veal trimmed to 0 fat	1 oz (28 g)
Dark meat skinless poultry or white meat chicken with skin	1 oz (28 g)
Oysters, salmon, catfish, sardines, tuna canned in oil	1 oz (28 g)
Cheese and deli sandwich meat with 3 grams of fat	1 oz (28 g)
Parmesan cheese	1 oz (28 g)
Medium-fat	
Most styles of beef, pork, lamb, veal—trimmed of fat, dark meat poultry with skin	1 oz (28 g)
Ground turkey or chicken	1 oz (28 g)
Cheese with 5 grams of fat	1 oz (28 g)
Cottage cheese 4.5% fat	1/4 c (56 g)
Whole egg	1 each
Tempeh	4 oz or 1/2 c (113 g)
Tofu	4 oz or 1/2 c (113 g)

*One portion counts as 1 very lean protein and 1 starch.

Added Sugar

There is no way that I could give you an exhaustive list of all the added sugar in foods. No food manufacturer puts that information on the label. But you can figure it out yourself, just like I do, by following these basic guidelines. Every 1 tsp (4 g), or serving, of sugar contains 4 g of carbohydrate and 16 calories (no protein or fat).

Cereals and grains

Grains do not contain any sugar. If you look at the Nutrition Facts label on the side of a box of cereal like Shredded Wheat, you'll see 0 g of sugar in a serving. Therefore, the manufacturer adds any sugar contained in a cereal. Most sweetened cereals contain 8 g of sugar per serving, which is the equivalent of 2 tsp of added sugar, and many contain much more. The exception is cereals with added fruit. Some of the sugar will come from the fruit. Look at the ingredient label. If any kind of sugar is listed ahead of the fruit, you know that the greatest proportion of the added sugar is not from the fruit. The same concept goes for breads, crackers, and other grain products. Any sugar on the label is added in processing.

Yogurt and milk

One cup (8 oz, or 237 ml) of milk contains 12 g of natural milk sugar, or lactose. If you look at the Nutrition Facts label on a carton of milk, you will see that one serving (1 cup) contains 12 g of sugar. Any amount of sugar above that is added, as in chocolate milk and other flavored milks.

Yogurt cartons are generally 6 oz (170 g). A carton of plain yogurt will contain about 12 g of natural milk sugar. Anything above that is added sugar. Most yogurts are sweetened with at least 4 tsp (16 g) of added sugar, and many use 6 (24) or more.

Fruit and fruit juices

A medium-sized piece of fruit contains about 15 g of carbohydrate. Some of that is fiber, often 2-3 g, and the rest is natural fruit sugar. When purchasing canned or frozen fruits and fruit juices, you must read the ingredients label to check for added sugar. Any amount of sugar above 13 g for 1/2 cup (122 g) of canned or frozen fruit or 1/2 cup (119 ml) of fruit juice is added to the product.

Vegetables, vegetable juices, and soups

A medium-sized vegetable contains 5 g of carbohydrate and no sugar. Any sugar listed on the Nutrition Facts label is added to the product.

Beverages

Water contains no natural sugar. If you're looking at the Nutrition Facts label on the side of a can of soft drink, all the sugar is added, and it usually amounts to about 10 tsp (40 g) per 12 oz (355 ml) can. Typical sport drinks contain about 12 g of sugar per cup, equivalent to 3 tsp (12 g) of added sugar per serving. This same principle can be applied to most bottled beverages that do not contain any milk or fruit juice. When it comes to fruit juice concentrates added as sweetners to beverages and foods, the juice is highly refined in the processing and is little more than sugar syrup. Ingredients like white grape juice concentrate are virtually the same as added sugar.

Fats and Oils

Each portion contains 45 calories.

Food	Size of portion
Diet margarine	1 tsp (5 g)
Cream cheese, cream, sour cream	1 tbsp (15 g)
Cream cheese, whipped cream, sour cream (low fat or nonfat)	1 tbsp (15 g)
Salad dressing (full fat)	1 tbsp (15 g)
Salad dressing (low fat or nonfat)	1 tbsp (15 g)
Avocado	1/8 medium (2 tbsp)
Olives, black	8 large
Nuts	6-10
Seeds	1 tbsp (9 g)
Peanut butter and other nut butters	1/2 tbsp (8 g)

Personalizing the Plan

In order to achieve the greatest strength and muscle-gain goals, follow these guidelines when designing your diet:

1. Assess Calorie Needs Based on Body Weight

As your weight changes, you must recalculate energy and nutrients. In chapters 12 through 15, I'll provide you with the calorie needs for each phase of the plan to help you do this.

• **Training to maintain muscle.** Men who train five or more times per week need 42 calories per kilogram of body weight a day (3,444 calories a day for a 180-pound [82-kilogram] man). Women who train five or more times per week may be able to increase muscle at 44 to 50 calories per kilogram of body weight a day (2,950 calories for a 130-pound [59-kilogram] woman) and maintain at about 38 to 40 calories per kilogram of body weight a day (2,360 calories). The larger and more muscular a woman, the more calories she can handle for maintenance.

Smaller women may need fewer than 38 calories per kilogram per day to maintain weight. There is a lot of trial and error with women, because all the research has been done on men and because levels of activity vary widely. For the rest of the phases, women should generally choose the lower end of the calorie ranges. This diet is great for bodybuilders, powerlifters, and weightlifters, as well as for recreational strength trainers. Novice trainers should follow the novice guidelines.

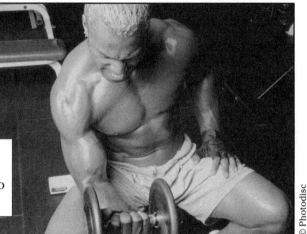

Competitive bodybuilders can use the losing fat diet to help them begin to sculpt their physiques.

© Photodisc

• **Building.** This plan requires 44 to 52 or more calories per kilogram of body weight a day, depending on intensity of training (4,264 or more calories for a 180-pound [82-kilogram] man; 2,596 to 2,950 calories for a 130-pound [59-kilogram] woman). Start low and add calories as needed. As stated earlier, women will likely be able to build at 44 calories per kilogram of body weight a day. Smaller women should try slightly fewer calories when beginning a building program and work up from there. This diet is good for all competitive and recreational strength trainers. Novice trainers should follow the novice guidelines.

• **Losing fat** (10-12 weeks of precontest dieting). To lose fat and begin to sculpt, you'll need 35 to 38 calories per kilogram of body weight a day (3,116 calories for a 180-pound [82-kilogram] man; 2,065 calories for a 130-pound [59-kilogram] woman). Because it's more difficult for women to lose fat than it is for men, women should choose the lower calorie range and increase aerobic exercise in order to burn 300 to 400 calories a day. Again, smaller women may need fewer calories. This recommendation is primarily for bodybuilders. Novice trainers should follow the novice guidelines.

• **Cutting** (7-14 days maximum). This plan requires 29 calories per kilogram of body weight a day for women (1,711 calories for a 130-pound [59-kilogram] woman) and 32 calories per kilogram of body weight a day for men (2,624 calories for a 180-pound [82-kilogram] man). If you are a smaller woman who has been losing fat on a lower calorie level, decrease recommended calories here as well. Use this approach only when absolutely necessary. This diet is only for bodybuilders or others trying to make a weight class—not for powerlifters or Olympic weightlifters.

• **Powerlifters and weightlifters trying to make a weight class.** After dieting to build muscle, go back to the maintenance diet for two weeks before your meet and use your goal weight for the calculations. This will allow for loss of body fat without loss of muscle, strength, or power. This strategy is also a good basic diet for overweight strength trainers who want to lose body fat.

2. Calculate Your Protein Needs

Protein needs change with both energy intake and training goals. Although the menu plans in chapters 12-15 provide grams per pound of body weight, you can easily convert your weight from pounds to kilograms by dividing your weight by 2.2. Make sure to cover your protein needs during all four diet strategies. If you are a vegan, add 10 percent more protein to all of the plans.

    Maintenance: 1.4 grams per kilogram of body weight a day

    Building: 2 grams per kilogram of body weight a day

    Losing fat: 2.2 grams per kilogram of body weight a day

    Cutting: 2.3 grams per kilogram of body weight a day (2.2 for those eating mostly vegetarian)

3. Calculate Your Carbohydrate Needs

Calculate your carbohydrate needs as 5 to 7 grams per kilogram of body weight a day. Strength trainers need closer to 5 to 6 grams per kilogram of body weight a day for maintenance and 6.5 to 7 grams per kilogram of body weight a day for building. Cross-trainers who do an intense ultra type of sport like an Ironman event need closer to 8 to 10 grams per kilogram of body weight a day. Novice athletes need less carbohydrate at all levels of training, but the amount will increase as they increase their training intensity.

    During losing fat and cutting phases, women and men need different amounts of carbohydrate. Here is the amount of carbohydrate needed per kilogram of body weight per day.

Losing Fat	Women: 2.5 to 3.5 grams per kilogram Men: 3 to 4 grams per kilogram
Cutting	Women: 1.8 to 2.9 grams per kilogram Men: 2.3 to 3 grams per kilogram

4. Calculate Your Fat Needs

The rest of your calories will be 25 to 30 percent of the total. Fat sources should be predominantly monounsaturated and polyunsaturated, including omega-3 fats, with much less saturated fat.

    To find the number of fat grams you need in your plan, first determine the calories of protein and carbohydrate that you have calculated for yourself (1 gram protein = 4 calories; 1 gram carbohydrate = 4 calories). Then subtract those calories from the total number of calories needed for your weight and training phase, and you have the number of fat calories that you need. Fat contains 9 calories per gram, so if you divide the fat calories by 9, you have your grams of fat.

Here's an example of a maintenance diet for a novice 180-pound (82-kilogram) man.

Calories:	33 calories per kilogram
	33×82 kg = 2,706 calories
Protein:	1.4 grams per kilogram
	1.4×82 kg = 115 g protein
Carbohydrate:	4.5 grams per kilogram
	4.5×82 kg = 369 g carbohydrate
Fat:	The leftover calories, or about 1 gram per kilogram

Calculate the calories in the protein and carbohydrate grams:

115 g protein $\times$ 4 calories/g = 460 protein calories.

369 g carbohydrate $\times$ 4 calories/g = 1,476 carbohydrate calories.

460 + 1,476 = 1,936 protein and carbohydrate calories.

Then, calculate the fat calories and grams.

2,706 total calories – 1,936 protein and carbohydrate calories = 770 fat calories.

$$\frac{770 \text{ fat calories}}{9 \text{ calories}} = 86 \text{ g of fat.}$$

So, the diet consists of 2,706 calories, 115 grams of protein, 369 grams of carbohydrate, and 86 grams of fat. Then, by using the chart of the nutritional content of food groups (page 200), you can write your own diet. Use the menus that I have written as your guide. An easy solution is to add or subtract por-

---

Power Profiles: A Winning Formula

A championship high school football team in Pennsylvania was accused by the local newspaper of taking creatine—even performance-enhancing drugs—because the players had gotten so big. But when confronted with these accusations, the coach replied, "All we are using is Dr. Susan Kleiner's Power Eating diet. That is our winning formula."

This high school won five district football championships and four state championships through 2000. In 2004 they were the Suburban One League American Conference Champs. They just won their fourth championship in a row. Since 1998, I have been working with the strength coach on nutrition strategies for the players. The players have more energy, endurance, muscle, and power during training, practices, and games. The team is always ranked in the top 20 in the nation or among those to watch nationwide.

tions from the menus that I have already written for you. For instance, if you need to subtract carbohydrate grams, remove some servings of sugar; if you need to subtract fat grams, remove some servings of fat, and so on.

Adjusting the Plan for Competitive Bodybuilders

If you're preparing for a contest, begin the losing fat phase 10 to 12 weeks before your contest. Decrease calories and increase aerobic exercise. The more aerobically fit you are, the more fat you'll burn. Aerobic exercise should be part of your all-around program, but it's even more important now. During the losing fat phase, reduce calories by primarily reducing carbohydrate and fat. Avoid carbohydrate three to four hours before aerobic exercise in order to maximize your fat-burning potential.

If you're not looking as ripped as you would like, follow the cutting program for one or two weeks before your contest. Consume 29 to 32 calories per kilogram per body weight a day for this phase. This will allow for a final loss of 3 to 4 pounds (1-2 kilograms), as long you keep your aerobic training intense. Make sure to increase your protein intake to 2.3 grams per kilogram of body weight a day.

Sticking to Your Plan

For these strategies to work, you have to stick to your Power Eating plan. Design your diet with foods that you like. Use the sample diets in chapters 12 through 15 to help you design your personal plan. If you don't like the foods you're supposed to eat, you won't stick to the plan. If you're using liquid supplements, try different brands and flavors to find supplements that you like.

Pay attention to your body and plan to eat when you're hungry. You might want to pick specific times of the day to eat rather than depending on the pace of each day. But also be aware of whether you are hungry or thirsty; sometimes we confuse thirst with hunger. Keep food and drink on hand wherever you go. The most successful strength trainers always have a backpack full of food and drink that goes with them everywhere. This way, they can stick to their timed eating patterns, and if they get hungry, they're not dependent on vending machines or other snack foods that are high in fat and sodium.

When you're trying to lose fat, you might find it difficult to eat at restaurants and it might be especially difficult to travel. If you must do either, try to find restaurants that specialize in healthy fare. They should be able to easily adjust their menu to meet your personal needs. Don't forget to ask what's in the recipe. A menu description may be misleading. You can even ask for foods that aren't on the menu—restaurants may be able to accommodate your request.

Remember to always recalculate your requirements based on your present weight. If you have gained weight during a building or bulking phase and now want to lose weight, use your new weight rather than that of the prebulking phase.

No one can do this for you. You know that to get big and strong, you have to work your body hard. You also have to fuel your body to grow, and this is the best way. Plan your diet and stick to it. You'll be thrilled with how you feel, how you look, and how you perform.

Power Profiles: Yo-Yo Dieting

Here's a familiar story: Melody B., a 35-year-old female executive, was a yo-yo dieter who could never keep her lost weight off, despite a regular program of strength training and aerobic exercise. At 5 feet, 6 inches (168 centimeters) and 150 pounds (68 kilograms), Melody had tried every fad diet, product, and diet drug there was, all to no avail. She was muscular, but her body-fat percentage was too high.

In just six weeks on the Power Eating diet, Melody lost 1 percent of her body fat and one whole dress size. After this experience, she became so excited about fitness and nutrition that she started her own health and fitness promotion company. After going on the diet, Melody had this to say: "Susan saved my life. Before, I couldn't go on any longer thinking about food all the time. Now I just know what to do and I do it, because it feels good."

Sport Nutrition Fact Versus Fiction:
Fast-Food Nutrition

If yours is an on-the-go lifestyle, you probably have to order fast food every now and then. The key is to make the right choices—those that are low in fat and high in nutrition. Fortunately, fast-food restaurants today cater to the low-fat preferences of consumers. To help you make healthy choices, the appendix on page 287 lists some best bets at fast-food restaurants.

Here are some additional fast-food tips to keep you on track:

- Always order the regular-sized sandwiches, because they are lower in fat.
- Instead of ordering a bigger sandwich, order a salad, low-fat milk, and low-fat frozen yogurt to complete your meal.
- Stay away from fried foods.
- Don't eat the high-fat tortilla shells from taco salads.
- Request that sour cream and secret sauces be left off your order.
- Top your baked potato with chili instead of fatty cheese sauce.
- Whatever you order, order just one!

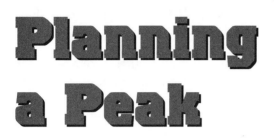

Planning a Peak

Perhaps you've decided to fine-tune your physique to look more trim, fit, and muscular. Maybe you desire to take your strength training up a notch—to competitive bodybuilding, powerlifting, or weightlifting. Or perhaps you're already a competitive strength trainer who's searching for that extra edge. No matter what your ambition, proper nutrition is the key.

You may not realize it, but the same nutritional techniques that work for bodybuilders and other athletes can also be applied to recreational exercisers and strength trainers. That's because the goals are generally the same: increasing muscularity (degree of muscular bulk), etching in definition (absence of body fat), and training for symmetry (shape and size of muscles in proportion to each other).

Whether you're trying to get in shape for swimsuit season, preparing for a bodybuilding competition, cross-training to support another sport, or building strength for your sport, you strive to reduce body fat without sacrificing muscle mass so as to reveal as much muscular definition as possible. Or perhaps one of your chief goals is building strength and muscle mass, either for looks and health or because you're a competitive powerlifter and weightlifter. In these cases, your goal is to lift as much weight as possible when you train and compete.

If you're a competitor, you'll be required to make weight to qualify for a specific weight class. You must focus on gaining and preserving muscular weight and losing body fat to achieve your contest weight. Diet therefore plays a critical role in precontest preparation for all competitive strength trainers who want to achieve peak shape.

Until recently, most strength athletes partitioned their diets into two distinct phases: a bulking phase, in which the competitor eats huge amounts of food without much regard to sound nutrition practices or to the type of calories taken in from food, and a cutting phase, in which drastic measures such as starvation dieting and drugs are used to lose weight rapidly in the weeks before a contest. Even if you're not a competitor, you've probably done something similar: bulking up in the winter, then crash dieting to get in shape for summer.

Unless sound nutritional practices are followed, the cutting phase, much like a crash diet, can be unhealthy, rigid, monotonous, and damaging to performance. And bulking up tends to pile on fat pounds, which are that much harder to lose when it comes time to get in shape or prepare for competition.

Today, though, more strength athletes choose to stay in competition shape year-round. That way, it's easier to lose body fat because there's less to lose, and the process of cutting is much safer and more successful.

This chapter discusses a step-by-step diet strategy called *tapering* that lets you lose maximum body fat, retain hard-earned muscle, and perform at your best. This strategy works for exercisers, bodybuilders, and strength athletes—anyone who wants to become lean and muscular. The end of the chapter covers key issues for bodybuilders, powerlifters, and weightlifters.

A Strategy for Losing Fat

If you follow these guidelines as best you can, you'll be amazed by how easy dieting can be. Within just a few months, you'll achieve superb condition. So get started—off with the body fat, and on with the muscle!

Step 1: Plan Your Start Date

The length of time you spend dieting depends on how out of shape you are to begin with. If you've let yourself get too fat by bulking up, then you'll really have to stretch your dieting out by several months.

A caution for bodybuilding competitors: Don't start your dieting too close to your contest. You'll be too tempted to resort to crash dieting, which can result in loss of muscle, decreased strength and power, low energy, moodiness and irritability, and low immunity. Losing lots of fat in a short period of time is virtually impossible for most people, anyway. Physiologically, no one can lose more than 4 pounds (2 kilograms) of fat a week even by total fasting. Instead, take a gradual approach to dieting.

Start your diet or contest preparation about 10 to 12 weeks before your competition. During this period, make slight adjustments to your calorie and nutrient intake, as well as to your aerobic exercise level. In addition, supplement with creatine and drink one of my muscle-building formulas (see pages 263 to 266).

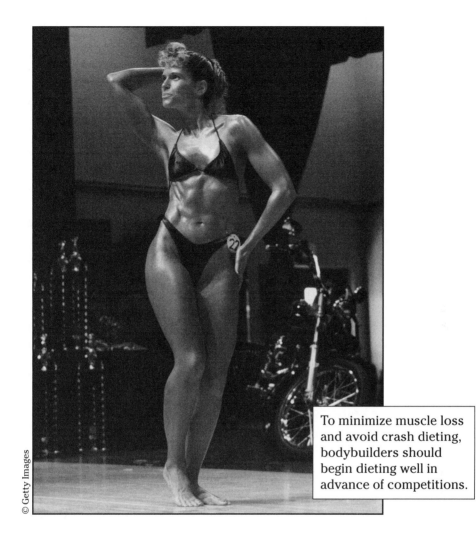

© Getty Images

To minimize muscle loss and avoid crash dieting, bodybuilders should begin dieting well in advance of competitions.

Step 2: Determine a Safe Reduction in Calories

Getting cut is essential for achieving physique perfection, as well as for achieving competitive success in a sport such as bodybuilding. One way to begin this process is by slightly reducing your caloric intake. By consuming fewer calories, you can gradually reduce body fat to lower levels. However, you don't want to cut calories too much. A drastic reduction in calories will slow down your RMR for two reasons. The first has to do with the thermic effect of food (TEF), the increase in RMR after you eat a meal as food is digested and metabolized. Eating more calories increases the thermic effect of food and along with it, the RMR. Likewise, cutting calories decreases the TEF as well as the RMR. Without enough calories to drive your metabolic processes, it becomes harder for your body to burn calories to lose body fat.

Second, long periods of calorie deprivation—that is, diets under 1,200 calories a day—lower your RMR as a result of the starvation adaptation response. This response simply means that your metabolism has slowed down to accommodate your lower caloric intake. Your body is stockpiling dietary fat and calories rather than burning them for energy. You can actually gain body fat on a diet of fewer than 1,200 calories a day.

The starvation adaptation response has been observed frequently in undernourished endurance athletes. In a study of triathletes, researchers found that these athletes weren't consuming enough calories to fuel themselves for training and competition. When calories were increased, the athletes' weight stayed the same. This occurred because their RMRs returned to normal with the introduction of ample calories. To keep your metabolism running in high gear, you have to eat enough calories to match your energy requirements.

When you drastically cut calories, you also slash your fat intake too much. That's a problem because you starve your brain of the fat it requires for nourishment. Consequently, your brain sends messages to your body to hang onto fat rather than burn it.

While dieting, reduce your calories by up to 300 each day if you are a woman and 400 each day if you are a man. This is the ideal metabolic window for fat burning and will not adversely affect your RMR. (See Chapter 5 for a discussion of this metabolic window.) At the same time, increase your aerobic exercise to burn up to 300 to 400 calories a day. This type of caloric manipulation will help you burn fat efficiently. You'll lose more fat in the initial weeks, and then you'll need to increase your exercise and probably lower your calories as you continue to shed body weight. I've designed the Power Eating losing fat (chapter 14) and cutting (chapter 15) plans with exactly these scientific concepts in mind.

You might wonder, Why can't I just crash diet for a few weeks to get in shape? After all, I'm training hard with weights. Shouldn't strength training protect me from losing muscle?

As logical as the argument sounds, scientific research proves otherwise. Case in point: In one study, overweight women were divided into two groups: a group that only dieted and a group that dieted and strength trained. The diet provided only 800 calories a day, and the study lasted four weeks. The results revealed that both groups lost the same amount of weight (11 pounds, or 5 kilograms). Even the composition of the lost weight was the same. All the women lost 8 pounds (3.5 kilograms) of fat and 3 pounds (1 kilogram) of muscle. The bottom line is that strength training does not preserve muscle under these low-calorie dieting conditions, but it does when caloric restriction isn't so severe.

The implications are clear: In just four short weeks, you can lose precious muscle if you crash diet. Watch how low you go in decreasing your caloric intake. Research with bodybuilders confirms that you can lose muscle in just seven days on calories as low as 18 per kilogram of body weight a day.

Step 3: Increase Aerobic Exercise

To sculpt a fit physique, increase the intensity and duration of your aerobic exercise. Aerobic exercise stimulates the activity of a fat-burning enzyme called *hormone-sensitive lipase,* which breaks down stored fat and moves it into circulation to be burned for energy. Aerobic exercise also increases $\dot{V}O_2$max—the capability to process oxygen and transport it to body tissues. Fat is burned most efficiently when sufficient oxygen is available.

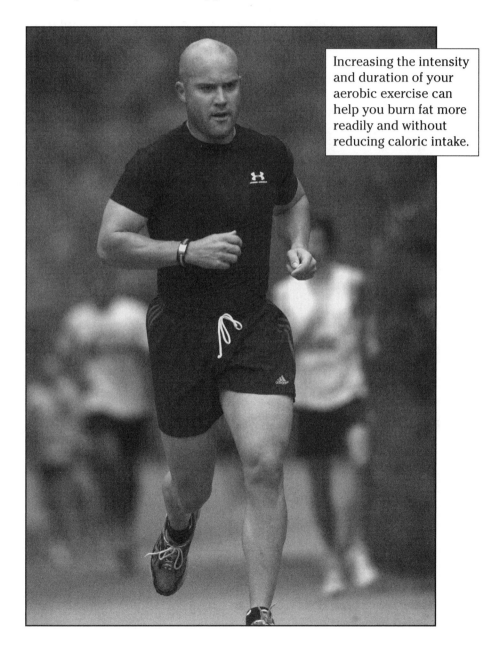

Increasing the intensity and duration of your aerobic exercise can help you burn fat more readily and without reducing caloric intake.

If you put a lot of effort into your aerobic exercise, you may not have to reduce your calories. That's the conclusion of a recent study from West Virginia University. Women of normal weight were able to decrease their body fat within three months simply by exercising aerobically four days a week for about 45 minutes each time at a heart rate between 80 and 90 percent of their maximum. They didn't have to cut calories, yet still lost plenty of body fat.

Here's some more good news: The better trained you are aerobically—and the leaner you are—the better your body can burn fat for energy. By increasing $\dot{V}O_2$max and thus available oxygen to tissues, aerobic exercise enhances the ability of your muscles to combust fat as fuel. At the cellular level, the breakdown of fat speeds up, and it's released faster from storage sites in fat and muscle tissue.

In addition, focus on interval training, which alternates short bursts (1-2 minutes) of high-intensity exercise with short bursts (1-2 minutes) at a lower intensity. Research has shown this form of exercise to keep your metabolic rate elevated for many hours following your workout and is thus an effective fat-burning strategy. Plus, it maximizes your time in the gym and gives you a great whole-body workout.

There's no doubt about it: Aerobic exercise, particularly when organized into intervals, is a miracle worker when it comes to fat burning. Stay aerobically fit year-round and you'll have no trouble shedding those last few pounds of pudge.

Step 4: Eat More Protein

To shed body fat, you should be eating at least 2.2 to 2.5 grams of protein per kilogram of body weight a day. This level will help you maintain muscle mass. Increasing your protein intake during a time of calorie reduction helps protect against muscle loss; the extra protein can be used as a backup energy source in case your body needs it.

Step 5: Time Your Meals and Exercise

When you are well fueled throughout the day, you can train harder and burn more calories. Eat a preworkout snack. Don't skip it—it will fuel your workout and help you burn more fat. After your workout, be sure to take in protein, carbohydrate, and fat in order to replenish glycogen and create a hormonal environment in your body that is conducive to building muscle.

Step 6: Don't Neglect Carbohydrate

As far as the rest of your diet is concerned, don't cut too much carbohydrate, or you're going to be really sluggish and out of sorts—lack of carbohydrate will adversely affect your energy levels and mood. It's critical to have some carbohydrate in your diet throughout the tapering phase.

With the recommended increase in your protein intake, for the peaking diet your total calories might look something like this: protein, 30 to 35 percent; carbohydrate, 40 percent; and fat, 25 to 30 percent. As long as you do not cut calories too drastically, you'll still have enough carbohydrate to support your training requirements. You can even have a minimal amount of added sugar and still meet the 40 percent carbohydrate requirement, although I prefer that you use your carbohydrate calories to eat nutritionally dense foods like milk, vegetables, and fruits.

Some of the very low-carbohydrate diets can hinder your training. Case in point: A study published in the *Journal of the International Society of Sports Nutrition* pointed out that the Atkins diet decreased exercise capacity in nine exercisers. Yes, they lost weight; however, they had a significant drop in their blood glucose levels, and this caused them to fatigue very early on during their workouts. This type of diet and others like it are neither appropriate nor necessary if you are active.

Step 7: Control Fat Intake

When your goal is to build lean muscle mass (the building diet), there is plenty of room in your plan for the right types of dietary fat. However, when you are trying to peak in a losing fat or cutting diet, there isn't any room for the wrong kinds of fat. Fat is critical to your success and should be eaten in the right proportions with protein and the right types of carbohydrate.

The key is to focus on healthy monounsaturated fat, including fat from vegetable oils, olives, nuts, and avocados. Continue to obtain your omega-3 fats from fatty fish and a little flaxseed meal. If you do not eat fish, supplement with omega-3 supplements. Always avoid saturated and trans fats from processed snack foods, commercially baked goods, and fried foods, since they will sabotage your progress.

Step 8: Space Your Meals

Your body will better use its calories for energy, rather than deposit them as fat, if you eat several small meals throughout the day. Most bodybuilders and other strength athletes eat five, six, or more meals a day. Spacing meals in this manner keeps you fueled throughout the day. Plus, the more times you eat, the higher your metabolism stays, thanks to the thermic effect of food. In other words, every time you eat, your metabolism accelerates. Eating multiple meals throughout the day is a good dietary practice regardless of whether you're dieting for competition.

Step 9: Include Anti-Inflammatory Foods

Exercise can increase free radical production and inflammation in the body. However, you can mitigate these processes by choosing anti-inflammatory foods and immune-boosting foods, all of which are loaded with antioxidants. The key is to choose bright, colorful vegetables and fruits (I'm not talking about Fruit Loops or Trix cereals, either!), from green spinach to sweet oranges. You can also get many of these healing nutrients from dairy products, eggs, and fish. Fish is especially high in omega-3 fatty acids, which have very effective anti-inflammatory properties.

Here is a list of healing foods to consider:

Citrus fruits	Broccoli	Tomatoes
Carrots	Pineapple	Apples
Oranges	Bananas	Star fruits
Papayas	Mangos	Kiwi fruits
Blood oranges	Passion fruits	Prickly pears
Strawberries	Cherries	Cranberries
Raspberries	Blueberries	Red grapes
Black currants	Green tea	

At the same time, stay away from or limit certain foods that activate inflammation in the body. These are mainly omega-6 fats, such as safflower oil, sunflower oil, soybean oil, cottonseed oil, and corn oil, as well as processed foods and commercially baked goods.

Step 10: Supplement Prudently

There are some real nutritional horror stories among people who crash diet or diet stringently for contests. They tend to suffer deficiencies in calcium, magnesium, zinc, vitamin D, and other nutrients. Generally, these deficiencies occur because dieters and bodybuilders eliminate dairy foods and red meat while dieting. However, you don't need to shy away from these foods. You can include red meat in your diet as long as it's lean and cooked appropriately. You can also include nonfat dairy foods, an important source of body-strengthening minerals and fat-burning whey protein. Neither of these foods will make you gain fat, as long as you eat them in moderation.

Because calories are cut during diets, supplement with an antioxidant vitamin and mineral formula that contains 100 percent of the DRI for all essential nutrients. This type of supplement will help cover your nutritional bases. See chapters 7, 8, and 9 for additional supplement recommendations.

Step 11: Watch Water Intake

Fitness-conscious people live in dread of water retention, medically known as edema. Water retention can keep you from looking lean even after you've pared down to physique perfection. Water swells up in certain areas, and you look like you have body fat even though it's only water weight.

How can you prevent water retention? Ironically, the best defense is to drink plenty of water throughout your tapering period. This means drinking between 8 and 12 cups (2-3 liters) of water or more daily. With ample fluid, your body automatically flushes itself of extra water. Not drinking enough water can make your body cling to as much fluid as it can, and you'll end up bloated. Dehydration can sap your energy, and you won't be able to work out as intensely.

Besides drinking plenty of water, follow these strategies to prevent water retention.

• **Moderate your sodium intake.** Sodium has gained a bad reputation, but it's an essential element in our diets. Our bodies have a minimum requirement of 500 milligrams a day. The body tightly regulates its electrolyte levels, including sodium. Decreasing sodium levels really doesn't have much of an effect; your body holds on to the exact amount of sodium it needs, even if you reduce your intake. It's essential to consume the minimum requirement to maintain fluid balance and electrolyte balance. Otherwise, nerve and muscle function will be impaired, and exercise performance will definitely diminish. Some bodybuilders have passed out just before their competition because of dehydration and possible electrolyte imbalance.

If you're sodium sensitive—that is, sodium causes you to retain water—you probably should reduce your intake slightly. Don't go to extremes, though. Simply avoid high-sodium foods, such as snack foods, canned foods, salted foods, pickled foods, cured foods, and lunch meats. Certainly don't add any extra salt to your food. But eliminating natural, whole foods because of their sodium content is usually unnecessary. Concentrate your food choices on whole grains, fresh fruits and vegetables, nonfat dairy foods, and unprocessed meats.

• **Eat naturally diuretic vegetables.** Some foods naturally help the body eliminate water, including asparagus, cucumbers, and watercress. You might try eating these while dieting, especially if water retention is a concern. Add a serving or two of these foods to your diet every day. Avoid pharmacologic forms of diuretics at all cost. Diuretic drugs flush sodium and other electrolytes from your body, causing life-threatening imbalances.

• **Continue aerobic exercise.** Aerobic exercise improves the resiliency and tone of blood vessels. Unless blood vessels are resilient, water can seep from them and collect in the tissues, and water retention is the result. A regular program of aerobics helps prevent this.

For Powerlifters and Weightlifters Only

As a powerlifter or weightlifter, you probably don't care much about getting ripped. Rather, you want to be as strong and as powerful as possible in your weight class. Here's what you should do to get strong for training and competition.

• **Load your muscles with energy sources.** Carbohydrate and creatine are your best bets. Stay on a carbohydrate-dense diet, supplemented with creatine. Take your creatine with carbohydrate, as recommended in chapter 8, to supercharge your muscles with energy. Numerous studies now published on creatine have shown that this supplement is a sure thing for boosting strength and power.

You don't need to carbohydrate load. There's no scientific evidence that this method has any performance-enhancing benefit for strength athletes. Simply maintain a high-carbohydrate diet throughout your training and competition preparation. Going into competition well fueled is critical.

• **Manipulate your aerobics and carbohydrate.** Increase your aerobics and slightly lower your carbohydrate intake if you need to make weight. This will help you lose fat to qualify for your weight class. You may need to decrease your calories slightly, and you can do this by cutting carbohydrate. However, try to go no lower than 40 to 50 percent of your total calories. That way, you can reduce weight but maintain strength.

Give yourself plenty of time to make weight—at least 10 to 12 weeks. If your contest is fast approaching, you can cut your calories down to 30 per kilogram of body weight a day. That will result in a loss of 3 to 4 pounds (1-2 kilograms) a week. But keep in mind that you may lose some muscle mass too.

If you do cut to 30 calories per kilogram of body weight a day, stay on this regimen for no longer than seven days. Prolonged restrictive dieting slows your RMR—and your ability to burn fat.

• **Avoid dangerous practices for making weight.** Before a meet, it's fairly common for some lifters to exercise in rubberized suits or sit in steam and sauna baths for extended periods—all without drinking much water. This practice can lead to dehydration so severe that it can harm the kidneys and heart. Dehydrated lifters also usually do poorly in competition.

Fasting isn't a good idea, either, even for a day or two. You'll lose water rapidly, and with it, you'll gain the health problems caused by dehydration. Glycogen depletion sets in, too, making it virtually impossible to perform well on competition day.

Sport Nutrition Fact Versus Fiction:

Is Insulin a Magic Bullet?

One of the most powerful and multifunctional hormones in the human body is insulin. It increases the uptake and use of glucose by cells, including muscle cells. It has an anabolic (tissue-building) effect on the body by promoting protein formation. It joins forces with GH to promote growth. And, on the downside, it promotes fat synthesis.

Medically, insulin is used to treat diabetes, a complex disease in which either the pancreas does not produce enough insulin (type I diabetes) or the body doesn't use it properly (type II diabetes). Type I diabetic patients require injections of insulin, and some people with poorly controlled type II diabetes may also require injections. Diabetes is the seventh leading cause of death in the United States, and about 11 million people have it.

In bodybuilding circles, insulin got a lot of attention in the 1980s when an insulin-dependent diabetic bodybuilder won several major contests and came to prominence. Nondiabetic, healthy bodybuilders started experimenting with insulin to see whether it would spark muscle growth. Thus, insulin joined the ranks of chemical muscle-building aids.

Bodybuilders and other strength athletes assumed that if insulin increased the body's use of glucose, then it could maximize glycogen storage. But they were wrong—there is no scientific evidence backing this belief. Besides, it is well known that you can stockpile plenty of glycogen with a high-carbohydrate diet. In addition, there's no evidence that insulin promotes muscle growth.

Fooling around with insulin is downright dangerous. Injections of insulin, or any other synthetic hormone for that matter, can throw your natural hormonal balance out of whack and lead to a whole host of medical problems. Plus, there's the danger of insulin shock, which occurs when too much insulin is injected. You could become unconscious or have a seizure. Another complication is hypoglycemia, in which blood sugar drops dangerously low. Symptoms include tremors and sweating, and, in extreme cases, convulsions and loss of consciousness.

Unless you are being treated for diabetes, leave insulin alone. Combined with hard training in the gym, the nutritional discoveries now available to strength trainers and other athletes are all you need to build a winning physique.

12

Maintaining Physique Menu Plans

The following Power Eating maintenance diet is designed for exercisers; bodybuilders; and novice and recreational strength trainers, powerlifters, and weightlifters. Often during training you may not be trying to gain or lose weight. Sometimes, it's a timing issue; you're just too busy in the rest of your life to spend more time in the gym. Sometimes, it is a planned part of your training schedule, like after the competitive season. Whatever the reason, this menu plan will keep you right where you want to be.

Power Eating Maintenance Diet

	Man		Woman	
Workouts per week	3-4	5 or more	3-4	5 or more
Calories/kg	33	42	29-33	38-40
Calories/lb	15	19	13-15	17-18
Protein				
g/kg	1.4	1.4	1.4	1.4
g/lb	.64	.64	.64	.64
Carbohydrate				
g/kg	4.5	6.0	3.5	5.5
g/lb	2.0	2.7	1.75	2.3
Fat*				
g/kg	~1.0	~1.4	~.85-1.0	~1.0-1.3
g/lb	~.45	~.64	~.39-.45	~.45-.59

*Total fat is variable based on total calories. To find your fat grams, determine your total calories, protein grams, and carbohydrate grams. Add your protein and carbohydrate calories (1 g protein = 4 calories, 1 g carbohydrate = 4 calories), subtract this total from the total calories, and divide by 9 (1 g fat = 9 calories). See page 207 for more information.

1,690 calories (29 calories per kilogram); 83 grams protein; 228 grams carbohydrate; 50 grams fat

Food groups	Number of servings
Bread	5
Fruit	5
Nonfat milk	3
Tsp added sugar	3
Vegetable	5
Protein sources	
Very lean	4
Lean	3
Medium fat	1
Fat	6

Food group servings	Menu
Breakfast	
	Water
1 bread	1/2 c (25 g) Shredded Wheat cereal
1 milk	1 c (237 ml) fat-free milk
2 fruit	1/2 c (119 ml) orange juice
	2 tbsp (18 g) raisins for cereal
1 medium-fat protein	1 whole egg, scrambled in nonstick skillet
1 fat	1 tbsp (12 g) ground flaxseed sprinkled on cereal
Snack	
	Green tea (or other tea)
1 fruit	4 dried apricots
1 vegetable	1 c (128 g) mini carrots
1 fat	6 almonds

Lunch

	Water
3 bread	6 in. (15 cm) Subway sandwich (choose from "6 grams of fat or less" list)
2 vegetable	Fill sandwich with vegetable choices
2 very lean protein	2 oz (57 g) meat included in sandwich
2 fat	2 tsp (10 ml) olive oil or 2 tbsp (30 ml) salad dressing

Pre-workout Snack

	Water
1 milk	1 c plain yogurt
1 fruit	3/4 c blueberries
	Sweeten with Splenda or low-calorie sweetener

Workout

	Water

Postworkout smoothie

1 fruit	1 1/4 c (180 g) whole strawberries
1 milk	1 c (237 ml) fat-free milk
3 tsp added sugar	1 tbsp (21 g) honey
2 very lean protein	14 g isolated whey protein

Dinner

	Green tea (or other tea)
1 bread	1/2 baked sweet potato
2 vegetable	1/2 c (90 g) steamed asparagus
	1 c (28 g) mixed green salad
3 lean protein	3 oz (85 g) wild salmon, grilled
2 fat	1 tsp (5 ml) olive oil for salmon
	1 tsp (4 g) butter or Heart Smart Omega margarine for potato
	2 tbsp (30 ml) reduced-fat salad dressing

2,340 calories (40 calories per kilogram); 83 grams protein; 325 grams carbohydrate; 79 grams fat

Food groups	Number of servings
Bread	7
Fruit	6
Nonfat milk	3
Tsp added sugar	16
Vegetable	6
Protein sources	
Very lean	4
Lean	3
Medium fat	1
Fat	11

Food group servings	Menu
Breakfast	
	Water
2 bread	2 slices whole-grain bread
1 milk	1 c (237 ml) fat-free milk
2 fruit	1 c (237 ml) orange juice
4 tsp added sugar	4 tsp (24 g) 100% fruit spread for bread
1 medium-fat protein	1 whole egg, scrambled
2 fats	1/8 avocado, sliced and cooked with eggs
	1 tsp (4 g) Heart Smart Omega margarine for cooking eggs
Snack	
	Green tea (or other tea)
1 fruit	4 dried apricots
1 tsp added sugar	1 tsp sugar (4 g) or honey (7 g)
3 fat	18 almonds

Lunch

	Water
3 bread	6 in. (15 cm) Subway sandwich (choose from "6 grams of fat or less" list)
2 vegetable	Fill sandwich with vegetable choices
2 very lean protein	2 oz (57 g) meat included in sandwich
2 fat	2 tsp (10 ml) olive oil or 2 tbsp (30 ml) salad dressing

Preworkout snack

	Water
1 milk	1 c (245 g) plain yogurt
1 fruit	¾ c (109 g) blueberries
3 tsp added sugar	1 tbsp (21 g) honey

Workout

	Water
8 tsp added sugar	16 oz (473 ml) sport drink

Postworkout smoothie

1 fruit	1-1/4 c (180 g) whole strawberries
1 milk	1 c (237 ml) fat-free milk
2 very lean protein	14 g isolated whey protein

Dinner

	Green tea (or other tea)
2 bread	1 baked sweet potato
1 fruit	3 oz (85 g, or about 15) red grapes
4 vegetable	1 c (180 g) steamed asparagus
	2 c (56 g) mixed green salad
3 lean protein	3 oz (85 g) wild salmon, grilled
4 fat	1 tsp (5 ml) olive oil for salmon
	1 tsp (4 g) butter or Heart Smart Omega margarine for potato
	4 tbsp (60 ml) reduced-fat salad dressing

2,700 calories (33 calories per kilogram); 115 grams protein; 360 grams carbohydrate; 89 grams fat

Food groups	Number of servings
Bread	8
Fruit	7
Nonfat milk	3
Tsp added sugar	16
Vegetable	6
Protein sources	
Very lean	6
Lean	4
Medium-fat	1
Fat	11

Food group servings	Menu
Preworkout snack	
	Water
1 milk	1 c (245 g) plain yogurt
1 fruit	3/4 c (109 g) blueberries
3 tsp added sugar	1 tbsp (21 g) honey
Workout	
	Water
8 tsp added sugar	16 oz (473 ml) sport drink
Breakfast	
	Water
1 bread	1 slice whole-grain bread
1 milk	1 c (237 ml) fat-free milk
2 fruit	1 c (237 ml) orange juice
3 tsp added sugar	1 tbsp (18 g) 100% fruit spread for bread

1 medium-fat protein	1 whole egg, scrambled
2 very lean protein	4 egg whites, cooked with whole egg
2 fat	1/8 avocado, sliced and cooked with eggs
	1 tsp (4 g) Heart Smart Omega margarine for cooking eggs

Snack

1 vegetable	1 c (124 g) celery sticks
3 fat	1 1/2 tbsp (24 g) natural peanut butter

Lunch

5 bread	Foot-long (30 cm) Subway sandwich (choose from "6 grams of fat or less" list)
2 vegetable	Fill sandwich with vegetable choices
1 fruit	Banana
4 very lean protein	4 oz (113 g) meat included in sandwich
2 fat	2 tsp (10 ml) olive oil or 2 tbsp (30 ml) salad dressing

Snack

2 fruit	8 dried apricots
1 milk	1 tall nonfat latte
1 tsp added sugar	1 tsp (4 g) sugar
2 fat	12 almonds

Dinner

	Green tea (or other tea)
2 bread	1 baked sweet potato
1 fruit	3 oz (85 g, or about 15) red grapes
1 tsp added sugar	1 tsp sugar (4g) or honey (7 g) for tea
3 vegetable	1/2 c (90 g) steamed asparagus
	2 c (56 g) mixed green salad
4 lean protein	4 oz (113 g) wild salmon, grilled
2 fat	1 tsp (5 ml) olive oil for salmon
	2 tbsp (30 ml) reduced-fat salad dressing

3,420 calories (42 calories per kilogram); 115 grams protein; 486 grams carbohydrate; 113 grams fat

Food groups	Number of servings
Bread	11
Fruit	9
Nonfat milk	3
Tsp added sugar	29
Vegetable	6
Protein sources	
Very lean	5
Lean	4
Medium-fat	1
Fat	18

Food group servings	Menu
Preworkout snack	
	Water
1 milk	1 c (245 g) plain yogurt
1 fruit	3/4 c (109 g) blueberries
3 tsp added sugar	1 tbsp (21 g) honey
Workout	
	Water
16 tsp added sugar	32 oz (946 ml) sport drink
Breakfast	
	Water
2 bread	2 slices whole-grain bread
1 milk	1 c (237 ml) fat-free milk
3 fruit	1 c (237 ml) orange juice
	1 c (170 g) melon cubes

6 tsp added sugar	2 tbsp (36 g) 100% fruit spread for bread
1 medium-fat protein	1 whole egg, scrambled
1 very lean protein	2 egg whites, cooked with whole egg
5 fat	1/2 avocado, sliced and cooked with eggs
	1 tsp (4 g) Heart Smart Omega margarine for cooking eggs

Snack

2 bread	8 whole-wheat crackers
1 vegetable	1 c (124 g) celery sticks
6 fat	3 tbsp (48 g) natural peanut butter

Lunch

5 bread	Foot-long (30 cm) Subway sandwich (choose from "6 grams of fat or less" list)
2 vegetable	Fill sandwich with vegetable choices
1 fruit	Banana
4 very lean protein	4 oz (113 g) meat included in sandwich
2 fat	2 tsp (10 ml) olive oil or 2 tbsp (30 ml) salad dressing

Snack

2 fruit	8 dried apricots
1 milk	1 tall nonfat latte
2 tsp added sugar	2 tsp (8 g) sugar in latte
2 fat	12 almonds

Dinner

	Green tea (or other tea)
2 bread	1 baked sweet potato
2 fruit	6 oz (170 g, or about 30) red grapes
2 tsp added sugar	2 tsp sugar (8 g) or honey (14 g) in tea
3 vegetable	½ c (90 g) steamed asparagus
	2 c (56 g) mixed green salad
4 lean protein	4 oz (113 g) wild salmon, grilled
3 fat	4 tbsp (60 ml) reduced-fat salad dressing

13

Building Muscle Menu Plans

My Power Eating diet for building muscle is designed for novice or experienced exercisers, bodybuilders, powerlifters, weightlifters, and other serious strength trainers who are interested in building quality muscle. The larger you are and the greater your muscle mass, the more calories it will take for you to build muscle. If you are not seeing gains at these levels, increase your calories by 300 to 400 per day by primarily increasing carbohydrate (75 percent of the calorie increase) and secondarily increasing fat (25 percent of the increase). If you are cross-training with intense aerobic exercise, increase your carbohydrate intake by another 1 to 2 grams per kilogram of body weight per day.

Power Eating Building Muscle Diet

	Man		Woman	
Workouts per week	3-4	5 or more	3-4	5 or more
Calories/kg	42	52+	35-38	44-50
Calories/lb	19	24+	16-17	20-23
Protein				
g/kg	2.0	2.9	2.0	2.0
g/lb	.9	.9	.9	.9
Carbohydrate				
g/kg	5.5	7.0	4.5	6.5
g/lb	2.5	3.2	2.1	3.0
Fat*				
g/kg	~1.33	~1.77	~1.0-1.3	~1.0-1.77
g/lb	~.6	~.8	~.45-.59	~.5-.8

*Total fat is variable based on total calories. To find your fat grams, determine your total calories, protein grams, and carbohydrate grams. Add your protein and carbohydrate calories (1 g protein = 4 calories, 1 g carbohydrate = 4 calories), subtract this total from the total calories, and divide by 9 (1 g fat = 9 calories). See page 207 for more information.

2,080 calories (35 calories per kilogram); 118 grams protein; 266 grams carbohydrate; 60 grams fat

Food groups	Number of servings
Bread	7
Fruit	5
Nonfat milk	3
Tsp added sugar	3
Vegetable	6
Protein sources	
Very lean	5
Lean	3
Medium fat	1
Fat	9

Food group servings	Menu
Breakfast	
	Water
2 bread	1 c (49 g) Shredded Wheat cereal
1 milk	1 c (237 ml) fat-free milk
2 fruit	1/2 c (119 ml) orange juice
	2 tbsp (18 g) raisins for cereal
1 medium-fat protein	1 whole egg, scrambled in a nonstick skillet
1 fat	1 tbsp (12 g) ground flaxseed sprinkled on cereal
Snack	
	Green tea (or other tea)
1 fruit	4 dried apricots
1 vegetable	1 c (128 g) mini carrots
2 fat	12 almonds

BUILDING MUSCLE

Lunch

	Water
3 bread	6 in. (15 cm) Subway sandwich (choose from "6 grams of fat or less" list)
2 vegetable	Fill sandwich with vegetable choices
3 very lean protein	2 oz (57 g) meat included in sandwich
	1 oz (28 g) cheese included in sandwich
3 fat	1 fat included in cheese
	2 tsp (10 ml) olive oil or 2 tbsp (30 ml) salad dressing

Preworkout snack

	Water
1 milk	1 c (245 g) plain yogurt
1 fruit	3/4 c (109 g) blueberries
	Sweeten with Splenda or other low-calorie sweetener

Workout

	Water

Postworkout smoothie

1 fruit	1-1/4 c (180 g) whole strawberries
1 milk	1 c (237 ml) fat-free milk
3 tsp added sugar	1 tbsp (21 g) honey
2 very lean protein	14 g isolated whey protein

Dinner

	Green tea (or other tea)
2 bread	1 baked sweet potato
2 vegetable	1/2 c (90 g) steamed asparagus
	2 c (56 g) mixed green salad
3 lean protein	3 oz (85 g) wild salmon, grilled
3 fat	1 tsp (5 ml) olive oil for salmon
	1 tsp (4 g) butter or Heart Smart Omega margarine for potato
	2 tbsp (30 ml) reduced-fat salad dressing

2,950 calories (50 calories per kilogram); 118 grams protein; 384 grams carbohydrate; 105 grams fat

Food groups	Number of servings
Bread	8
Fruit	8
Nonfat milk	3
Tsp added sugar	18
Vegetable	7
Protein sources	
Very lean	5
Lean	3
Medium fat	1
Fat	18

Food group servings	Menu
Breakfast	
	Water
2 bread	2 slices whole-grain bread
1 milk	1 c (237 ml) fat-free milk
2 fruit	1 c (237 ml) orange juice
4 tsp added sugar	4 tsp (24 g) 100% fruit spread for bread
1 vegetable	1/2 c (28 g) sautéed mushrooms added to egg
1 medium-fat protein	1 whole egg, scrambled
4 fat	1/4 avocado, sliced and cooked with egg
	2 tsp (8g) Heart Smart Omega margarine for cooking mushrooms and eggs
Snack	
	Green tea (or other tea)
2 fruit	8 dried apricots
3 fat	18 almonds
Lunch	
	Water

3 bread	6 in. (15 cm) Subway Sandwich (choose from "6 grams of fat or less" list)
2 vegetable	Fill sandwich with vegetable choices
2 very lean protein	2 oz (57 g) meat included in sandwich
	1 oz (28 g) cheese included in sandwich
3 fat	1 fat included in cheese
	2 tsp (10 ml) olive oil or 2 tbsp (30 ml) salad dressing

Preworkout snack

	Water
1 milk	1 c (245 g) plain yogurt
1 fruit	3/4 c (109 g) blueberries
3 tsp added sugar	1 tbsp (21 g) honey

Workout

	Water
8 tsp added sugar	16 oz (473 ml) sport drink

Postworkout smoothie

1 fruit	1-1/4 c (180 g) whole strawberries
1 milk	1 c (237 ml) fat-free milk
3 tsp added sugar	1 tbsp (21 g) honey
2 very lean protein	14 g isolated whey protein
1 fat	1 tbsp (10 g) ground flaxseed

Dinner

	Green tea (or other tea)
3 bread	1 baked sweet potato
	1 slice French bread
2 fruit	6 oz (170 g, or about 30) red grapes
4 vegetable	1 c (180 g) steamed asparagus
	2 c (56 g) mixed green salad
3 lean protein	3 oz (85 g) wild salmon, grilled
7 fat	4 tsp (20 ml) olive oil: 1 tsp (5 ml) to rub on salmon, 3 tsp (15 ml) for dipping bread
	1 tsp (4 g) butter or Heart Smart Omega margarine for potato
	4 tbsp (30 ml) reduced-fat salad dressing

3,420 calories (42 calories per kilogram); 162 grams protein; 450 grams carbohydrate; 108 grams fat

Food groups	Number of servings
Bread	11
Fruit	8
Nonfat milk	3
Tsp added sugar	24
Vegetable	6
Protein sources	
Very lean	8
Lean	5
Medium fat	1
Fat	17

Food group servings	Menu
Preworkout snack	
	Water
1 milk	1 c (245 g) plain yogurt
1 fruit	1-3/4 c (109 g) blueberries
3 tsp added sugar	1 tbsp (21 g) honey
Workout	
	Water
16 tsp added sugar	32 oz (946 ml) sport drink
Breakfast	
	Water
2 bread	2 slices whole-grain bread
1 milk	1 c (237 ml) fat-free milk
2 fruit	1 c (237 ml) orange juice
4 tsp added sugar	4 tsp (24 g) 100% fruit spread for bread

1 medium-fat protein	1 whole egg, scrambled
2 very lean protein	4 egg whites, cooked with whole egg
5 fat	1/2 avocado, sliced and cooked with eggs
	1 tsp (4 g) Heart Smart Omega margarine for cooking eggs

Snack

2 bread	8 whole-wheat crackers
1 vegetable	1 c (124 g) celery sticks
4 fat	2 tbsp (32 g) natural peanut butter

Lunch

5 bread	Foot-long (30 cm) Subway sandwich (choose from "6 grams of fat or less" list)
2 vegetable	Fill sandwich with vegetable choices
1 fruit	Banana
6 very lean protein	4 oz (113 g) meat included in sandwich
	2 oz (57 g) cheese included in sandwich
4 fat	2 fat servings included in cheese
	2 tsp (10 ml) olive oil or 2 tbsp (30 ml) salad dressing

Snack

2 fruit	8 dried apricots
1 milk	1 tall nonfat latte
1 tsp added sugar	1 tsp (4 g) sugar for latte
2 fat	12 almonds

Dinner

	Green tea (or other tea)
2 bread	1 baked sweet potato
2 fruit	6 oz (170 g, or about 30) red grapes
3 vegetable	1/2 c (90 g) steamed asparagus
	2 c (56 g) mixed green salad
5 lean protein	5 oz (142 g) wild salmon, grilled
2 fat	1 tsp (5 ml) olive oil for salmon
	2 tbsp (30 ml) reduced-fat salad dressing

4,245 calories (52 calories per kilogram); 162 grams protein; 576 grams carbohydrate; 145 grams fat

Food groups	Number of servings
Bread	13
Fruit	12
Nonfat milk	3
Tsp added sugar	30
Vegetable	9
Protein sources	
Very lean	7
Lean	5
Medium-fat	1
Fat	24

Food group servings	Menu
Preworkout snack	
	Water
1 milk	1 c (245 g) plain yogurt
1 fruit	3/4 c (109 g) blueberries
3 tsp added sugar	1 tbsp (21 g) honey
Workout	
	Water
16 tsp added sugar	32 oz (946 ml) sport drink
Breakfast	
	Water
2 bread	2 slices whole-grain bread
1 milk	1 c (237 ml) fat-free milk
3 fruit	1 c (237 ml) orange juice
	1 c (170 g) melon cubes
6 tsp added sugar	2 tbsp (36 g) 100% fruit spread for bread
2 vegetable	1 c (156 g) sautéed mushrooms and red peppers
1 medium-fat protein	1 whole egg, scrambled
1 very lean protein	2 egg whites, cooked with whole egg
6 fat	1/2 avocado, sliced and cooked with eggs
	2 tsp (8 g) Heart Smart Omega margarine for cooking eggs and vegetables

Snack

2 bread	8 whole-wheat crackers
2 fruit	2/3 c (156 ml) Concord grape juice (make a spritzer by mixing with sparkling water)
1 vegetable	1 c (124 g) celery sticks
6 fat	3 tbsp (48 g) natural peanut butter

Lunch

5 bread	Foot-long (30-cm) Subway sandwich (choose from "6 grams of fat or less" list)
2 vegetable	Fill sandwich with vegetable choices
1 fruit	Banana
6 very lean protein	4 oz (113 g) meat included in sandwich
	2 oz (57 g) cheese included in sandwich
4 fat	2 fat servings included in cheese
	2 tsp (10 ml) olive oil or 2 tbsp (30 ml) salad dressing

Snack

2 fruit	8 dried apricots
1 milk	1 tall nonfat latte
2 tsp added sugar	1 tsp (4 g) sugar
2 fat	12 almonds

Dinner

	Green tea (or other tea)
4 bread	1 baked sweet potato
	2 slices French bread
3 fruit	1 c (124 g) raspberries and 1 c (165 g) cubed mango on top of ice cream
3 tsp added sugar	1/2 c light ice cream
4 vegetable	1 c (180 g) steamed asparagus
	2 c (56 g) mixed green salad
5 lean protein	5 oz (142 g) wild salmon, grilled
6 fat	1 fat included in ice cream
	1 tsp (5 ml) olive oil for salmon
	1 tbsp (15 ml) olive oil for dipping bread
	2 tbsp (30 ml) reduced-fat salad dressing
Free	1 tbsp (15 ml) whipped cream to top fruit and ice cream

Power Profile: Weight Gain

Are you a hard gainer—unable to put on any appreciable muscle weight no matter how hard you try?

That was the case of Scott E., a 44-year-old business executive who at 6 feet, 3 inches (191 centimeters) and 177 pounds (80 kilograms) had not been able to gain weight in 20 years. To make matters worse, he had no appetite, plus he had stomach problems caused by stress, infections, and overtreatment with antibiotics. I placed him on my Power Eating building diet.

Before beginning this diet, Scott was consuming only about 2,800 calories a day and not enough vitamins, minerals, or fluids. I increased his calories to 3,560 calories daily, plus added more protein (113 grams daily) and carbohydrate (570 grams daily). He started supplementing with a good antioxidant, eating multiple meals throughout the day, and consuming healthier fat from fish and plant sources. He also decreased his alcohol intake.

In addition, I recommended that Scott supplement with Kleiner's Easy Muscle-Building Formula, take 400 milligrams of vitamin E, and continue taking acidophilus, a supplement that restores intestinal flora after antibiotic treatment. I also suggested that Scott try a natural supplement, Prelief, to help reduce stomach irritation.

In only six weeks, Scott's energy levels soared, and he felt energetic enough to begin a regular exercise program. He gained 15 pounds (7 kilograms) of pure muscle—with no increase in his waist measurement. Scott felt that the Prelief helped him eat the extra calories without stomach irritation.

As Scott put it, "In the first three weeks, I gained 14 pounds [6 kilograms], from 180 [82 kilograms] to 194 [88 kilograms]. To put this in perspective, I have not weighed over 184 [83 kilograms] in 20 years and have been trying to gain weight for the past two to three years."

What's more, most of his stomach problems were resolved.

14

Losing Fat Menu Plans

The following diet for losing fat is designed for novice and experienced exercisers, bodybuilders, athletes, and virtually anyone who wants to lose body fat in a safe, controlled manner—without losing precious muscle. Caloric levels differ for men and women because it is more difficult for women to lose fat than it is for men.

Power Eating Losing Fat Diet				
	Man		**Woman**	
Workouts per week	**3-4**	**5 or more**	**3-4**	**5 or more**
Calories/kg	28	38	25	35
Calories/lb	12.7	17.3	11.4	16.0
Protein				
g/kg	2.2	2.2	2.2	2.2
g/lb	1.0	1.0	1.0	1.0
Carbohydrate				
g/kg	3.0	4.0	2.5	3.5
g/lb	1.4	1.8	1.1	1.6
Fat*				
g/kg	~.8	~1.5	~.7	~1.4
g/lb	~.36	~.68	~.32	~.64

*Total fat is variable based on total calories. To find your fat grams, determine your total calories, protein grams, and carbohydrate grams. Add your protein and carbohydrate calories (1 g protein = 4 calories, 1 g carbohydrate = 4 calories), subtract this total from the total calories, and divide by 9 (1 g fat = 9 calories). See page 207 for more information.

1,475 calories (25 calories per kilogram); 130 grams protein; 148 grams carbohydrate; 40 grams fat

Food groups	Number of servings
Bread	3
Fruit	3
Nonfat milk	3
Tsp added sugar	0
Vegetable	4
Protein sources	
Very lean	7
Lean	5
Medium fat	1
Fat	4

Food group servings	Menu
Breakfast	
	Water
1 bread	1/2 c (25 g) Shredded Wheat cereal
1 milk	1 c (237 ml) fat-free milk
1 fruit	2 tbsp (18 g) raisins for cereal
1 medium-fat protein	1 whole egg, scrambled in nonstick skillet
1 very lean protein	2 egg whites, scrambled with whole egg
1 fat	1 tbsp (12 g) ground flaxseed sprinkled on cereal
Snack	
	Green tea (or other tea)
1 vegetable	1 c (128 g) mini carrots
1 fat	6 almonds

LOSING FAT

Lunch

	Water
1 bread	Subway turkey breast wrap
2 vegetable	Fill wrap with vegetable choices
4 very lean protein	3 oz (85 g) turkey included in wrap
	1 oz (28 g) cheese included in wrap
1 fat	1 fat included in cheese
Free	Dijon mustard

Preworkout snack

	Water
1 milk	1 c (245 g) plain yogurt
1 fruit	3/4 c (109 g) blueberries
	Sweeten with Splenda or low-calorie sweetener

Workout

	Water

Postworkout smoothie

1 fruit	1-1/4 c (180 g) whole strawberries
1 milk	1 c (237 ml) fat-free milk
2 very lean protein	14 g isolated whey protein

Dinner

	Green tea (or other tea)
1 bread	1/2 baked sweet potato
1 vegetable	1/2 c (90 g) steamed asparagus
5 lean protein	5 oz (142 g) wild salmon, grilled
1 fat	1 tsp (5 ml) olive oil for salmon

2,065 calories (35 calories per kilogram); 130 grams protein; 207 grams carbohydrate; 80 grams fat

Food groups	Number of servings
Bread	6
Fruit	4
Nonfat milk	3
Tsp added sugar	0
Vegetable	5
Protein sources	
Very lean	6
Lean	4
Medium-fat	1
Fat	11

Food group servings	Menu
Breakfast	
	Water
2 bread	2 slices whole-grain bread
1 milk	1 c (237 ml) fat-free milk
1 fruit	1/2 c (119 ml) orange juice
1 medium-fat protein	1 whole egg, scrambled
2 fat	1/8 avocado, sliced and cooked with eggs
	1 tsp (4 g) Heart Smart Omega margarine for cooking eggs
Snack	
	Green tea (or other tea)
1 fruit	4 dried apricots
3 fat	18 almonds

Lunch

	Water
1 bread	Subway turkey breast wrap
2 vegetable	Fill wrap with vegetable choices
4 very lean protein	3 oz (85 g) turkey included in wrap
	1 oz (28 g) cheese included in wrap
2 fat	1 fat included in cheese
	1 tsp (5 ml) olive oil or 1 tbsp (30 ml) salad dressing

Preworkout snack

	Water
1 bread	3/4 oz (21 g) whole-wheat pretzels
1 milk	1 c (245 g) plain yogurt
1 fruit	3/4 c (109 g) blueberries
	Sweeten with Splenda or low-calorie sweetener

Workout

	Water

Postworkout smoothie

1 fruit	1 1/4 c (180 g) whole strawberries
1 milk	1 c (237 ml) fat-free milk
2 very lean protein	14 g isolated whey protein

Dinner

	Green tea (or other tea)
2 bread	1 baked sweet potato
3 vegetable	1/2 c (90 g) steamed asparagus
	2 c (56 g) mixed green salad
4 lean protein	4 oz (113 g) wild salmon, grilled
4 fat	1 tsp (5 ml) olive oil for salmon
	1 tsp (4 g) butter or Heart Smart Omega margarine for potato
	4 tbsp (60 ml) reduced-fat salad dressing

2,290 calories (28 calories per kilogram); 180 grams protein; 245 grams carbohydrate; 66 grams fat

Food groups	Number of servings
Bread	7
Fruit	5
Nonfat milk	3
Tsp added sugar	0
Vegetable	6
Protein sources	
Very lean	11
Lean	6
Medium-fat	1
Fat	8

Food group servings	Menu
Preworkout snack	
	Water
1 milk	1 c (245 g) plain yogurt
1 fruit	3/4 c (109 g) blueberries
	Sweeten with Splenda or low-calorie sweetener
Workout	
	Water
Breakfast	
1 bread	1 slice whole-grain bread
1 milk	1 c (237 ml) fat-free milk
2 fruit	1 c (237 ml) orange juice
1 medium-fat protein	1 whole egg, scrambled in nonstick skillet
5 very lean protein	4 egg whites, cooked with whole egg
	21 g isolated whey protein added to milk and orange juice and blended with 3 to 4 ice cubes
1 fat	1/8 avocado, sliced and cooked with eggs

LOSING FAT

Snack

1 bread	Included in the edamame or Genisoy crisps
1 vegetable	1 c (124 g) celery sticks
1 very lean protein	1/2 c (90 g) edamame or 1 serving (about 1/3 bag) of Genisoy crisps
2 fat	1 tbsp (16 g) natural peanut butter

Lunch

3 bread	6 in. (15 cm) Subway sandwich (choose from "6 grams of fat or less" list)
2 vegetable	Fill sandwich with vegetable choices
1 fruit	Banana
5 very lean protein	2 oz (57 g) included in sandwich; request double meat
	1 oz (28 g) cheese included in sandwich
1 fat	1 fat included in cheese
Free	Dijon mustard

Snack

1 fruit	4 dried apricots
1 milk	1 tall nonfat latte
	Sweeten with Splenda or other low-calorie sweetener
2 fat	12 almonds

Dinner

	Green tea (or other tea)
2 bread	1 baked sweet potato
1 fruit	3 oz (85 g, or about 15) red grapes
3 vegetable	1/2 c (90 g) steamed asparagus
	2 c (56 g) mixed green salad
6 lean protein	6 oz (170 g) wild salmon, grilled
2 fat	1 tsp (5 ml) olive oil for salmon
	2 tbsp (30 ml) reduced-fat salad dressing

3,108 calories (38 calories per kilogram); 180 grams protein; 327 grams carbohydrate; 120 grams fat

Food groups	Number of servings
Bread	9
Fruit	8
Nonfat milk	3
Tsp added sugar	0
Vegetable	6
Protein sources	
Very lean	10
Lean	6
Medium fat	1
Fat	19

Food group servings	Menu
Preworkout snack	
	Water
1 milk	1 c (245 g) plain yogurt
1 fruit	3/4 c (109 g) blueberries
	Sweeten with Splenda or other low-calorie sweetener
Workout	
	Water
Breakfast	
	Water
2 bread	2 slices whole-grain bread
1 milk	1 c (237 ml) fat-free milk
3 fruit	1 c (237 ml) orange juice
	1 c (170 g) melon cubes
1 medium-fat protein	1 whole egg, scrambled
4 very lean protein	4 egg whites, cooked with whole egg
	14 g isolated whey protein added to milk and orange juice and blended with 3 to 4 ice cubes
5 fat	1/2 avocado, sliced and cooked with eggs

	1 tsp (4 g) Heart Smart Omega margarine for cooking eggs
Snack	
2 bread	Included in edamame or Genisoy crisps
1 vegetable	1 c (124 g) celery sticks
2 very lean protein	1 c (180 g) edamame or 2 servings (about 2/3 bag) of Genisoy crisps
6 fat	3 tbsp (48 g) natural peanut butter
Lunch	
3 bread	6 in. (15 cm) Subway sandwich (choose from "6 grams of fat or less" list)
2 vegetable	Fill sandwich with vegetable choices
1 fruit	Banana
4 very lean protein	2 oz (57 g) meat included in sandwich; request double meat and no cheese
2 fat	2 tsp (10 ml) olive oil or 2 tbsp (30 ml) salad dressing
Snack	
2 fruit	8 dried apricots
1 milk	1 tall nonfat latte
2 fat	12 almonds
Dinner	
	Green tea (or other tea)
2 bread	1 baked sweet potato
1 fruit	3 oz (85 g, or about 15) red grapes
3 vegetable	1/2 c (90 g) steamed asparagus
	2 c (56 g) mixed green salad
6 lean protein	6 oz (170 g) wild salmon, grilled
6 fat	8 large black olives
	2 tsp (10 ml) olive oil for rubbing on salmon and drizzling on asparagus
	1 tsp (4 g) butter or Heart Smart Omega margarine for potato
	4 tbsp (60 ml) reduced-fat salad dressing

Power Profile: Fat Loss

Several years ago, I was asked to work with a 28-year-old basketball player after his physical conditioning and performance had markedly diminished over a period of a year.

At our initial meeting, the 6-foot, 11-inch (211-centimeter) player weighed 276 pounds (125 kilograms) and had 23 percent body fat. Seriously concerned about his condition and his performance, he reported that he had been desperately trying to lose weight, particularly because his contract required him to maintain a certain weight and body fat; his ultimate goal was 257 pounds (166.5 kilograms) or 13 percent body fat.

His diet consisted of 1,700 calories, with 30 percent coming from protein, 27 percent from carbohydrate, 32 percent from fat, and 11 percent from alcohol. These are clearly not optimal percentages for an athlete, particularly one who is trying to lose weight and retain muscle.

Because of his poor diet, he was fatigued, even unable to eat when he got home from practice. What's more, he was afraid to eat, fearing that food would show up the next day on the scale. He truly was in the beginning stages of an eating disorder. And the less he ate, the higher his body-fat percentage climbed.

With only five weeks to go until his first goal-weight deadline, I placed him on the Power Eating diet for losing fat. This initially included 4,019 calories (33 calories per kilogram), 222 grams of protein, 603 grams of carbohydrate, and 80 grams of fat. In addition, he drank a gallon (4 liters) of fluid a day and supplemented with 500 milligrams of vitamin E. During his workout, he sipped 48 ounces (1,420 milliliters) of a glucose–electrolyte solution; after his workout, he consumed a serving of Kleiner's Essential Muscle-Building Formula for Men or Kleiner's Muscle-Building Formula.

After several weeks and some success, I discontinued the glucose–electrolyte solution during his aerobic workouts to enhance fat-burning during exercise since he was required to make weight by a contract deadline. This was the only major change that I made. I also decreased his daily calories by 100 to activate further weight loss.

In five weeks, he made amazing progress, reaching 263.5 pounds (119.5 kilograms) and 12.75 percent body fat. A few weeks later, he weighed in at 261 pounds (118 kilograms) and 12.9 percent body fat.

15

Getting Cut Menu Plans

To lean out—either for additional body-fat reduction or for a bodybuilding competition—tweak your diet using my Power Eating seven-day cutting diet. (It's particularly useful for bodybuilders who must lean out the week before a competition.) The distribution of nutrients for the cutting plan is based on getting enough protein and fat within the restricted number of calories. This forces a limited amount of carbohydrate, which allows for rapid weight loss. Use this approach only when absolutely necessary. Because women have more difficulty losing fat than men do, calorie levels are different. Stay on this diet no longer than 14 days.

Power Eating Getting Cut Diet				
	Man		Woman	
Workouts per week	3-4	5 or more	3-4	5 or more
Calories/kg	25	32	22	29
Calories/lb	11.4	14.5	10	13.2
Protein				
g/kg	2.3	2.3	2.3	2.3
g/lb	1.05	1.05	1.05	1.05
Carbohydrate				
g/kg	2.3	3.0	1.8	2.9
g/lb	1.05	1.36	0.82	1.32
Fat*				
g/kg	~0.7	~1.2	~0.6	~0.9
g/lb	~0.32	~0.55	~0.27	~0.41

*Total fat is variable based on total calories. To find your fat grams, determine your total calories, protein grams, and carbohydrate grams. Add your protein and carbohydrate calories (1 g protein = 4 calories, 1 g carbohydrate = 4 calories), subtract this total from the total calories, and divide by 9 (1 g fat = 9 calories). See page 207 for more information.

1,300 calories (22 calories per kilogram); 136 grams protein; 106 grams carbohydrate; 37 grams fat

Food groups	Number of servings
Bread	1
Fruit	2
Nonfat milk	3
Tsp added sugar	0
Vegetable	5
Protein sources	
Very lean	10
Lean	4
Medium-fat	1
Fat	4

Food group servings	Menu
Breakfast	
	Water
1 bread	1/2 c (25 g) Shredded Wheat cereal
1 milk	1 c (237 ml) fat-free milk
1 fruit	2 tbsp (18 g) raisins for cereal
1 medium-fat protein	1 whole egg, scrambled in nonstick skillet
2 very lean protein	4 egg whites, scrambled with whole egg
1 fat	1 tbsp (12 g) ground flaxseed sprinkled on cereal

Snack

	Green tea (or other tea)
1 vegetable	1 c (128 g) mini carrots
1 fat	6 almonds

Lunch

	Water
2 vegetable	Subway grilled chicken breast and spinach salad
6 very lean protein	3 oz (85 g) chicken included in salad; request double meat
1 fat	2 tbsp (30 ml) reduced-fat dressing

Preworkout snack

	Water
1 milk	1 c (245 g) plain yogurt
1 fruit	3/4 c (109 g) blueberries
	Sweeten with Splenda or other low-calorie sweetener

Workout

	Water

Postworkout smoothie

1 milk	1 c (237 ml) nonfat milk
2 very lean protein	14 g isolated whey protein, blended with milk and 3 or 4 ice cubes

Dinner

	Green tea (or other tea)
2 vegetable	1/2 c (90 g) steamed asparagus
	1 c (28 g) mixed green salad
4 lean protein	4 oz (113 g) wild salmon, grilled
1 fat	1 tsp (5 ml) olive oil for salmon
Free	2 tbsp (30 ml) fat-free Italian dressing

1,711 calories (29 calories per kilogram); 136 grams protein; 171 grams carbohydrate; 54 grams fat

Food groups	Number of servings
Bread	3
Fruit	4
Nonfat milk	3
Tsp added sugar	0
Vegetable	6
Protein sources	
Very lean	8
Lean	5
Medium-fat	1
Fat	7

Food group servings	Menu
Breakfast	
	Water
1 bread	1 slice whole-grain bread
1 milk	1 c (237 ml) fat-free milk
1 fruit	1/2 c (119 ml) orange juice
1 medium-fat protein	1 whole egg, scrambled in nonstick skillet
2 very lean protein	4 egg whites, cooked with whole egg
1 fat	1/8 avocado, sliced and cooked with eggs
Snack	
	Green tea (or other tea)
1 fruit	4 dried apricots
1 vegetable	1 c (128 g) mini carrots
2 fat	12 almonds

Lunch

	Water
1 bread	Subway turkey breast wrap
2 vegetable	Fill wrap with vegetable choices
4 very lean protein	3 oz (85 g) turkey included in wrap
	1 oz (28 g) cheese included in wrap
2 fat	1 fat included in cheese
	1 tsp (5 ml) olive oil or 1 tbsp (15 ml) salad dressing

Preworkout snack

	Water
1 milk	1 c (245 g) plain yogurt
1 fruit	1 c (109 g) blueberries
	Sweeten with Splenda or low-calorie sweetener

Workout

	Water

Postworkout smoothie

1 fruit	1 1/4 c (180 g) whole strawberries
1 milk	1 c (237 ml) fat-free milk
2 very lean protein	14 g isolated whey protein

Dinner

	Green tea (or other tea)
1 bread	1/2 sweet potato
3 vegetable	1/2 c (90 g) steamed asparagus
	2 c (56 g) mixed green salad
5 lean protein	5 oz (142 g) wild salmon, grilled
2 fat	1 tsp (5 ml) olive oil for salmon
	2 tbsp (30 ml) reduced-fat salad dressing

MAN: 3 TO 4 WORKOUTS/WEEK

2,045 calories (25 calories per kilogram); 188 grams protein; 188 grams carbo-hydrate; 60 grams fat

Food Groups	Number of servings
Bread	5
Fruit	3
Nonfat milk	3
Tsp added sugar	0
Vegetable	6
Protein sources	
Very lean	11
Lean	8
Medium-fat	1
Fat	8

Food group servings	Menu
Preworkout snack	
	Water
1 milk	1 c (245 g) plain yogurt
1 fruit	3/4 c (109 g) blueberries
	Sweeten with Splenda or low-calorie sweetener
Workout	
	Water
Breakfast	
	Water
1 bread	1 slice whole-grain bread
1 milk	1 c (237 ml) fat-free milk
1 fruit	1/2 c (119 ml) orange juice

1 medium-fat protein	1 whole egg, scrambled in nonstick skillet
5 very lean protein	4 egg whites, cooked with whole egg
	21 g isolated whey protein, added to milk and orange juice and blended with 3 or 4 ice cubes
1 fat	1/8 avocado, sliced and cooked with eggs

Snack

2 bread	Included in the edamame or Genisoy soy crisps
1 vegetable	1 c (124 g) celery sticks
2 very lean protein	1 c (180 g) edamame or 2 servings (about 2/3 bag) of Genisoy soy crisps
2 fat	1 tbsp (16 g) natural peanut butter

Lunch

1 bread	Subway turkey breast wrap
2 vegetable	Fill wrap with vegetable choices
4 very lean protein	3 oz (85 g) turkey included in wrap
	1 oz (28 g) cheese included in wrap
1 fat	1 fat included in cheese
Free	Dijon mustard

Snack

1 fruit	4 dried apricots
1 milk	1 tall nonfat latte
	Sweeten with Splenda or low-calorie sweetener
2 fat	12 almonds

Dinner

	Green tea (or other tea)
1 bread	1/2 baked sweet potato
3 vegetables	1/2 c (90 g) steamed asparagus
	2 c (56 g) mixed green salad
8 lean protein	8 oz (227 g) wild salmon, grilled
2 fat	1 tsp (5 ml) olive oil for salmon
	2 tbsp (30 ml) reduced-fat salad dressing

2,618 calories (32 calories per kilogram); 188 grams protein; 245 grams carbohydrate; 98 grams fat

Food groups	Number of servings
Bread	6
Fruit	6
Nonfat milk	3
Tsp added sugar	0
Vegetable	6
Protein sources	
Very lean	10
Lean	8
Medium-fat	1
Fat	14

Food group servings	Menu
Preworkout snack	
	Water
1 milk	1 c (245 g) plain yogurt
1 fruit	3/4 c (109 g) blueberries
	Sweeten with Splenda or low-calorie sweetener
Workout	
	Water
Breakfast	
	Water
1 bread	1 slice whole-grain bread
1 milk	1 c (237 ml) fat-free milk
3 fruit	1 c (237 ml) orange juice
1 medium-fat protein	1 whole egg, scrambled

4 very lean protein	4 egg whites, cooked with whole egg
	14 g isolated when protein, added to milk and orange juice and blended with ice cubes
5 fat	1/2 avocado, sliced and cooked with eggs
	1 tsp (4 g) Heart Smart Omega margarine for cooking eggs
Snack	
2 bread	Included in edamame or Genisoy soy crisps
1 vegetable	1 c (124 g) celery sticks
2 very lean protein	1 c (180 g) edamame or 2 servings (about 2/3 bag) of Genisoy soy crisps
4 fat	2 tbsp natural peanut butter
Lunch	
1 bread	Subway turkey breast wrap
2 vegetable	Fill wrap with vegetable choices
4 very lean protein	3 oz (85 g) turkey included in wrap
	1 oz (28 g) cheese included in wrap
1 fat	1 fat included in cheese
Free	Dijon mustard
Snack	
2 fruit	8 dried apricots
1 milk	1 tall nonfat latte
2 fat	12 almonds
Dinner	
	Green tea (or other tea)
2 bread	1 baked sweet potato
1 fruit	3 oz (85 g, or about 15) red grapes
3 vegetable	1/2 c (90 g) steamed asparagus
	2 c (56 g) mixed green salad
8 lean protein	8 oz (227 g) wild salmon, grilled
2 fat	8 large black olives
	1 tsp (5 ml) olive oil for salmon
Free	2 tbsp (30 ml) fat-free Italian salad dressing

Special Advice to Competitors

Many strength athletes worry about being too full just as they go into competition. However, it's critical to have enough fluid, calories, and nutrients to feel strong and look great. Probably the best way to do this is to supplement your diet with liquid meal replacements. These will charge you up but pass through your digestive system more quickly than solid foods.

Because each serving of meal replacement is about the same number of calories as a small meal or snack, you should drink it two and a half to three hours before your competition. If you feel comfortable, you can also add some low-fiber foods throughout the day to increase your nutritional intake and avoid the boredom of just drinking. Then, eat a variety of foods after the competition to round out your nutrition for the day.

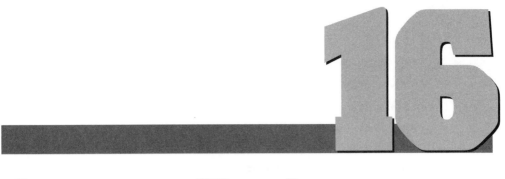

Power Eating Recipes

Although there are many supplements on the market, I always like to use fresh ingredients whenever possible. These recipes have been designed for my strength-training clients and teams over many years. Try them all to find out which ones are your favorites. If you've been a reader of earlier editions of Power Eating, you'll notice that some of the recipes have been updated, using new formulations and new ingredients.

Power Drinks

Kleiner's Essential Muscle-Building Formula for Women

> 1 cup (237 ml) nonfat milk
>
> 1/4 cup (59 ml) calcium-fortified orange juice
>
> 1/4 cup (37 g) frozen strawberries
>
> 14 g isolated whey protein powder
>
> 1 tsp (5 ml) (rounded) omega-3 brain booster powder*

Blend until smooth.

One serving contains:

Nutrients	Food Group Servings
242 calories	1 fruit serving
29 grams carbohydrate	1/2 lean protein serving
27 grams protein	2 very lean protein servings
2 grams fat	1 nonfat milk serving
<1 gram dietary fiber	

*Available at www.omega3brainbooster.com.

Kleiner's Essential Muscle-Building Formula for Men

1 cup (237 ml) nonfat milk

1/2 cup (119 ml) calcium-fortified orange juice

1 tbsp (21 g) honey

1/4 cup (37 g) frozen strawberries

21 g isolated whey protein powder

1 tsp (5 ml) (rounded) omega-3 brain booster powder*

Blend until smooth.

One serving contains:

Nutrients	Food Group Servings
378 calories	1 1/2 fruit servings
54 grams carbohydrate	1/2 lean protein serving
36 grams protein	3 very lean protein servings
2 grams fat	1 nonfat milk serving
1 gram dietary fiber	4 tsp added sugar

* Available at www.omega3brainbooster.com.

Kleiner's Easy Muscle-Building Formula

1 cup (237 ml) nonfat milk

1 packet instant breakfast

1 banana

1 tbsp (16 g) peanut butter

(Optional: Add 25 g isolated whey protein and 100 calories.)

Blend until smooth.

One serving contains:

Nutrients	Food Group Servings
438 calories	1 nonfat milk serving
70 grams carbohydrate	2 fruit servings
17 grams protein	1 very lean protein serving
10 grams fat	2 fat servings
6 grams fiber	6 tsp added sugar

Kleiner's Muscle-Building Formula

1 cup (149 g) frozen strawberries

1 cup (245 g) nonfat strawberry yogurt

15 g isolated whey protein powder

1 tbsp (21 g) honey

1 cup (237 ml) nonfat milk

1 cup (237 ml) calcium-fortified orange juice

Blend until smooth.

One serving contains:

Nutrients	Food Group Servings
529 calories	3 fruit servings
100 grams carbohydrate	2 very lean protein servings
31 grams protein	2 nonfat milk servings
1 gram fat	6 tsp added sugar
4 grams dietary fiber	

Kleiner's Muscle Formula Plus

24 g bovine colostrum or isolated whey protein

1 cup (149 g) frozen unsweetened strawberries

1 medium banana

1 cup (237 ml) nonfat vanilla soy milk fortified with calcium and vitamins A and D

1 cup (237 ml) orange juice fortified with calcium and vitamin C

Blend until smooth.

One serving contains:

Nutrients	Food Group Servings
436 calories	4 fruit servings
86 grams carbohydrate	3 very lean protein servings
27 grams protein	1 nonfat milk serving
0 grams fat	3 tsp added sugar
8 grams dietary fiber	

Kleiner's Muscle Formula Plus Light

21 g bovine colostrum or isolated whey protein

1 cup (149 g) frozen unsweetened strawberries

1/2 medium banana

1 cup (237 ml) nonfat vanilla soy milk fortified with calcium and vitamins A and D

1/2 cup (119 ml) orange juice fortified with calcium and vitamin C

Blend until smooth.

One serving contains:

Nutrients	Food Group Servings
316 calories	2 1/2 fruit servings
58 grams carbohydrate	3 very lean protein servings
26 grams protein	1 nonfat milk serving
0 grams fat	3 tsp added sugar
6 grams dietary fiber	

Bone-Builder Smoothie

One serving contains 750 milligrams of calcium.

1 cup (237 ml) nonfat milk

1/2 cup (119 ml) calcium-fortified orange juice

1/2 cup (123 g) nonfat vanilla yogurt

1 cup (149 g) mixture of frozen mango, blueberries, strawberries

1 tbsp (15 ml) nonfat dry milk powder

14 g isolated whey protein powder

Blend until smooth.

One serving contains:

Nutrients	Food Group Servings
440 calories	3 fruit servings
80 grams carbohydrate	2 very lean protein servings
30 grams protein	2 nonfat milk servings
0 grams fat	3 tsp added sugar
5 grams dietary fiber	

Mocha Breakfast Smoothie

1 cup (237 ml) nonfat milk

1/2 cup (119 ml) strongly brewed coffee

2 tbsp (32 g) natural peanut butter

1/2 large banana

1 envelope chocolate instant breakfast mix

10 ice cubes

Blend until smooth.

One serving contains:

Nutrients	Food Group Servings
485 calories	1 fruit serving
62 grams carbohydrate	3 very lean protein servings
21 grams protein	2 nonfat milk servings
17 grams fat	3 fat servings
5 grams dietary fiber	4 tsp added sugar

Soyful Smoothie (Lactose Free)

1/3 block soft tofu (5 oz, or 142 g)

3/4 cup (112 g) frozen strawberries

1/2 medium banana

1/2 cup (119 ml) vanilla nonfat soy milk fortified with vitamins A and D and calcium

1/2 cup (119 ml) calcium-fortified orange juice

2 tsp (14 g) honey

Cream tofu in blender until smooth. Add the next five ingredients and blend until smooth.

One serving contains:

Nutrients	Food Group Servings
321 calories	3 fruit servings
61 grams carbohydrate	1 medium-fat protein serving
11 grams protein	1/2 nonfat milk serving
5 grams fat	2 tsp added sugar
4 grams dietary fiber	

Phytochemical Phenomenon II

    1 cup (149 g) frozen mixture of mango and papaya

    1/2 medium kiwifruit, peeled and quartered

    1/2 cup (115 g) plain nonfat yogurt

    1/3 cup (78 ml) pomegranate juice

    2/3 cup (156 ml) pineapple juice

    1 cup (237 ml) nonfat milk or unflavored soy milk

Blend until smooth.

One serving contains:

Nutrients	**Food Group Servings**
383 calories	5 fruit servings
83 grams carbohydrate	3 very lean protein servings
16 grams protein	1 1/2 nonfat milk servings
<1 gram fat	
4 grams dietary fiber	

Zesty Citrus Smoothie

This smoothie will help replenish fluids and electrolytes, particularly on hot days.

    2 in. (5 cm) piece of fresh ginger

    Zest of 1 large lemon (about 2 tbsp, or 30 ml)

    1 cup (148 g) lemon sorbet

    2 cups (473 ml) cold unflavored sparkling water

    2 tbsp (30 ml) fresh lemon juice

    1 tbsp (15 ml) lime juice

    1/8 tsp salt

    2 tbsp (25 g) sugar

    2 tbsp (1 g) Splenda

    15 ice cubes

Grate the ginger and squeeze the juice from the grated ginger. Blend the ginger juice with the remaining ingredients until mixture reaches the consistency of a frozen margarita drink. For a lower-calorie beverage, make one recipe for two servings.

One serving contains:

Nutrients	**Food Group Servings**
150 calories	9 1/2 tsp added sugar
38 grams carbohydrate	
<1 gram protein	
0 grams fat	
<1 gram dietary fiber	

Piña Colada Smoothie

1 cup (237 ml) nonfat milk

1 envelope vanilla instant breakfast powder

6 oz (170 g) low-fat piña colada yogurt (or other coconut and
pineapple yogurt)

1/2 cup (119 ml) crushed pineapple in natural juice

2 tbsp (30 ml) light coconut milk

1/2 tsp (3 ml) rum extract

4 ice cubes

Blend until smooth.

One serving contains:

Nutrients	Food Group Servings
455 calories	1 fruit serving
82 grams carbohydrate	3 nonfat milk servings
21 grams protein	1 fat serving
5 grams fat	6 tsp added sugar
1 gram dietary fiber	

Antioxidant Advantage

1 cup (237 ml) nonfat milk

1/3 cup (78 ml) Concord grape juice

1 tbsp (15 ml) lime juice

1/2 cup (115 g) plain nonfat yogurt

1/2 cup (75 g) frozen strawberries

1/4 cup (37 g) frozen blueberries

5 g creatine monohydrate

1 tsp (5 ml) (rounded) omega-3 brain booster supplement*

Blend until smooth.

One serving contains:

Nutrients	Food Group Servings
273 calories	2 fruit servings
50 grams carbohydrate	1/2 lean protein serving
18 grams protein	1 1/2 nonfat milk servings
2 grams fat	
3 grams dietary fiber	

* Available at www.omega3brainbooster.com.

Morning Pick-Me-Up

2 tsp (10 ml) chai tea leaves

2 cups (473 ml) nonfat milk

1/3 cup (40 g) nonfat dry milk powder

1 1/2 tbsp (32 g) honey

1/8 tsp (.5 ml) nutmeg

4 ice cubes

Simmer the tea in milk for 5 to 8 minutes. Cool in the refrigerator. Pour the milk into a blender, straining out the tea leaves. Add the remaining ingredients. Blend until smooth.

One serving contains:

Nutrients	Food Group Servings
350 calories	3 nonfat milk servings
62 grams carbohydrate	6 tsp added sugar
25 grams protein	
1 gram fat	
0 grams dietary fiber	

Caribbean Crush

11.5 oz (340 ml, or 1 can) papaya juice

1/3 cup crushed pineapple in natural juice

1/2 banana

21 g isolated whey protein powder

6 ice cubes

Blend until smooth.

One serving contains:

Nutrients	Food Group Servings
364 calories	4 1/2 fruit servings
69 grams carbohydrate	3 very lean protein servings
23 grams protein	
<1 gram fat	
4 grams dietary fiber	

Apple Pie à la Mode

1 cup (237 ml) unfiltered apple juice

1/2 cup (119 ml) unsweetened applesauce

1/3 cup (48 g) vanilla nonfat frozen yogurt

2 tbsp (30 ml) toasted wheat germ

1/3 cup (40 g) nonfat dry milk powder

10 g isolated whey protein powder

Blend until smooth.

One serving contains:

Nutrients	Food Group Servings
399 calories	3 fruit servings
74 grams carbohydrate	2 very lean protein servings
25 grams protein	1 nonfat milk serving
2 grams fat	3 tsp added sugar
4 grams dietary fiber	

Lemon-Lime Zinger Sport Drink

To fuel and hydrate your body, drink this power booster within two hours before exercise. It's also a great fluid replenisher during or after exercise or anytime during an active day.

1 in. (3 cm) piece of fresh ginger

2 cups (473 ml) cold unflavored sparkling water

1 tbsp (15 ml) lemon juice

2 tsp (10 ml) lime juice

2 tbsp (25 g) sugar

Scant 1/8 tsp (.75 g) salt

Grate the ginger and squeeze out the juice. Blend the ginger juice with the remaining ingredients for 20 seconds. Serve immediately.

One serving contains:

Nutrients	Food Group Servings
109 calories	7 tsp added sugar
28 grams carbohydrate	
0 grams protein	
0 grams fat	
0 grams dietary fiber	

Easy Main Courses

Chicken in Orange Sauce With Pistachios

8 skinless, boneless chicken breast halves

4 tbsp (34 g) cake flour

Salt and pepper to taste

1 1/2 cups (355 ml) fresh orange juice

1/4 cup (59 ml) white wine

1/4 cup (59 ml) white wine vinegar

1/2 cup (119 ml) minced shallots

2 tbsp (28 g) brown sugar

2 tbsp (30 ml) olive oil

2 tbsp (28 g) unsalted butter, cut into small pieces

3 tbsp (64 g) honey

8 orange slices and 8 tbsp (62 g) unsalted pistachio nuts to garnish

Wax paper

1. Trim chicken breasts and pound thick ends under wax paper to cook evenly. Combine salt, pepper, and cake flour. Dust on chicken breasts.

2. In a saucepan, bring orange juice, wine, vinegar, shallots, and brown sugar to a boil. Simmer and reduce to about 1 cup. Keep warm.

3. Heat olive oil in a large skillet over medium heat. Sauté chicken breasts in batches until springy to the touch, 4 minutes per side. Transfer to an ovenproof casserole dish and set aside.

4. Remove sauce from heat and whisk in cold butter pieces. Pour over chicken and keep chicken warm in oven set at 250 degrees F (121 degrees C). Chicken may be chilled or frozen at this point.

5. To serve, thoroughly reheat chicken in oven at 325 degrees F (150 degrees C), basting well with the sauce.

6. Heat honey with 2 tbsp (30 ml) of the orange sauce. Sprinkle each breast with 1 tbsp (8 g) of pistachios. Coat orange slice to garnish chicken.

Makes 8 servings.

Each serving contains:

Nutrients	Food Group Servings
334 calories	4 very lean protein servings
22 grams carbohydrate	2 fat servings
30 grams protein	1/2 fruit serving
13 grams fat	1 tsp added sugar
2 grams dietary fiber	

Here are two recipes that give you the mood-boosting effects of omega-3 fats and the metabolism-boosting benefits of cayenne pepper. If you can stand the heat, add cayenne to your diet on a daily basis and it may help you stay lean, but not mean.

Pan-Fried Cajun Catfish

1/2 cup (69 g) cornmeal

1 tsp (.3 g) dried parsley flakes

1/2 tsp (1 g) paprika

1/8 tsp (.2 g) cayenne pepper (or to taste)

1/8 tsp (.2 g) white pepper

1/8 tsp (.2 g) black pepper

1/2 tsp (3 g) salt

1/4 tsp (.4 g) thyme

1/2 tsp (1.4 g) garlic powder

1/4 tsp (.6 g) onion powder

1 egg

2 1/2 tbsp (37 ml) water

12 oz (340 g) catfish fillets

Nonstick cooking spray

Lemon wedges

1. Mix together the cornmeal, herbs, and spices in a flat dish. In a separate dish, beat the egg with the water.

2. Heat a nonstick frying pan over medium-high heat for 30 seconds. Generously spray the pan with cooking spray. Dip each fillet in the egg–water mixture and then coat generously in the cornmeal mixture. Place skin side down in the frying pan for 5 to 6 minutes, or until the bottom is golden brown. Turn the fish and cook another 6 to 7 minutes. Turn again if needed and remove promptly. Watch the fish closely as it cooks. Do not let the oil smoke or the coating burn. Fish should be tender inside, crisp and brown on the outside. Serve hot with lemon wedges.

Makes 3 servings.

Each serving contains:

Nutrients	Food Group Servings
281 calories	4 lean protein servings
18 grams carbohydrate	1 bread serving
25 grams protein	
11 grams fat	
2 grams dietary fiber	

Lemon Sole With Mustard Sauce

This is a great fish recipe for those who don't love fish, as well as for those who do.

1 lb (454 g) lemon sole fillets

1/4 cup (59 ml) lemon juice

1/4 cup (59 ml) white wine

1 tsp (5 ml) cornstarch dissolved in 1/8 cup (31 ml) cold water

1 cup (237 ml) water

1/4 cup (59 ml) apple juice

2 tsp (10 ml) dry white wine

1 tsp (3 g) minced garlic

1 tbsp (15 ml) lime juice sweetened with 1 tsp (4 g) sugar

2 tsp (10 g) prepared yellow mustard

1 tsp (5 ml) Worcestershire sauce

1/8 tsp (.2 g) cayenne pepper (or to taste)

1. Place the fish, lemon juice, and 1/4 cup (59 ml) white wine in a pan and bake at 400 degrees F (200 degrees C) for 20 minutes, or until the fish is flaky and white.

2. Combine the dissolved cornstarch, water, apple juice, dry white wine, and garlic in a saucepan. Heat over medium heat to thicken, stirring often.

3. In a small bowl, whisk together the sweetened lime juice, mustard, Worcestershire sauce, and cayenne pepper. Add the mustard mixture to the cornstarch mixture and whisk until well blended. Allow the mixture to continue cooking until thickened.

4. Place the fish on a platter, pour the mustard sauce over it, and serve.

Makes 4 servings.

Each serving contains:

Nutrients

170 calories
6 grams carbohydrate
26 grams protein
2 grams fat
0 grams dietary fiber

Food Group Servings

1/2 fruit serving
4 very lean protein servings

Ready-to-Serve Vegetables

Irene's Marinated Broccoli

This is the easiest recipe to prepare for yourself or for entertaining. It makes the best-tasting raw broccoli you could imagine! It's great alone, or you could add the optional dip for a special occasion.

1 bunch broccoli, cut into small florets (about 3 cups, or 213 g)

Marinade

1/4 cup (59 ml) cider or wine vinegar

3/4 cup (178 ml) virgin olive oil

2 cloves garlic, split (or more if desired)

1 tsp (4 g) sugar

2 tsp (2 g) fresh dill

Put broccoli in resealable bag and cover with marinade. Marinate in bag, refrigerated, overnight. Drain.

Optional Dip*

2 cups (448 g) light mayonnaise (also works with half mayo and half plain yogurt)

1 1/2 tsp (3 g) curry powder

1 tsp (5 g) ketchup

1/4 tsp (1 ml) Worcestershire sauce

Mix together. Serve with drained broccoli. Makes 6 servings.

One serving without dip contains:

Nutrients	Food Group Servings
90 calories	1/2 vegetable serving
2 grams carbohydrate	2 fat servings
1 gram protein	
9 grams fat	
1 gram dietary fiber	

*Add 1 fat serving for every 1 tbsp dip

Alotta Onions Soup

Whenever I've shared this recipe with anyone, the description has always started out with "a lot of onions." The water and electrolyte content makes it a great fluid replacer after exercise. This recipe, which serves only two or three, is pared down from the army-sized version we make at home.

2 cloves fresh garlic, minced

1 tbsp (15 ml) canola oil

1/2 tbsp (7 ml) sesame oil

1 1/2 large yellow onions, thinly sliced

6 cups (1,420 ml) water

1 1/2 tbsp (22 ml) soy sauce

1/4 tsp (1 ml) freshly ground black pepper

4-6 tsp (8-12 g) freshly grated Parmesan cheese

1. Sauté the garlic in the oils in a shallow nonstick pan over medium heat until slightly soft, about 3 to 5 minutes. Add onions and cook, stirring occasionally, until slightly caramelized, about 20 minutes.

2. Transfer the onions and garlic to a soup pot. Add the water, soy sauce, and pepper. Bring to a low boil over high heat, then reduce the heat to low and simmer uncovered for 15 minutes.

3. Serve in full bowls sprinkled with 2 tsp of Parmesan cheese.

Makes 3 servings.

Each serving contains:

Nutrients	Food Group Servings
109 calories	1 1/2 vegetable servings
8 grams carbohydrate	1 1/2 fat servings
2 grams protein	
8 grams fat	
1 gram dietary fiber	

Great Grains

Easy Energy Couscous

4 tbsp (27 g) slivered almonds

4 tbsp (36 g) golden raisins

12 dried apricots, quartered

8 dried figs, quartered

1/2 tsp (1.2 g) cinnamon

1/2 cup (119 ml) fresh orange juice

1 1/2 cups (355 ml) water

1/4 tsp (1 ml) salt

1 tbsp (14 g) butter

1 cup (173 g) whole-wheat couscous

1. Place the almonds, raisins, apricots, and figs in a bowl with the cinnamon. Cover with the orange juice and refrigerate for a minimum of 30 minutes and up to overnight.

2. In a saucepan, bring the water, salt, and butter to a boil. Stir in the couscous. Cover and simmer over low heat for 5 minutes. Remove from heat and let stand 5 minutes. Fluff the couscous lightly with a fork.

3. Transfer the fruit and nut mixture to a saucepan and warm thoroughly over medium-low heat. Turn into a mixing bowl and add the cooked couscous. Mix well. Couscous can be served warm or cold.

Makes 6 servings.

Each serving contains:

Nutrients

258 calories
49 grams carbohydrate
5 grams protein
5 grams fat
7 grams dietary fiber

Food Group Servings

2 fruit servings
1 bread serving
1 fat serving

Seashore Buckwheat

2/3 cup whole-wheat pasta shells (70 g)

1 tbsp (15 ml) canola oil

1 cup (70 g) sliced mushrooms

1 small onion, diced

2 cups (473 ml) chicken stock

1 whole egg, slightly beaten

1 cup (164 g) preroasted buckwheat kernels or groats

Pinch of white pepper and salt to taste

1. Cook the pasta shells until al dente according to package directions; drain and set aside.

2. Heat the oil in a nonstick pan over medium heat. Add the mushrooms and onion and sauté until the onion is translucent, about 7 minutes. Set aside.

3. Heat the stock to boiling. In a small mixing bowl, combine the egg with the buckwheat until the kernels are coated. Turn the buckwheat into a medium-sized skillet. Stir the egg and buckwheat mixture over medium-high heat for 3 to 4 minutes until it is hot and slightly toasted and the egg-coated kernels are well separated. Reduce the heat to low and carefully stir in the boiling stock, sautéed mushrooms and onions, and pepper and salt. Cover tightly and simmer 10 to 12 minutes, or until the buckwheat kernels are tender and all the liquid has been absorbed.

4. Turn into an oven-safe casserole dish and mix in the pasta shells. Place uncovered under an oven broiler for 3 to 5 minutes, just to brown the top. Watch closely and remove promptly.

Makes 4 servings.

Each serving contains:

Nutrients	**Food Group Servings**
232 calories	2 bread servings
39 grams carbohydrate	2 vegetable servings
9 grams protein	1/2 very lean protein serving
6 grams fat	1/2 fat serving
5 grams dietary fiber	

Power Breakfasts

Indian Breakfast Salad

This delicious salad is served as a side dish in India but makes a fast and fabulous breakfast. It is spiced with cardamom, but because cardamom is expensive, you may prefer to use cinnamon.

1/2 tsp (2 g) butter

2 tbsp (14 g) slivered almonds

2 medium bananas, thinly sliced

4 tbsp (61 g) low-fat plain yogurt

3 tbsp (45 g) light sour cream

1 tbsp (21 g) honey

1/8 tsp (.25 g) ground cardamom or 1/4 tsp (.6 g) ground cinnamon

1. Melt the butter in a small nonstick skillet over medium heat. Toast almonds, stirring frequently, until golden, about 3 minutes.

2. Meanwhile, in a medium bowl, mix bananas with yogurt, sour cream, honey, and cardamom. Add almonds and enjoy.

Makes 2 servings.

One serving contains:

Nutrients	Food Group Servings
250 calories	2 fruit servings
42 grams carbohydrate	1 lean protein serving
6 grams protein	1 fat serving
8 grams fat	3 tsp added sugar
4 grams dietary fiber	

Breakfast Parfait

Make this artistic, high-powered breakfast portable by using plastic drinking cups with lids.

2 cups (490 g) low-fat strawberry yogurt
1 cup (110 g) low-fat granola
1 1/4 cup (208 g) fresh berries (whatever is in season)

1. In two 16 oz (473 ml) glass or plastic cups, layer the ingredients by adding 1/4 of the yogurt, 1/4 of the granola, and 1/4 of the berries.
2. Repeat step 1, reserving a dollop of the yogurt for the top.

Makes 2 servings.

One serving contains:

Nutrients	Food Group Servings
448 calories	1 bread serving
90 grams carbohydrate	1 fruit serving
13 grams protein	1/2 lean protein serving
5 grams fat	1 nonfat milk serving
5 grams dietary fiber	1/2 fat serving
	12 tsp added sugar

Peach Melba Yogurt Pops

These delicious pops can be prepared the night before to make a great light breakfast that you can easily hit the road with on a warm summer morning. If you don't want to bother with adding the sticks, just poke a fork into the pop when you're ready to eat.

1 cup (247 g) sliced canned peaches in light syrup
1 cup (245 g) low-fat raspberry yogurt
1 cup (237 ml) orange juice

1. Blend ingredients until smooth. Pour into four 10 oz (296 ml) plastic cups. Place in the freezer.
2. When mixture is partly frozen, insert sticks or plastic spoons.

Makes 2 servings.

One serving contains:

Nutrients	Food Group Servings
280 calories	2 fruit servings
64 grams carbohydrate	1 nonfat milk serving
6 grams protein	5 tsp added sugar
1 gram fat	
3 grams dietary fiber	

Orange Cinnamon French Toast

This toast takes only slightly longer to prepare than the standard version that pops out of the toaster.

2 large eggs, lightly beaten
2 tbsp (30 ml) orange juice
1/4 tsp (.6 g) ground cinnamon
4 slices whole-wheat bread
Vegetable cooking spray

1. In a shallow bowl, combine eggs, orange juice, and cinnamon.
2. Spray a nonstick skillet and heat over medium heat for 1 to 2 minutes, until hot. Dip bread into the mixture to coat both sides. Place bread slices in the skillet, pouring any extra egg mixture over them. Cook for about 2 minutes on each side or until browned.

Makes 2 servings.

One serving contains:

Nutrients	Food Group Servings
220 calories	2 bread servings
28 grams carbohydrate	1 medium-fat protein serving
12 grams protein	
7 grams fat	
4 grams dietary fiber	

Pineapple Cheese Danish

4 slices raisin bread
4 tbsp (62 g) canned unsweetened crushed pineapple, drained
1/2 cup (4 oz, or 113 g) part-skim ricotta cheese
1 tsp (5 g) brown sugar
Dash ground cinnamon

1. Spread each slice of bread with 1 oz of cheese and top with pineapple. Combine brown sugar and cinnamon and sprinkle on top of the pineapple.
2. Broil in toaster oven or under the broiler until sugar starts to bubble, about 2 minutes.

Makes 2 servings.

One serving contains:

Nutrients	Food Group Servings
246 calories	2 bread servings
35 grams carbohydrate	1/3 fruit serving
11 grams protein	1/2 medium-fat protein serving
7 grams fat	1/2 fat serving
3 grams dietary fiber	

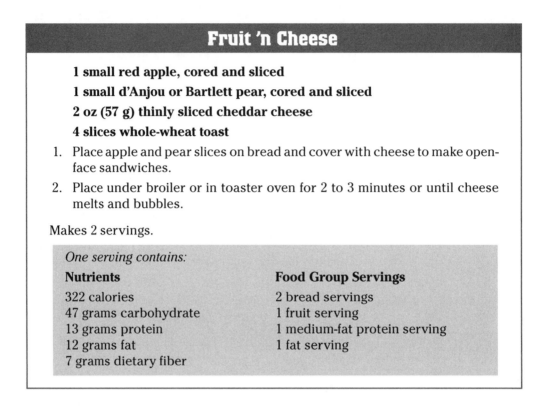

Fruit 'n Cheese

1 small red apple, cored and sliced

1 small d'Anjou or Bartlett pear, cored and sliced

2 oz (57 g) thinly sliced cheddar cheese

4 slices whole-wheat toast

1. Place apple and pear slices on bread and cover with cheese to make open-face sandwiches.
2. Place under broiler or in toaster oven for 2 to 3 minutes or until cheese melts and bubbles.

Makes 2 servings.

One serving contains:

Nutrients	Food Group Servings
322 calories	2 bread servings
47 grams carbohydrate	1 fruit serving
13 grams protein	1 medium-fat protein serving
12 grams fat	1 fat serving
7 grams dietary fiber	

Pump Up Your Power Drink

You can create your own designer drink by adding certain natural ingredients and nutritional supplements. Here's a rundown:

Fiber. With a goal of 25 to 35 grams per day, getting enough fiber is often difficult. Commercial juices and smoothies are usually devoid of fiber, but they don't have to be. Increase the fiber content of your powder drinks by using fruit, fruit with skins or seeds, ground flaxseed, and wheat germ. You can also eat whole-wheat crackers or breads with your drink to easily increase fiber.

Protein. Protein powders boost the protein content of your drink when you don't want to increase any other nutrients. Nonfat dry milk and whey powder are easy ways to supplement drinks with protein, carbohydrate, calcium, and riboflavin.

Energy. To pack in energy and nutrients, instant breakfast powders work well. If you are lactose intolerant, choose a lactose-free energy-boosting supplement powder.

Creatine monohydrate. If you participate in power sports or strength train, add creatine to your diet to enhance your performance. Especially after exercise, a power drink is a great way to get in one of your four daily 5-milligram doses.

Appendix A

Three-Day Food Record

Choose at least three days that will represent your typical schedule (work days and nonwork days, training days and rest days, or home days and travel days) and record your food intake for those days in a 24-hour diet log. You can make copies of the diet log that follows. Try to record the food as you eat it or just afterward; it is often difficult to remember in the evening exactly what you ate eight hours before. Record everything you eat and drink, including water, and be as detailed as possible.

When you are done recording, translate all the foods from a single day into food groups, and then into calories and grams of protein, carbohydrate, and fat by plugging them into the diet analysis table that follows. Use the food group tables from chapter 10 to get the nutrient details about each food group.

Sample Entry for 24-Hour Diet Log

Time of day	Food eaten	Description	Quantity	Location	Why you ate
12 noon	Chicken breast, no skin	Broiled	4 ounces	Home	Hungry
	Broccoli	Steamed	4 stalks		

24-Hour Diet Log

Time of day	Food eaten	Description	Quantity	Location	Why you ate

Diet Analysis Table

Diet Record Date _____

Food groups	Number of servings	Carbohydrate (g)	Protein (g)	Fat (g)	Calories
Bread/Starch					
Fruit					
Milk					
Nonfat					
Low fat					
Tsp of added sugar					
Vegetables					
Protein					
Very lean					
Lean					
Medium-fat					
Fat					
Totals					

Appendix B

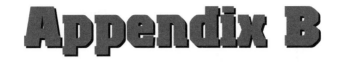

Healthy Fast Food

Food	Calories	Percent fat
Burger King		
Tendergrill chicken sandwich (no sauce)	450	20
McDonald's		
Premium grilled chicken classic sandwich	420	19
Bacon ranch salad with grilled chicken	260	31
Fruit and yogurt parfait	160	13
Apple dippers (without caramel)	35	0
Low-fat caramel dip (2 tsp added sugar)	70	7
Pizza Hut		
Chicken supreme medium thin and crispy (1 slice)	200	30
Veggie Lover's medium thin and crispy (1 slice)	180	33
Cheese-only medium hand-tossed style (1 slice)	240	29
Quartered ham medium hand-tossed style (1 slice)	220	23
Chicken supreme medium hand-tossed style (1 slice)	230	26
Veggie Lover's medium hand-tossed style (1 slice)	220	27

Food	Calories	Percent fat
Taco Bell (Order all items fresco style.)		
Ranchero chicken soft taco	170	21
Grilled steak soft taco	170	26
Gordita Baja chicken	230	22
Gordita Baja steak	230	26
Tostada	200	25
Enchirito chicken	250	20
Enchirito steak	250	24
Bean burrito	370	24
Fiesta chicken burrito	370	27
Fiesta steak burrito	370	29
Wendy's		
Broccoli and cheese baked potato	340	8
Sour cream and chives baked potato	320	11
Subway		
Choose from their extensive menu of items containing 6 grams of fat or less.		

Works Consulted

Abramowicz, W.N., et al. 2005. Effects of acute versus chronic L-carnitine L-tartrate supplementation on metabolic responses to steady state exercise in males and females. *International Journal of Sport Nutrition and Exercise Metabolism* 15: 386-400.

Akermark, C., I. Jacobs, M. Rasmusson, and J. Karlsson. 1996. Diet and muscle glycogen concentration in relation to physical performance in Swedish elite ice hockey players. *International Journal of Sport Nutrition* 6: 272-284.

Alkhenizan, A.H., et al. 2004. The role of vitamin E in the prevention of coronary events and stroke. Meta-analysis of randomized controlled trials. *Saudi Medical Journal* 25: 1808-14.

Allen, J.D. et al. 1998. Ginseng supplementation does not enhance healthy young adults' peak aerobic exercise performance. *Journal of the American College of Nutrition* 17: 462-466.

American Dietetic Association. 1995. Position of the American Dietetic Association: Phytochemicals and functional foods. *Journal of the American Dietetic Association* 95: 493-496.

American Dietetic Association. 1998. Position of the American Dietetic Association: Use of nutritive and non-nutritive sweeteners. *Journal of the American Dietetic Association* 98: 580-588.

Andersson, B., X. Xuefan, M. Rebuffe-Scrive, K. Terning, et al. 1991. The effects of exercise training on body composition and metabolism in men and women. *International Journal of Obesity* 15: 75-81.

Anomasiri, W., et al. 2004. Low dose creatine supplementation enhances sprint phase of 400 meters swimming performance. *Journal of the Medical Association of Thailand* 87: S228-32.

Antonio, J., 2000. The effects of Tribulus terrestris on body composition and exercise performance in resistance-trained males. *International Journal of Sports Nutrition and Exercise Metabolism* 10: 208-215.

Antonio, J. et al. 1999. Glutamine: A potentially useful supplement for athletes. *Canadian Journal of Applied Physiology* 24: 1-14.

Applegate, L. 1992. Protein power. *Runner's World*, June, 22-24.

Armstrong, L.E. 2002. Caffeine, body fluid-electrolyte balance, and exercise performance. *International Journal of Sport Nutrition and Exercise Metabolism* 12: 189-206.

Avery, N.G., et al. 2003. Effects of vitamin E supplementation on recovery from repeated bouts of resistance exercise. *Journal of Strength and Conditioning Research* 17: 801-809.

Backhouse, S.H., et al. 2005. Effect of carbohydrate and prolonged exercise on affect and perceived exertion. *Medicine and Science in Sports and Exercise* 37: 1768-1773.

Bahrke, M.S., et al. 2004. Abuse of anabolic androgenic steroids and related substances in sport and exercise. *Current Opinion in Pharmacology* 4: 614-620.

Bahrke, M.S., et al. 1994. Evaluation of the ergogenic properties of ginseng. *Sports Medicine* 18: 229-248.

Balon, T.W., J.F. Horowitz, and K.M. Fitzsimmons. 1992. Effects of carbohydrate loading and weight-lifting on muscle girth. *International Journal of Sports Nutrition* 2: 328-334.

Balsom, P.D., et al. 1998. Carbohydrate intake and multiple sprint sports: With special reference to football (soccer). *International Journal of Sports Medicine* 20: 48-52.

Baranov, A.I. 1982. Medicinal uses of ginseng and related plants in the Soviet Union: Recent trends in the Soviet literature. *Journal of Ethnopharmacology* 6: 339-353.

Barth, C.A., and U. Behnke. 1997. Nutritional physiology of whey components. *Nahrung* 41: 2-12.

Bazzarre, T.L., et al. 1992. Plasma amino acid responses of trained athletes to two successive exhaustive trials with and without interim carbohydrate feeding. *Journal of the American College of Nutrition* 11 (5): 501-511.

Bean, A. 1996. Here's to your immunity. *Runner's World*, February, 23.

Bellisle, F., and C. Perez. 1994. Low-energy substitutes for sugars and fats in the human diet: Impact on nutritional regulation. *Neuroscience Behavioral Review* 18: 197-205.

Bemben, M.G., et al. 2005. Creatine supplementation and exercise performance: Recent findings. *Sports Medicine* 35: 107-125.

Bent, S., et al. 2006. Saw palmetto for benign prostatic hyperplasia. *New England Journal of Medicine* 354: 557-566.

Benton, D., et al. 2001. The influence of phosphatidylserine supplementation on mood and heart rate when faced with an acute stressor. *Nutritional Neuroscience* 4: 169-178.

Biolo, G., et al. 1997. An abundant supply of amino acids enhances the metabolic effect of exercise on muscle protein. *American Journal of Physiology* 273: E122-E129.

Bird, S.P., et al. 2006. Effects of liquid carbohydrate/essential amino acid ingestion on acute hormonal response during a single bout of resistance exercise in untrained men. *Nutrition* 22: 367-375.

Bjorntorp, P. 1991. Importance of fat as a support nutrient for energy: Metabolism of athletes. *Journal of Sports Sciences* 9: 71-76.

Blankson, H., et al. 2000. Conjugated linoleic acid reduces body fat mass in overweight and obese humans. *Journal of Nutrition* 130: 2943-2948.

Blomstrand, E. 2006. A role for branched-chain amino acids in reducing central fatigue. *Journal of Nutrition* 136: 544S-547S.

Blomstrand, E., et al. 2006. Branched-chain amino acids activate key enzymes in protein synthesis after physical exercise. *Journal of Nutrition* 136: 269S-273S.

Bloomer, R.J., et al. 2000. Effects of meal form and composition on plasma testosterone, cortisol, and insulin following resistance exercise. *International Journal of Sport Nutrition and Exercise Metabolism* 10: 415-424.

Blumenthal, M. (ed.). 1998. *The Complete German Commission E Monographs*. Austin, Texas: American Botanical Council.

Borsheim, E., et al. 2004. Effect of an amino acid, protein, and carbohydrate mixture on net muscle protein balance after resistance exercise. *International Journal of Sport Nutrition and Exercise Metabolism* 14: 255-271.

Borsheim, E., et al. 2002. Essential amino acids and muscle protein recovery from resistance exercise. *American Journal of Physiology, Endocrinology, and Metabolism* 2002: E648-E657.

Boullata, J.I., et al. 2003. Anaphylactic reaction to a dietary supplement containing willow bark. *The Annals of Pharmacotherapy* 37: 832-5.

Brass, E.P. 2004. Carnitine and sports medicine: Use or abuse? *Annals of the New York Academy of Sciences* 1033: 67-78.

Bremner, K., et al. 2002. The effect of phosphate loading on erythrocyte 2,3-bisphosphoglycerate levels. *Clinica Chimica Acta* 323: 111-114.

Brilla, L.R., and V. Conte. 1999. Effects of zinc-magnesium (ZMA) supplementation on muscle attributes of football players. *Medicine and Science in Sports and Exercise* 31 (5 Supplement): Abstract No. 483.

Brilla, L.R., and T.F. Haley. 1992. Effect of magnesium supplementation on strength training in humans. *Journal of the American College of Nutrition* 11: 326-329.

Brown, G.A., et al. 2000. Effects of anabolic precursors on serum testosterone concentrations and adaptations to resistance training in young men. *International Journal of Sports Nutrition and Exercise Metabolism* 10: 340-359.

Brown, J., M.C. Crim, V.R. Young, and W.J. Evans. 1994. Increased energy requirements and changes in body composition with resistance training in older adults. *The American Journal of Clinical Nutrition* 60: 167-175.

Bryner, R.W., R.C. Toffle, I.H. Ullrich, and R.A. Yeager. 1997. The effects of exercise intensity on body composition, weight loss, and dietary composition in women. *Journal of the American College of Nutrition* 16: 68-73.

Bucci, L.R. 2000. Selected herbals and human exercise performance. *The American Journal of Clinical Nutrition* 72 (2 Supplement): 624S-636S.

Buckley, J.D., et al. 1998. Effect of an oral bovine colostrum supplement (Intact) on running performance. Abstract, 1998 Australian Conference of Science and Medicine in Sport, Adelaide, South Australia.

Buckley, J.D., et al. 1999. Oral supplementation with bovine colostrum (Intact) increases vertical jump performance. Abstract, 4th Annual Congress of the European College of Sport Science, Rome.

Bujko, J., et al. 1997. Benefit of more but smaller meals at a fixed daily protein intake. *Zeitschrift Fur Ernahrungswissenschaft* 36: 347-349.

Burke, E.R. 1999. *D-ribose: What you need to know*. Garden City Park, New York: Avery Publishing Group.

Burke, L.M. 1997. Nutrition for post-exercise recovery. *International Journal of Sports Nutrition* 1: 214-224.

Burke, L.M., et al. 1998. Carbohydrate intake during prolonged cycling minimizes effect of glycemic index of preexercise meal. *Journal of Applied Physiology* 85: 2220-2226.

Butterfield, G., et al. 1991. Amino acids and high protein diets. In D. Lamb and M. Williams (Eds.). *Perspectives in exercise science and sports medicine.* Vol. 4, Brown & Benchmark, 87-122.

Campbell, B.I., et al. 2004. The ergogenic potential of arginine. *Journal of the International Society of Sports Nutrition* 1: 35-38.

Campbell, W.W., M.C. Crim, V.R. Young, et al. 1995. Effects of resistance training and dietary protein intake on protein metabolism in older adults. *American Journal of Physiology* 268: E1143-E1153.

Carli, G., et al. 1992. Changes in exercise-induced hormone response to branched chain amino acid administration. *European Journal of Applied Physiology* 64: 272-277.

Castell, L.M. 1996. Does glutamine have a role in reducing infections in athletes? *European Journal of Applied Physiology* 73: 488-490.

Chandler, R.M., H.K. Byrne, J.G. Patterson, and J.L. Ivy. 1994. Dietary supplements affect the anabolic hormones after weight-training exercise. *Journal of Applied Physiology* 76: 839-845.

Charley, H. 1982. *Food science.* New York: John Wiley & Sons, Inc.

Chilibeck, P.D., et al. 2005. Creatine monohydrate and resistance training increase bone mineral content and density in older men. *The Journal of Nutrition, Health & Aging* 9: 352-353.

Chilibeck, P.D., et al. 2004. Effect of creatine ingestion after exercise on muscle thickness in males and females. *Medicine and Science in Sports and Exercise* 36: 1781-1788.

Clancy, S.P., P.M. Clarkson, M.E. DeCheke, et al. 1994. Effects of chromium picolinate supplementation on body composition, strength, and urinary chromium loss in football players. *International Journal of Sport Nutrition* 4: 142-153.

Clark, N. 1993. Athletes with amenorrhea. *The Physician and Sportsmedicine* 21: 45-48.

Clarkson, P.M. 1991. Nutritional ergogenic aids: Chromium, exercise, and muscle mass. *International Journal of Sport Nutrition* 1: 289-293.

Clarkson, P.M. 1996. Nutrition for improved sports performance: Current issues on ergogenic aids. *Sports Medicine* 21: 393-401.

Coleman, E. 1997. Carbohydrate unloading: A reality check. *The Physician and Sportsmedicine* 25: 97-98.

Collomp, K. 1991. Effects of caffeine ingestion on performance and anaerobic metabolism during the Wingate Test. *International Journal of Sports Medicine* 12: 439-443.

Collomp, K., A. Ahmaidi, M. Audran, and C. Prefaut. 1992. Benefits of caffeine ingestion on sprint performance in trained and untrained swimmers. *European Journal of Applied Physiology* 64: 377-380.

Colson, S.N., et al. 2005. Cordyceps sinensis- and Rhodiola rosea-based supplementation in male cyclists and its effect on muscle tissue oxygen saturation. *Journal of Strength and Conditioning Research* 19: 358-363.

Convertino, V.A., et al. 1996. ACSM position stand. Exercise and fluid replacement. *Medicine and Science in Sports and Exercise* 28: i-vii.

Coyle, E.F. 1991. Timing and method of increased carbohydrate intake to cope with heavy training, competition and recovery. *Journal of Sports Sciences* 9 Spec No: 29-51.

Coyle, E.F. 1995. Fat metabolism during exercise. *Sports Science Exchange* 8: 1-7.

Coyle, E.F. 1997. Fuels for sport performance. In D. Lamb and R. Murray (Eds.). *Perspectives in exercise science and sports medicine.* Carmel, Indiana: Cooper Publishing Group.

Craciun, A.M., et al. 1998. Improved bone metabolism in female elite athletes after vitamin K supplementation. *International Journal of Sports Medicine* 19: 479-484.

Dalton, R.A., et al. 1999. Acute carbohydrate consumption does not influence resistance exercise performance during energy restriction. *International Journal of Sport Nutrition* 9: 319-332.

Davis, J.M., et al. 1999. Effects of branched-chain amino acids and carbohydrate on fatigue during intermittent, high-intensity running. *International Journal of Sports Medicine* 20: 309-314.

DeMarco, H.M., et al. 1999. Pre-exercise carbohydrate meals: Application of glycemic index. *Medicine and Science in Sports and Exercise* 31: 164-170.

Deschenes, M.R., and W.J. Kraemer. 1989. The biochemical basis of muscular fatigue. *National Strength and Conditioning Association Journal* 11: 41-44.

Dimeff, R.J. 1993. Steroids and other performance enhancers. In R.N. Matzen and R.S. Lang (Eds.). *Clinical preventive medicine.* St. Louis: Mosby–Year Book, Inc.

Dimeff, R.J. May 19, 1996. Drugs and sports: Prescription and non-prescription. Presented at Sports Medicine for the Rheumatologist, American College of Rheumatology, Phoenix, Arizona.

Doherty, M., et al. 2005. Effects of caffeine ingestion on rating of perceived exertion during and after exercise: A meta-analysis. *Scandinavian Journal of Medicine & Science in Sports* 15: 69-78.

Dowling, E.A., et al. 1996. Effect of Eleutherococcus senticosus on submaximal and maximal performance. *Medicine and Science in Sports and Exercise* 28: 482-489.

Dulloo, A.G. 1999. Efficacy of a green tea extract rich in catechin polyphenols and caffeine in increasing 24-h energy expenditure and fat oxidation in humans. *The American Journal of Clinical Nutrition* 70: 1040-1045.

Earnest, C.P., et al. 2004. Effects of a commercial herbal-based formula on exercise performance in cyclists. *Medicine and Science in Sports and Exercise* 36: 504-509.

Editor. 2006. Choosing safer beef to eat. Web site: www.cspinet.org/foodsafety/saferbeef.html.

Editor. 2001. Conjugated linoleic acid overview. Professional Monographs: Herbal, Mineral, Vitamin, Nutraceuticals. Intramedicine, March 1.

Editor. 2006. The hoopla about hoodia. Web site: bestdietforme.com.

Editor. 1996. The new diet pills: Fairly but not completely safe. *Harvard Heart Letter.* 7: 1-2.

Editor. 2006. The triad. Web site: www.femaleathletetriad.org.

Editor. 2006. Vitamin E pills: Now it's thumbs down. Web site: consumerreports.org.

Editor. Winter 1997. Ergogenic aids: Reported facts and claims. *Scan's Pulse Supplement*: 15-19.

Editor. 2000. Smart waters™. BevNet. Internet Web site: bevnet.com/reviews/smartwater/index/asp.

Editor. 2000. Vitamin drink. *Nutritional Outlook* 3: 70.

Engels, H.J., et al. 1997. No ergogenic effects of ginseng (Panax C.A. Meyer) during graded maximal aerobic exercise. *Journal of the American Dietetic Association* 97: 1110-1115.

Essen-Gustavsson, B., and P.A. Tesch. 1990. Glycogen and triglyceride utilization in relation to muscle metabolic characteristics in men performing heavy-resistance exercise. *European Journal of Applied Physiology* 61: 5-10.

Evans, W. 1996. The protective role of antioxidants in exercise induced oxidative stress. Keynote address, 13th Annual SCAN Symposium, April 28, Scottsdale, Arizona.

Fairfield, K.M., and R.H. Fletcher. 2002. Vitamins for chronic disease prevention in adults. *Journal of the American Medical Association* 287: 3116-3126.

Fawcett, J.P., S.J. Farquhar, R.J. Walker, et al. 1996. The effect of oral vanadyl sulfate on body composition and performance in weight-training athletes. *International Journal of Sport Nutrition* 6: 382-390.

Ferreira, M., et al. 1997. Effects of conjugated linoleic acid supplementation during resistance training on body composition and strength. *Journal of Strength and Conditioning Research* 11: 280.

Fogelholm, M. 1992. Micronutrient status in females during a 24-week fitness-type exercise program. *Annals of Nutrition and Metabolism* 36: 209-218.

Fogt, D.L., et al. 2000. Effects of post exercise carbohydrate-protein supplement on skeletal muscle glycogen storage. *Medicine and Science in Sports and Exercise* 2 (Supplement): Abstract No. 131.

Foley, D. 1984. Best health bets from the B team. *Prevention*, April, 62-67.

Food and Nutrition Board. 1989. National Research Council: *Recommended dietary allowances*. 10th Edition. National Academy Press.

Frentsos, J.A., and J.R. Baer. 1997. Increased energy and nutrient intake during training and competition improves elite triathletes' endurance performance. *International Journal of Sport Nutrition* 7: 61-71.

Frey-Hewitt, K.M., K.M. Vranizan, D.M. Dreon, and P.D. Wood. 1990. The effect of weight loss by dieting or exercise on resting metabolic rate in overweight men. *International Journal of Obesity* 14: 327-334.

Friedl, K.E., R.J. Moore, L.E. Martinez-Lopez, et al. 1994. Lower limit of body fat in healthy active men. *Journal of Applied Physiology* 77: 933-940.

Gerster, H. 1989. The role of vitamin C in athletic performance. *Journal of the American College of Nutrition* 8: 636-643.

Gerster, H. 1991. Function of vitamin E in physical exercise: A review. *Zeitschrift fur Ernahrungswissenschaft* 30: 89-97.

Gillette, C.A., R.C. Bullough, and C.L. Melby. 1994. Postexercise energy expenditure in response to acute aerobic or resistive exercise. *International Journal of Sport Nutrition* 4: 347-360.

Gillman, M.W., L.A. Cupples, D. Gagnon, et al. 1995. Protective effect of fruits and vegetables on development of stroke in men. *Journal of the American Medical Association* 273: 1113-1117.

Giovannuci, E., A. Ascherio, E.B. Rimm, et al. Intake of carotenoids and retinol in relation to risk of prostate cancer. *Journal of the National Cancer Institute* 87: 1767-1776.

Gisolfi, C.V., et al. 1992. Guidelines for optimal replacement beverages for different athletic events. *Medicine and Science in Sports and Exercise* 24: 679-687.

Goldfarb, A.H. 1999. Nutritional antioxidants as therapeutic and preventive modalities in exercise-induced muscle damage. *Canadian Journal of Applied Physiology* 24: 249-266.

Gornall, J., and R.G. Villani. 1996. Short-term changes in body composition and metabolism with severe dieting and resistance exercise. *International Journal of Sport Nutrition* 6: 285-294.

Goulet, E.D., et al. 2005. Assessment of the effects of eleutherococcus senticosus on endurance performance. *International Journal of Sport Nutrition and Exercise Metabolism* 15: 75-83.

Green, A.L., E. Hultman, I.A. MacDonald, D.A. Sewell, and P.L. Greenhaff. 1996. Carbohydrate ingestion augments skeletal muscle creatine accumulation during creatine supplementation in humans. *American Journal of Physiology* 271: E821-E826.

Green, N.R., and A.A. Ferrando. 1994. Plasma boron and the effects of boron supplementation in males. *Environmental Health Perspective Supplement* 7: 73-77.

Gross, M., et al. 1991. Ribose administration during exercise: Effects on substrates and products of energy metabolism in healthy subjects and a patient with myoadenylate deaminase deficiency. *Klinische Wochenschrift* 69: 151-155.

Groeneveld, G.J., et al. 2005. Few adverse effects of long-term creatine supplementation in a placebo-controlled trial. *International Journal of Sports Medicine* 26: 307-313.

Habeck, M. 2002. A succulent cure to end obesity. *Drug Discovery Today* 7: 280-281.

Haaz, S., et al. 2006. Citrus aurantium and synephrine alkaloids in the treatment of overweight and obesity: An update. *Obesity Reviews* 7: 79-88.

Haff, G.G., et al. 1999. The effect of carbohydrate supplementation on multiple sessions and bouts of resistance exercise. *Journal of Strength and Conditioning Research* 13: 111-117.

Haff, G.G., et al. 2000. Carbohydrate supplementation attenuates muscle glycogen loss during acute bouts of resistance exercise. *International Journal of Sport Nutrition and Exercise Metabolism* 10: 326-339.

Harberson, D.A. 1988. Weight gain and body composition of weightlifters: Effect of high-calorie supplementation vs. anabolic steroids. In W.E. Garrett Jr. and T.E. Malone (Eds.). *Report of the Ross Laboratories Symposium on muscle development: Nutritional alternatives to anabolic steroids.* Columbus, Ohio: Ross Laboratories, 72-78.

Hargreaves, M. 2000. Skeletal muscle metabolism during exercise in humans. *Clinical and Experimental Pharmacology and Physiology* 27: 225-228.

Hartung, G.H., J.P. Foreyt, R.S. Reeves, et al. 1990. Effect of alcohol dose on plasma lipoprotein subfractions and lipolytic enzyme activity in active and inactive men. *Metabolism* 39: 81-86.

Hasler, C.M. 1996. Functional foods: The western perspective. *Nutrition Reviews* 54 (11 Part 2): S6-S10.

Hassmen, P., et al. 1994. Branched-chain amino acid supplementation during 30-km competitive run: Mood and cognitive performance. *Nutrition* 10: 405-410.

Health, M.K. (Ed.). 1982. Diet manual, including a vegetarian meal plan, 6th edition. Seventh Day Adventist Dietetic Association, P.O. Box 75, Loma Linda, CA 92345.

Heaney, R.P. 1993. Protein intake and the calcium economy. *Journal of the American Dietetic Association* 93: 1259-1260.

Hegewald, M.G., et al. 1991. Ribose infusion accelerates thallium redistribution with early imaging compared with late 24-hour imaging without ribose. *Journal of the American College of Cardiology* 18: 1671-1681.

Heinonen, O.J. 1996. Carnitine and physical exercise. *Sports Medicine* 22: 109-132.

Hemila, H. 1996. Vitamin C and common cold incidence: A review of studies with subjects under heavy physical stress. *International Journal of Sports Medicine* 17: 379-383.

Henderson, S., et al. 2005. Effects of coleus forskohlii supplementation on body composition and hematological profiles in mildly overweight women. *Journal of the International Society of Sports Nutrition* 2: 54-62.

Herbert, V., and K.C. Dos. 1994. Folic acid and vitamin B12. In M. Shils, J. Olson, and M. Shike (Eds.). *Modern nutrition in health and disease.* Philadelphia: Lea & Febiger, 1430-1435.

Hickson, J.F., et al. 1987. Nutritional intake from food sources of high school football athletes. *Journal of the American Dietetic Association* 87: 1656-1659.

Hitchins, S., et al. 1999. Glycerol hyperhydration improves cycle time trial performance in hot humid conditions. *European Journal of Applied Physiology and Occupational Physiology* 80: 494-501.

Hoffman, J.R., et al. 2004. Effects of beta-hydroxy beta-methylbutyrate on power performance and indices of muscle damage and stress during high-intensity training. *Journal of Strength and Conditioning Research* 1: 747-752.

Holt, S.H., et al. 1999. The effects of high-carbohydrate vs high-fat breakfasts on feelings of fullness and alertness, and subsequent food intake. *International Journal of Food Sciences and Nutrition* 50: 13-28.

Hulmi, J.J., et al. 2005. Protein ingestion prior to strength exercise affects blood hormones and metabolism. *Medicine and Science in Sports and Exercise* 37: 1990-1997.

Ivy, J.L. 2002. Early postexercise muscle glycogen recovery is enhanced with a carbohydrate-protein supplement. *Journal of Applied Pphysiology* 93: 1337-1344.

Ivy, J.L., et al. 1988. Muscle glycogen storage after different amounts of carbohydrate ingestion. *Journal of Applied Physiology* 65: 2018-2023.

Jackman, M., P. Wendling, D. Friars, et al. 1994. Caffeine ingestion and high-intensity intermittent exercise. Abstract. Personal communication with Larry Spriet, University of Guelph, Ontario, Canada.

Jacobsen, B.H. 1990. Effect of amino acids on growth hormone release. *The Physician and Sportsmedicine* 18: 68.

Jennings, E. 1995. Folic acid as a cancer-preventing agent. *Medical Hypotheses* 45: 297-303.

Ji, L.L. 1996. Exercise, oxidative stress, and antioxidants. *The American Journal of Sports Medicine* 24: S20-S24.

Kalman, D., et al. 1999. The effects of pyruvate supplementation on body composition in overweight individuals. *Nutrition* 15: 337-340.

Kanarek, R. 1997. Psychological effects of snacks and altered meal frequency. *British Journal of Nutrition* 77 (Supplement): S105-S118.

Kanter, M.M., et al. 1995. Antioxidants, carnitine and choline as putative ergogenic aids. *International Journal of Sport Nutrition* 5: S120-S131.

Kanter, M.M., L.A. Nolte, and J.O. Holloszy. 1993. Effects of an antioxidant vitamin mixture on lipid peroxidation at rest and postexercise. *Journal of Applied Physiology* 74: 965-969.

Kaplan, S.A., et al. 2004. A prospective, 1-year trial using saw palmetto versus finasteride in the treatment of category III prostatitis/chronic pelvic pain syndrome. *Journal of Urology* 171: 284-288.

Kelly, G.S. 2001. Conjugated linoleic acid: A review. *Alternative Medicine Review* 6: 367-382.

Keim, N.L., T.F Barbieri, M.D. Van Loan, and B.L. Anderson. 1990. Energy expenditure and physical performance in overweight women: Response to training with and without caloric restriction. *Metabolism* 39: 651-658.

Keim, N.L., A.Z. Belko, and T.F. Barbieri. 1996. Body fat percentage and gender: Associations with exercise energy expenditure, substrate utilization, and mechanical work efficiency. *International Journal of Sport Nutrition* 6: 356-369.

Keith, R.E., K.A. O'Keefe, D.L. Blessing, and G.D. Wilson. 1991. Alterations in dietary carbohydrate, protein, and fat intake and mood state in trained female cyclists. *Medicine and Science in Sports and Exercise* 2: 212-216.

Kendrick, Z.V., M.B. Affrime, and D.T. Lowenthal. 1993. Effect of ethanol on metabolic responses to treadmill running in well-trained men. *Journal of Clinical Pharmacology* 33: 136-139.

Kerksick, C., et al. 2001. Bovine colostrum supplementation on training adaptations II: Performance. Abstract presented at 2001 FASEB meeting, Orlando, FL.

Kim, S.H., et al. 2005. Effects of Panax ginseng extract on exercise-induced oxidative stress. *The Journal of Sports Medicine and Physical Fitness* 45: 178-182.

Kingsley, M.I., et al. 2006. Effects of phosphatidylserine on exercise capacity during cycling in active males. *Medicine and Science in Sports and Exercise* 38: 64-71.

Kingsley, M.I., et al. 2005. Effects of phosphatidylserine on oxidative stress following intermittent running. *Medicine and Science in Sports and Exercise* 37: 1300-1306.

Kirkendall, D.T. 1998. Fluid and electrolyte replacement in soccer. *Clinics in Sports Medicine* 17: 729-738.

Kleiner, S.M. 1991. Performance-enhancing aids in sport: Health consequences and nutritional alternatives. *Journal of the American College of Nutrition* 10: 163-176.

Kleiner, S.M. 1999. Water: An essential but overlooked nutrient. *Journal of the American Dietetic Association* 99: 200-206.

Kleiner, S.M. 2000. Bodybuilding. In C.A. Rosenbloom (Ed.). *Sports nutrition: A guide for the professional working with active people.* (3rd edition). Chicago: SCAN, American Dietetic Association.

Kleiner, S.M., et al. 1989. Dietary influences on cardiovascular disease risk in anabolic steroid-using and non-using bodybuilders. *Journal of the American College of Nutrition* 8: 109-119.

Kleiner, S.M., et al. 1990. Metabolic profiles, diet, and health practices of championship male and female bodybuilders. *Journal of the American Dietetic Association* 90: 962-967.

Kleiner, S.M., et al. 1994. Nutritional status of nationally ranked elite bodybuilders. *International Journal of Sport Nutrition* 1: 54-69.

Kraemer, W.J., et al. 1998. Hormonal responses to consecutive days of heavy-resistance exercise with or without nutritional supplementation. *Journal of Applied Physiology* 85: 1544-1555.

Kreider, R.B. 1999. Dietary supplements and the promotion of muscle growth. *Sports Medicine* 27: 97-110.

Krieder, R.B. 2003. Effects of creatine supplementation on performance and training adaptations. *Molecular and Cellular Biochemistry* 244: 89-94.

Kreider, R.B. 2000. Nutritional considerations of overtraining. In J.R. Stout and J. Antonio (Eds.). *Sport supplements: A complete guide to physique and athletic enhancement.* Baltimore: Lippincott, Williams & Wilkins.

Kreider, R.B., R. Klesges, K. Harmon, et al. 1996. Effects of ingesting supplements designed to promote lean tissue accretion on body composition during resistance training. *International Journal of Sport Nutrition* 6: 234-246.

Kreider, R.B., V. Miriel, and E. Bertun. 1993. Amino acid supplementation and exercise performance: Analysis of the proposed ergogenic value. *Sports Medicine* 16: 190-209.

Kreider, R., et al. 1998. Effects of conjugated linoleic acid (CLA) supplementation during resistance training on bone mineral content, bone mineral density, and markers of immune stress. *FASEB Journal* 12: A244.

Kreider, R.B., et al. 1998. Effects of creatine supplementation on body composition, strength, and sprint performance. *Medicine and Science in Sports and Exercise* 30: 73-82.

Kreider, R.B., et al. (Eds.). 1998. *Overtraining in sport.* Champaign, IL: Human Kinetics.

Kreider, R.B., et al 1999. Effects of calcium b-hydroxy b-methylbutyrate (HMB) supplementation during resistance-training on markers of catabolism, body composition and strength. *International Journal of Sports Medicine* 22: 1-7.

Kreider, R.B., et al. 1999. Effects of protein and amino-acid supplementation on athletic performance. *Sportscience* 3: sportscie.org/jour/9901/rbk.html.

Kreider, R.B., et al. 2000. Nutrition in exercise and sport. In T. Wilson and N. Temple (Eds.). *Frontiers in nutrition.* Totowa, NJ: Humana Press, Inc.

Kreider, R.B., et al. 2001. Bovine colostrum supplementation on training adaptations I: Body Composition. Abstract presented at 2001 FASEB meeting, Orlando, FL.

Krochmal, R., et al. 2004. Phytochemical assays of commercial botanical dietary supplements. *Evidence-Based Complementary and Alternative Medicine* 1: 305-313.

Laaksonen, R., et al. 1995. Ubiquinone supplementation and exercise capacity in trained young and older men. *European Journal of Applied Physiology* 72: 95-100.

Lamb, D.R., K.F. Rinehardt, R.L. Bartels, et al. 1990. Dietary carbohydrate and intensity of interval swim training. *The American Journal of Clinical Nutrition* 52: 1058-1063.

Lambert, C.P., M.G. Flynn, J.B. Boone, et al. 1991. Effects of carbohydrate feeding on multiple-bout resistance exercise. *Journal of Applied Sport Science Research* 5: 192-197.

Lambert, C.P., et al. 2004. Macronutrient considerations for the sport of bodybuilding. *Sports Medicine* 34: 317-327.

Lambert, M.I., et al. 1993. Failure of commercial oral amino acid supplements to increase serum growth hormone concentrations in male body-builders. *International Journal of Sport Nutrition* 3: 298-305.

Lands, L.C., et al. 1999. Effect of supplementation with cysteine donor on muscular performance. *Journal of Applied Physiology* 87: 1381-1385.

Lane, L. 1999. Nutritionist calls for tighter regulation of supplements. *CNN.com News*, September 17.

Langfort, J., et al. 1997. The effect of a low-carbohydrate diet on performance, hormonal and metabolic responses to a 30-s bout of supramaximal exercise. *European Journal of Applied Physiology and Occupational Physiology* 76: 128-133.

Layman, D.K. 2002. Role of leucine in protein metabolism during exercise and recovery. *Canadian Journal of Applied Physiology* 27: 646-663.

Lefavi, R.G., R.A. Anderson, R.E. Keith, et al. 1992. Efficacy of chromium supplementation in athletes: Emphasis on anabolism. *International Journal of Sport Nutrition* 2: 111-122.

Lemon, P.W.R. 1991. Effect of exercise on protein requirements. *Journal of Sports Sciences* 9: 53-70.

Lemon, P.W.R. November 11-12, 1994. Dietary protein and amino acids. Presented at Nutritional Ergogenic Aids Conference sponsored by the Gatorade Sports Institute, Chicago.

Lemon, P.W.R. 2000. Beyond the Zone: Protein needs of active individuals. *Journal of the American College of Nutrition* 19: 513S-521S.

Lemon, P.W.R., et al. 1992. Protein requirements and muscle mass/strength changes during intensive training in novice bodybuilders. *Journal of Applied Physiology* 73: 767-775.

Lemon, P.W., et al. 2002. The role of protein and amino acid supplements in the athlete's diet: Does type or timing of ingestion matter? *Current Sports Medicine Reports* 1: 214-221.

Liang, M.T., et al. 2005. Panax notoginseng supplementation enhances physical performance during endurance exercise. *Journal of Strength and Conditioning Research* 19: 108-114.

Liberti, L.E., et al. 1978. Evaluation of commercial ginseng products. *Journal of Pharmaceutical Sciences* 67: 1487-1489.

Liese, A.D., et al. 2005. Dietary glycemic index and glycemic load, carbohydrate and fiber intake, and measures of insulin sensitivity, secretion, and adiposity in the Insulin Resistance Atherosclerosis Study. *Diabetes Care* 12: 2832-2838.

Linde, K., et al. 2006. Echinacea for preventing and treating the common cold. *Cochrane Database of Systematic Reviews* 2006 Jan 25: CD000530.

Louis-Sylvestre, J., et al. 2003. Highlighting the positive impact of increasing feeding frequency on metabolism and weight management. *Forum of Nutrition* 56: 126-128.

Lowe, B. 2000. Powerful products. *Nutritional Outlook* 3: 37-43.

Ludwig, D.S., et al. 2001. Relation between consumption of sugar-sweetened drinks and childhood obesity: A prospective, observational analysis. *Lancet* 357: 505-508.

Lukaski, H.C. 2000. Magnesium, zinc, and chromium nutriture and physical activity. *American Journal of Clinical Nutrition* 72 (2 Supplement): 585S-593S.

Lukaszuk, J.M., et al. 2005. Effect of a defined lacto-ovo-vegetarian diet and oral creatine monohydrate supplementation on plasma creatine concentration. *Journal of Strength and Conditioning Research* 19: 735-740.

MacLean, D.B., and L.G. Luo. 2004. Increased ATP content/production in the hypothalamus may be a signal for energy-sensing of satiety: Studies of the anorectic mechanism of a plant steroidal glycoside. *Brain Research* 1020: 1-11.

Malm, C., et al. 1996. Supplementation with ubiquinone-10 causes cellular damage during intense exercise. *Acta Physiologica Scandinavica* 157: 511-512.

Manore, M.M. 2000. *Sports nutrition for health and performance.* Champaign, IL: Human Kinetics.

Manore, M.M., J. Thompson, and M. Russo. 1993. Diet and exercise strategies of a world-class bodybuilder. *International Journal of Sport Nutrition* 3: 76-86.

Manore, M.M. 2000. Effect of physical activity on thiamine, riboflavin, and vitamin B-6 requirements. *American Journal of Clinical Nutrition* 72: 598S-606S.

Manson, J.E., W.C. Willett, M.J. Stampfer, et al. 1994. Vegetable and fruit consumption and incidence of stroke in women. *Circulation* 89: 932.

Marquezi, M.L., et al. 2003. Effect of aspartate and asparagine supplementation on fatigue determinants in intense exercise. *International Journal of Sport Nutrition and Exercise Metabolism* 13: 65-75.

Maughan, R.J., and D.C. Poole. 1981. The effects of a glycogen-loading regimen on the capacity to perform anaerobic exercise. *European Journal of Applied Physiology* 46: 211-219.

Mazer, E. 1981. Biotin—The little known lifesaver. *Prevention*, July, 97-102.

McNulty, S.R., et al. 2005. Effect of alpha-tocopherol supplementation on plasma homocysteine and oxidative stress in highly trained athletes before and after exhaustive exercise. *The Journal of Nutritional Biochemistry* 16: 530-537.

McAnulty, S.R., et al. 2005. Effect of resistance exercise and carbohydrate ingestion on oxidative stress. *Free Radical Research* 39: 1219-1224.

McNaughton, L.R., et al. 1997. Neutralize acid to enhance performance. *Sportscience Training & Technology:* www.sportsci.org/traintech/buffer/lrm.htm.

Mendel, R.W., et al. 2005. Effects of creatine on thermoregulatory responses while exercising in the heat. *Nutrition* 21: 301-307.

Mero, A. 1999. Leucine supplementation and intensive training. *Sports Medicine* 27: 347-358.

Meydani, M., et al. 1993. Protective effect of vitamin E on exercise-induced oxidative damage in young and older adults. *American Journal of Physiology* 264 (5 Part 2): R992-998.

Miller, W.C., M.G. Niederpruem, J.P. Wallace, and A.K. Lindeman. 1994. Dietary fat, sugar, and fiber predict body fat content. *Journal of the American Dietetic Association* 94: 612-615.

Mosoni, L., et al. 2003. Type and timing of protein feeding to optimize anabolism. *Current Opinion in Clinical Nutrition and Metabolic Care* 6: 301-306.

Morifuji, M., et al. 2005. Dietary whey protein downregulates fatty acid synthesis in the liver, but upregulates it in skeletal muscle of exercise-trained rats. *Nutrition* 21: 1052-1058.

National Cholesterol Education Program. 2006. ATP III guidelines at-a-glance quick desk reference.

National Research Council. 1989. *Diet and health: Implications for reducing chronic disease risk*. Washington, D.C.: National Academy Press.

Nazar, K., et al. 1996. Phosphate supplementation prevents a decrease of triiodothyronine and increases resting metabolic rate during low energy diet. *Journal of Physiology and Pharmacology* 47: 373-383.

Nelson, G. 2001. American Heart Association calls for eating fish twice per week—What's a vegetarian to do? *Vegetarian Journal*, September/October issue.

Newhouse, I.J., et al. 2000. The effects of magnesium supplementation on exercise performance. *Clinical Journal of Sport Medicine* 10: 195-200.

Neychev, V.K. 2005. The aphrodisiac herb Tribulus terrestris does not influence the androgen production in young men. *Journal of Ethnopharmacology* 101: 319-323.

Nicholas, C.W., et al. 1999. Carbohydrate-electrolyte ingestion during intermittent high-intensity running. *Medicine and Science in Sports and Exercise* 31: 1280-1286.

Nielsen, F.H., et al. 2004. A moderately high intake compared to a low intake of zinc depresses magnesium balance and alters indices of bone turnover in postmenopausal women. *European Journal of Clinical Nutrition* 58: 703-710.

Nissen, S., R. Sharp, M. Ray, et al. 1996. Effect of leucine metabolite beta-hydroxy-beta-methylbutyrate on muscle metabolism during resistance-exercise training. *Journal of Applied Physiology* 81: 2095-2104.

Oakley, G.P., M.J. Adams, and C.M. Dickinson. 1996. More folic acid for everyone, now. *Journal of Nutrition* 126: 751S-755S.

O'Connor, D.M., et al. 2003. The effects of beta-hydroxy-beta-methylbutyrate (HMB) and HMB/creatine supplementation on indices of health in highly trained athletes. *International Journal of Sport Nutrition and Exercise Metabolism* 13: 184-197.

Olney, J. Transcript from December 29, 1996, airing of *60 Minutes*, CBS, New York.

Parcells, A.C., et al. 2004. Cordyceps Sinensis (CordyMax Cs-4) supplementation does not improve endurance exercise performance. *International Journal of Sport Nutrition and Exercise Metabolism* 14: 236-242.

Parrott, S. 1999. Herbs said harmful before surgery. *AOL News*, October 14.

Peake, J., et al. 2004. Neutrophil activation, antioxidant supplements and exercise-induced oxidative stress. *Exercise Immunology Review* 10: 129-141.

Phillips, S.M., et al. Dietary protein to support anabolism with resistance exercise in young men. *Journal of the American College of Nutrition* 24: 134S-139S.

Pieralisi, G. 1991. Effects of standardized ginseng extract combined with dimethylaminoethanol bitartrate, vitamins, minerals, and trace elements on physical performance during exercise. *Clinical Therapeutics* 13: 373-382.

Pline, K.A., et al. 2005. The effect of creatine intake on renal function. *The Annals of Pharmacotherapy* 39: 1093-1096.

Poortmans, J.R., et al. 2000. Do regular high protein diets have potential health risks on kidney function in athletes? *International Journal of Sport Nutrition and Exercise Metabolism* 10: 28-38.

Rehrer, N.J. 2001. Fluid and electrolyte balance in ultra-endurance sport. *Sports Medicine* 31: 701-715.

Reilly, T. 1997. Energetics of high-intensity exercise (soccer) with particular reference to fatigue. *Journal of Sports Science* 15: 257-263.

Riserus, U., et al. 2001. Conjugated linoleic acid (CLA) reduced abdominal adipose tissue in obese middle-aged men with signs of the metabolic syndrome: A randomised controlled trial. *International Journal of Obesity and Related Metabolic Disorders* 25: 1129-1135.

Robergs, R.A. 1998. Glycerol hyperhydration to beat the heat? *Sportscience Training & Technology:* www.sportsci.org/traintech/buffer/lrm.htm.

Rolls, B.J., et al. 1988. The specificity of satiety: The influence of foods of different macro-nutrient content on the development of satiety. *Physiology and Behavior* 43: 145-153.

Roy, B.D., et al. 2005. Creatine monohydrate supplementation does not improve functional recovery after total knee arthroplasty. *Archives of Physical Medicine and Rehabilitation* 86: 1293-1298.

Roy, B.D., et al. 2002. The influence of post-exercise macronutrient intake on energy balance and protein metabolism in active females participating in endurance training. *International Journal of Sport Nutrition and Exercise Metabolism* 12: 172-188.

Sachan, D.S., et al. 2005. Decreasing oxidative stress with choline and carnitine in women. *Journal of the American College of Nutrition* 24: 172-176.

Sarubin, A. 2000. *The health professional's guide to popular dietary supplements.* The American Dietetic Association, pp. 184-188.

Saunders, M.J., et al. 2006. Effects of a carbohydrate/protein gel on exercise performance in male and female cyclists. Poster 26.

Schabort, E.J., et al. 1999. The effect of a preexercise meal on time to fatigue during prolonged cycling exercise. *Medicine and Science in Sports and Exercise* 31: 464-471.

Seaton, T.B., S.L. Welle, M.K. Warenko, and R.G. Campbell. 1986. Thermic effect of medium and long chain triglycerides in man. *The American Journal of Clinical Nutrition* 44: 630-634.

Seidle, R., et al. 2000. A taurine and caffeine-containing drink stimulates cognitive performance and well-being. *Amino Acids* 19: 635-642.

Shugarman, A.E. 1999. Trends in the sports nutrition industry. *Nutraceuticals World* 2: 56-59.

Simko, M.D., and J. Jarosz. 1990. Organic foods: Are they better? *Journal of the American Dietetic Association* 90: 367-370.

Singh, A., et al. 1994. Exercise-induced changes in immune function: Effects of zinc supplementation. *Journal of Applied Physiology* 76: 2298-2303.

Slavin, J.L. 1991. Assessing athletes' nutritional status. *The Physician and Sportsmedicine* 19: 79-94.

Somer, E. 1996. Maximum energy: How to eat and exercise for it. *Working Woman*, May, 72-76.

Speechly, D.P., et al. 1999. Greater appetite control associated with an increased frequency of eating in lean males. *Appetite* 33: 285-297.

Spriet, L.L. 1995. Caffeine and performance. *International Journal of Sport Nutrition* 5: S84-S99.

Spriet, L.L., et al. 2004. Nutritional strategies to influence adaptations to training. *Journal of Sports Sciences* 22: 127-141.

Stanko, R.T., et al. 1996. Inhibition of regain in body weight and fat with addition of 3-carbon compounds to the diet with hyperenergetic refeeding after weight reduction. *International Journal of Obesity Related Metabolic Disorders* 20: 925-930.

Steinmetz, K.A., et al. 1996. Vegetables, fruit, and cancer prevention: A review. *Journal of the American Dietetic Association* 96: 1027-1039.

Stephens, F.B., et al. 2006. Insulin stimulates L-carnitine accumulation in human skeletal muscle. *The FASEB Journal* 20: 377-379.

Stewart, A.M. 1999. Amino acids and athletic performance: A mini-conference in Oxford. *Sportscience Training & Technology:* www.sportsci.org/jour/9902/ams.html.

Stone, N. 1996. AHA Medical/Scientific Statement on fish consumption, fish oil, lipids, and coronary heart disease. Internet Web site: www.americanheart.org.

Stout, J.R., et al. Effects of 28 days of beta-alanine and creatine monohydrate supplementation on physical working capacity at neuromuscular fatigue threshold. Poster 27.

Stout, J.R., et al. Effects of resistance exercise and creatine supplementation on myasthenia gravis: A case study. *Medicine and Science in Sports and Exercise* 33: 869-872.

Stuessi, C., et al. 2005. L-Carnitine and the recovery from exhaustive endurance exercise: A randomised, double-blind, placebo-controlled trial. *European Journal of Applied Physiology* 95: 431-435.

Szlyk, P.C., R.P. Francesconi, M.S. Rose, et al. 1991. Incidence of hypohydration when consuming carbohydrate-electrolyte solutions during field training. *Military Medicine* 156: 399-402.

Tarnopolsky, M.A., 1998. Influence of differing macronutrient intakes on muscle glycogen resynthesis after resistance training. *Journal of Applied Physiology* 84: 890-896.

Tarnopolsky, M.A., et al. 1992. Evaluation of protein requirements for trained strength athletes. *Journal of Applied Physiology* 73: 1986-1995.

Tarnopolsky, M.A., et al. 1997. Postexercise protein-carbohydrate supplements increase muscle glycogen in men and women. *Journal of Applied Physiology* 83: 1877-1883.

Thomas, D.E., et al. 1991. Carbohydrate feeding before exercise: Effect of glycemic index. *International Journal of Sports Medicine* 12: 180-186.

Thornton, J.S. 1990. How can you tell when an athlete is too thin? *The Physician and Sportsmedicine* 18: 124-133.

Tiidus, P.M., et al. 1995. Vitamin E status and response to exercise training. *Sports Medicine* 20: 12-23.

Trimmer, R., et al. 2006. Effects of two naturally occurring aromatase inhibitors on male hormonal and blood chemistry profiles. Poster 21.

Trumbo, P., et al. 2001. Dietary reference intakes. *Journal of the American Dietetic Association* 101(3): 294-301.

Tsang. G. 2006. Which sweeteners are safe? Web site: www.healthcastle.com/sweeteners.shtml.

Tullson, P.C., et al. 1991. Adenine nucleotide synthesis in exercising and endurance-trained skeletal muscle. *American Journal of Physiology* 261(2 Part 1): C342-347.

Tyler, V.E. 1987. *The new honest herbal: A sensible guide to the use of herbs and related remedies*. Philadelphia: George F. Stickley Co.

U.S. Department of Agriculture. 1998. USDA urges consumers to use food thermometer when cooking ground beef patties. White paper, August 11.

U.S. Department of Agriculture and U.S. Department of Health and Human Services. 1995. Nutrition and your health: Dietary guidelines for Americans. Washington, D.C.: GPO.

Van Someren, K.A., et al. 2005. Supplementation with beta-hydroxy-beta-methylbutyrate (HMB) and alpha-ketoisocaproic acid (KIC) reduces signs and symptoms of exercise-induced muscle damage in man. *International Journal of Sport Nutrition and Exercise Metabolism* 15: 413-424.

Van Zyl, C.G., et al. 1996. Effects of medium-chain triglyceride ingestion on fuel metabolism and cycling performance. *Journal of Applied Physiology* 80: 2217-2225.

Viitala, P.E., et al. 2004. The effects of antioxidant vitamin supplementation on resistance exercise induced lipid peroxidation in trained and untrained participants. *Lipids in Health and Disease* 3: 14.

Viitala, P.E., et al. 2004. Vitamin E supplementation, exercise and lipid peroxidation in human participants. *European Journal of Applied Physiology* 93: 108-115.

Volpe, S.L., et al. 2001. Effect of chromium supplementation and exercise on body composition, resting metabolic rate and selected biochemical parameters in moderately obese women following an exercise program. *Journal of the American College of Nutrition* 20: 293-306.

Wagner, D.R. 1999. Hyperhydrating with glycerol: Implications for athletic performance. *Journal of the American Dietetic Association* 99: 207-212.

Wagner, D.R., et al. 1992. Effects of oral ribose on muscle metabolism during bicycle ergometer exercise in AMPD-deficient patients. *Annals of Nutrition and Metabolism* 35: 297-302.

Wagner, J.C. 1991. Enhancement of athletic performance with drugs: An overview. *Sports Medicine* 12: 250-265.

Walberg, J.L., et al. 1988. Macronutrient content of a hypoenergy diet affects nitrogen retention and muscle function in weight lifters. *International Journal of Sports Medicine* 9: 261-266.

Walberg-Rankin, J.L. November 11-12, 1994. Ergogenic effects of carbohydrate intake during long- and short-term exercise. Presented at Nutritional Ergogenic Aids Conference sponsored by the Gatorade Sports Institute, Chicago.

Walberg-Rankin, J.L. 1995. Dietary carbohydrate as an ergogenic aid for prolonged and brief competitions in sport. *International Journal of Sport Nutrition* 5: S13-S28.

Walberg-Rankin, J.L., et al. 1994. The effect of oral arginine during energy restriction in male weight lifters. *Journal of Strength and Conditioning Research* 8: 170-177.

Walton, R.G., R. Hudak, and R.J. Green-Waite. 1993. Adverse reactions to aspartame: Double-blind challenge in patients from a vulnerable population. *Biological Psychiatry* 34: 13-17.

Ward, R.J., et al. 1999. Changes in plasma taurine levels after different endurance events. *Amino Acids* 16 (1): 71-77.

Wardlaw, G.M., P.M. Insel, and M.F. Seyler. 1994. *Contemporary nutrition.* St. Louis: Mosby–Year Book, Inc.

Washington State Department of Agriculture. 1995. Organic food standards. Organic Food Program, Food Safety and Animal Health Division.

Watson S. 2006. How diet pills work. Web site: health.howstuffworks.com/diet-pill.htm.

Wesson, M., L. McNaughton, P. Davies, and S. Tristram. 1988. Effects of oral administration of aspartic acid salts on the endurance capacity of trained athletes. *Research Quarterly for Exercise and Sport* 59: 234-239.

Wilborn, C.D., et al. 2004. Effects of methoxyisoflavone, ecdysterone, and sulfopolysaccharide (CSP3) supplementation during training on body composition and training adaptations. White paper from Exercise and Sport Nutrition Laboratory, University, Waco, Texas.

Wilborn, C.D., et al. 2004. Effects of zinc magnesium aspartate (ZMA) supplementation on training adaptations and markers and anabolism and catabolism. *Journal of the International Society of Sports Nutrition* 1: 12-20.

Williams, C. 1995. Macronutrients and performance. *Journal of Sports Sciences* 13: S1-S10.

Williams, M.H. 2005. Dietary supplements and sports performance: Minerals. *Journal of the International Society of Sports Nutrition* 2: 43-49.

Williams, M.B., et al. 2003. Effects of recovery beverages on glycogen restoration and endurance exercise performance. *Journal of Strength and Conditioning Research* 17:12-19.

Williams, M.H. 1989. Vitamin supplementation and athletic performance. *International Journal for Vitamin and Nutrition Research, Supplement*, 30: 163-191.

Williams, M.H., et al. 1998. *The ergogenics edge.* Champaign, IL: Human Kinetics.

Williams, M.H., et al. 1999. *Creatine: The power supplement.* Champaign, IL: Human Kinetics.

Wilmore, J.H., and D.L. Costill. 1994. *Physiology of sport and exercise.* Champaign, IL: Human Kinetics, 392-395.

Winters, L.R., R.S. Yoon, H.J. Kalkwarf, J.C. Davies, et al. 1992. Riboflavin requirements and exercise adaption in older women. *The American Journal of Clinical Nutrition* 56: 526-532.

Yaspelkis, B.B., et al. 1999. The effect of a carbohydrate-arginine supplement on postexercise carbohydrate metabolism. *International Journal of Sports Nutrition* 9: 241-250.

Youl Kang, H., et al. 2002. Effects of ginseng ingestion on growth hormone, testosterone, cortisol, and insulin-like growth factor 1 responses to acute resistance exercise. *Journal of Strength and Conditioning Research* 16: 179-183.

Zawadzki, K.M., B.B. Yaselkis, and J.L. Ivy. 1992. Carbohydrate-protein complex increases the rate of muscle glycogen storage after exercise. *Journal of Applied Physiology* 72: 1854-1859.

Zhang, M., et al. 2004. Role of taurine supplementation to prevent exercise-induced oxidative stress in healthy young men. *Amino Acids* 26: 203-207.

Zhou, S., et al. 2005. Muscle and plasma coenzyme Q10 concentration, aerobic power and exercise economy of healthy men in response to four weeks of supplementation. *The Journal of Sports Medicine and Physical Fitness* 45: 337-346.

Ziegenfuss, T.N., et al. 2006. Safety and efficacy of a commercially available, naturally occurring aromatase inhibitor in healthy men. Poster 43.

Index

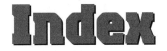

Note: The italicized *f* and *t* following pages numbers refer to figures and tables, respectively.

About the Authors

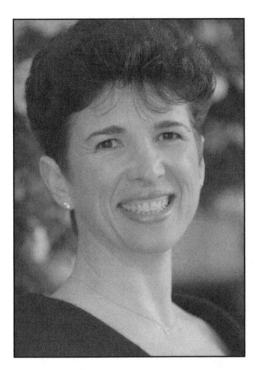

Susan M. Kleiner, PhD, RD, FACN, CNS, FISSN, is the nutrition authority on eating for strength, and her Power Eating program has reshaped the lives of thousands. She is the owner of High Performance Nutrition, a consulting firm based in Mercer Island, Washington.

Dr. Kleiner has worked as a nutrition consultant to the Seattle Seahawks (including quarterback Matt Hasselbeck), the Seattle SuperSonics, the Cleveland Browns, the Cleveland Cavaliers, and The Repertory Project Dance Company. She also worked with 2006 U.S. women's ice hockey Olympian Kelly Stephens and 2004-2006 U.S. women's master's Olympic weightlifting champion, Trish Zuccotti.

Dr. Kleiner is an advisory board member for *Can-Fit-Pro, Shape, Let's Live,* and *Physical* magazines and for Allrecipes.com. For her doctoral research on the cardiovascular disease risks of diet and anabolic steroid use in competitive male bodybuilders, Dr. Kleiner received a Young Investigator Award in 1987 from the American College of Nutrition. She is a fellow of the American College of Nutrition and the International Society of Sports Nutrition, as well as a member of the American College of Sports Medicine, the American Dietetic Association and its (SCAN) Practice Group, and the National Strength and Conditioning Association.

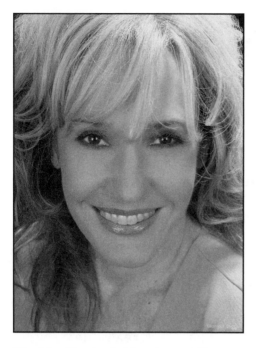

Maggie Greenwood-Robinson, PhD, is a leading health and medical writer in the United States. She has authored or coauthored more than 30 books on nutrition, exercise, weight loss, psychological health, and other health-related issues, among them *The Biggest Loser*, a *New York Times* bestseller that is the official diet and fitness book for NBC's hit reality show by the same name. Some of her most recent books are *20/20 Thinking, Good Carbs Versus Bad Carbs,* and *Foods That Combat Cancer.* Greenwood-Robinson has appeared on numerous television and radio shows, including the "Dr. Phil Show" and NBC's "Dateline." She has also written articles that have appeared in the magazines *Shape, Let's Live, Great Life, American Health, Physical, Muscle and Fitness,* and *MuscleMag International.* A frequent speaker on issues concerning health, anti-aging, nutrition, and exercise, Greenwood-Robinson is a member of the "Dr. Phil Show" advisory board and serves on the advisory board of *Physical* magazine.

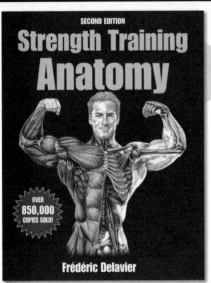
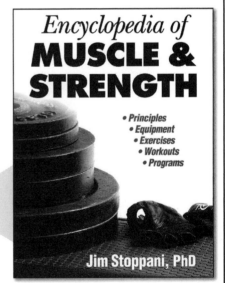

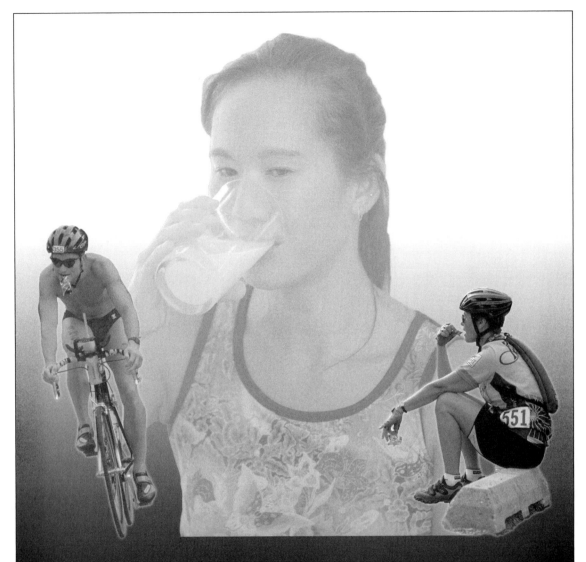